Macrobiotic Diet

Michio and Aveline Kushi

MACRBIOTIC DIET

Balancing Your Eating in Harmony with the Changing Environment and Personal Needs

Edited by Alex Jack

Japan Publications, Inc.

Note to the reader: Those with health problems are advised to seek the guidance of
a qualified medical or psychological professional in addition to a qualified macrobiotic
counselor before implementing any of the dietary and other approaches presented in
this book. It is essential that any readers who have any reason to suspect serious
illness in themselves or their family members seek appropriate medical, nutritional,
or psychological advice promptly. Neither this or any other health related book
should be used as a substitute for qualified care or treatment.

Published by JAPAN PUBLICATIONS, INC., Tokyo and New York

Distributors:
UNITED STATES: *Kodansha International/USA, Ltd., through Harper & Row,
Publishers, Inc., 10 East 53rd Street, New York, New York 10022.* SOUTH AMERICA:
Harper & Row, Publishers, Inc., International Department. CANADA: *Fitzhenry &
Whiteside Ltd., 195 Allstate Parkway, Markham, Ontario, L3R 4T8.* MEXICO AND
CENTRAL AMERICA: *HARLA S. A. de C. V., Apartado 30–546, Mexico 4, D. F.*
BRITISH ISLES: *International Book Distributors Ltd., 66 Wood Lane End, Hemel
Hempstead, Herts HP2 4RG.* EUROPEAN CONTINENT: *Fleetbooks, S. A., c/o Feffer
and Simons (Nederland) B. V., Rijnkade 170, 1382 GT Weesp, The Netherlands.*
AUSTRALIA AND NEW ZEALAND: *Bookwise International, 1 Jeanes Street, Beverley,
South Australia 5007.* THE FAR EAST AND JAPAN: *Japan Publications Trading Co., Ltd.,
1–2–1, Sarugaku-cho, Chiyoda-ku, Tokyo 101.*

First edition: July 1985

LCCC No. 84–080641
ISBN 0–87040–535–7

Printed in U.S.A.

Preface

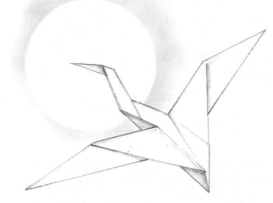

From an endless dream we have come,
In an endless dream we are living,
To an endless dream we shall return.

Toward the end and immediately following World War II, people in all countries aspired for world peace. Among various attempts to achieve peace, an effort was made to establish a world federal government either through amending the United Nations Charter or through the formation of worldwide conventions by people representing populations of different areas.

As a student of political science and international law at Tokyo University, I became earnestly interested in studying possible ways to realize world federation. At this time I received valuable guidance from Professor Shigeru Nanbara, Chancellor of Tokyo University, Toyohiko Hori, Senior Faculty Member of Political Science, other members of the Faculty of Law and Politics, Rev. Toyohiko Kagawa, the Christian evangelist, Morikatsu Inagaki, promoter of world federation, and many others who dreamt of an international federation of states as the most practical way to control the spread of atomic weapons and prevent future wars.

However, the person whose view of human society I was most deeply influenced by was George Ohsawa. Our meeting came about in a curious way. One of the groups with which I was in touch was the United World Federalists of North America. In a letter shortly after the end of the war, they advised me to visit a world government association near Tokyo. This small organization was headed by Yukikazu Sakurazawa, an Oriental philosopher who had traveled and lived abroad for many years, synthesizing the teachings of East and West. For simplification, he used the pen name George Ohsawa in French and English.

At our first meeting, Ohsawa asked me, "Have you ever thought about the dialectical application of dietary principles to the problem of world peace?" I was puzzled. Political science, and even social science at large, never addressed the

dietary practices of the human race except for some esoteric cultural and anthro-
pological studies. Back at the university, I discussed this matter with some of my
professors and elicited only disinterest.

In 1949 I journeyed to the United States to continue researching possible ways
of establishing world federation. At Columbia University in New York, I had the
opportunity to examine more than sixty drafts of proposed world constitutions
published during the twentieth century, as well as many debates, discussions, and
reports related to the formation of a world government. However, while studying
these documents and attending meetings related to world federation, I began to
wonder whether the structural change of society alone really could realize world
peace. It might control nuclear weapons and other destructive measures. But it
appeared difficult to alter hatred, fear, prejudice, and discrimination so deeply
rooted in the human mind.

The phrases "the reconstruction of humanity" and "medicine for humanity"
frequently entered my thoughts. I sought guidance from Albert Einstein, Thomas
Mann, Upton Sinclair, Robert M. Hutchins, Norman Cousins, and leading
world federalists. I also wrote letters to Indian Prime Minister Jawaharlal Nehru
and other leading figures devoted to the cause of world order and peace. Their
suggestions and advice were similar and led me to conclude that, although the
formation of world federation is absolutely necessary for avoiding future warfare,
it was not the ultimate answer for building a better world and enabling humanity
to realize its physical, mental, and spiritual potential. To realize universal peace
and happiness, it became apparent to me that the human race needed to be elevated
toward physical health, sound mind, and unlimited spiritual understanding. So long
as the quality of the human species remained at the present level there would continuously arise disputes, arguments, crimes, and conflicts that would again destroy
world order even if it were established through legal and political means.

I asked myself, What is the practical solution to this ultimate question? Religions? They have been offering solutions for the past several thousand years.
Modern education? Judicial, economic, and political systems? They all appear to
offer no lasting answer. Science and technology? I hoped studying medicine might
provide a solution for healing human minds and conduct. But the eminent figures
whom I contacted all noted that there were no colleges, no books, and no teachers
on this issue, and that even the modern medical system could not fundamentally
change the way people thought and behaved. I had to search and search.

The quest had to begin somewhere, so I stopped all my studies and began to
stand along Fifth Avenue and in Times Square in New York City. I watched one
by one thousands of people passing by. I watched their mannerisms and behavior,
their postures and figures, their expressions and habits. Days and weeks passed.
I discovered that although everyone shared basic human characteristics, individual
qualities were different, and these differences resulted from two major factors: 1)
environmental conditions, including the natural, social, and cultural environments
in which individuals were brought up and were now living and the background of
their parents and ancestors, and 2) food that individuals have been eating during
the present, in childhood, during the embryonic period, and the food consumed

by parents, grandparents, and ancestors that contributed to their inherited features and predispositions.

From these discoveries, I could really understand for the first time Ohsawa's words concerning "the dialectical application of dietary principles to the problem of world peace." I set aside my studies of political science and international law and began to study history, biology, chemistry, religion, philosophy, culture, the arts, literature, and other subjects to understand more clearly the relationship among humanity, environment, and food. I also continued to look at society around me, especially changing environmental and dietary patterns. I soon found that degenerative physical, mental, and social disorders were rapidly increasing in modern society. Closely connected with the rise in heart disease, cancer, and other chronic diseases was a rapid change of food quality which was taking place through refinement, mass production, chemicalization, artificialization, and other highly industrialized processes. I discovered that compared with even twenty years before, the food we were consuming was fundamentally different from that our parents ate, and compared to the early part of the century, it was totally different from that of our grandparents and ancestors.

Realizing the basic cause of modern degeneration, I felt sad at the prospects for humanity. Not only nuclear war but also biological disaster could lead to the decline and extinction of our species, *homo sapiens*. If degeneration continued unchecked, the end would probably come by the middle of the twenty-first century, even if we managed to avoid nuclear war. During this period, heart disease, cancer, diabetes, arthritis, sexual and reproductive disorders, allergies, and many other disorders would spread epidemically. Psychological disorders, including schizophrenia, paranoia, anxiety, and depression, would become common in daily life. Disputes, crimes, and conflicts within the family and community would increase. Religious and educational influences would be ignored. Economic and political systems would end in chaos. Poverty, disease, misery, and madness would spread through the entire modern world, with or without war.

To reverse this march toward biological degeneration and build a new era for the further development of human life on this planet, I realized that the following measures were essential:

1. Recovering genuine food, largely of natural, organic quality, and making it available to every family at reasonable cost.
2. Establishing proper dietary guidelines, reflecting both traditional practice and modern nutritional awareness, that could be easily understood by every family.
3. Restoring the natural environment and overcoming the adverse effects of chemical agriculture and modern industry.
4. Developing and embracing a new orientation for education, culture, and consciousness, directed toward the development of world family consciousness, with brotherhood and sisterhood transcending differences of sex, age, nationality, religion, class, tradition, and custom.
5. Strengthening of world community and the formation of world federal

government as quickly as possible to end the nuclear arms race and resolve disagreements and conflicts among states and nations peacefully.
6. Unifying the sciences, including medicine and technology, for the benefit of all humanity, based on a deep understanding of natural order.
7. Recognizing universal laws and principles—the infinite order of the universe—as the foundation of all existing world philosophies, religions, cultures, economic and political systems, and arts and sciences, and applying this understanding to daily life and the realization of personal growth and development, family health and happiness, community and social stability, and world peace.

Health, happiness, peace, and freedom are the natural birthright of every man, woman, and child. The cosmological principles leading to these goals are apprehended by native common sense and intuitive self-reflection. Down through the ages the universal laws of change have been described in many names and forms. In the Orient, the terms *yin* and *yang* were used to describe the dynamic ever-changing order of the cosmos and nature of which we are a small part. In the Occident, the concept *logos* conveyed a similar meaning. Over the centuries, as humanity's health and consciousness fluctuated, the universal laws of change were forgotten or remembered only partially. Modern society's political and economic systems, science and technologies, for example, are based on a fragmented or disjointed understanding of these principles.

The primary application of universal principles needed in our time is for the biological regeneration of modern society. Recovery of human physical and psychological health will create the environment in which world unity, including disarmament and world federal government, can be realized, as well as ensure further human evolution. With my wife Aveline Kushi and a handful of friends and associates, I began to secure the best natural quality of food—organic and naturally processed. To differentiate this type of food from "health food" which consisted mostly of supplements, vitamins, minerals, and enzymes, we named our orientation "natural food." Our movement began to alter entire dietary patterns with more natural quality food around 1960 and especially after 1965 when we decided to dedicate our full energies to this cause.

We talked with farmers, food processors, manufacturers, exporters, distributors, retailers, and consumers. We began constant lectures, seminars, and study sessions for the education of the food industry, government and social leaders, the medical profession, and the general public. Natural food industries began to spread, not only in North America, but also in Central and South America, Europe, Australia, and the Far East. Natural foods stores, restaurants, and coops spread rapidly, and organic farming and gardening became popular.

Along with securing the best possible natural quality of food, it was necessary to guide individuals and families in the direction of more healthy dietary patterns and cooking methods using these natural foods. By the early 1970s several hundred teaching centers were established all around the world by our associates, friends, students, and people who shared the same dream. These centers offered cooking instruction, as well as classes in East West philosophy, medicine for humanity, and personal development. Books, magazines, and pamphlets were published and continue to be published in many languages through a network of centers, associations, and publishers to bring these dietary and way of life teachings to a wider audience.

What should this way of life for the physical, mental, and spiritual development of humanity be called? In ancient Greece, Hippocrates, the father of Western medicine, followed the same approach, emphasizing environment and diet, and introduced the term *makrobios*, or macrobiotics, from the Greek words for "Great Life" and "Long Life." Since then, *macrobiotics* has come down through Western history to mean a natural way of life, including a simple, natural way of eating, leading to maximum health and longevity. The term was used by Herodotus, the historian of ancient cultures, by François Rabelais, the great French humanist and writer, and by Christoph W. Hufeland, an eighteenth century European medical doctor and philosopher who wrote a famous book, *Macrobiotics or the Art of Prolonging Life*.

The traditional Far Eastern approach to health and longevity, based on the principles of yin and yang, was translated by Professor Joseph Needham in his multivolume history, *Science and Civilization in China*, as "macrobiotics." In the late 1950s and early 1960s, during travels to France, Belgium, and the United States, George Ohsawa introduced the term "Zen Macrobiotics" to refer to his teachings since balanced dietary practices were traditionally kept by Zen practitioners.

I adopted "macrobiotics" in its original meaning, as the universal way of health and longevity which encompasses the largest possible view of not only diet but also all dimensions of human life, natural order, and cosmic evolution. Macrobiotics, embraces behavior, thought, breathing, exercise, relationships, customs, cultures, ideas, and consciousness, as well as individual and collective life-styles found throughout the world.

In this sense, macrobiotics is not simply or mainly a diet. Macrobiotics means the universal way of life with which humanity has developed biologically, psychologically, and spiritually and with which we will maintain our health, freedom, and happiness. Macrobiotics includes a dietary approach but its purpose is to ensure the survival of the human race and its further evolution on this planet.

Macrobiotics is not an abstract concept but a living reality. It has evolved from generation to generation from the time of the earliest human cultures and civilizations on this planet. It encompasses eating and sleeping, acting and resting, thinking and feeling. Macrobiotics involves respect for parents and ancestors, love and nurturing of children and offspring, caring and helping of brothers and sisters, admiring the beauty and miracle of flowers, trees, mountains, rivers, and stars, and marveling at the rhythmic order of nature and the universe. The macrobiotic spirit is inseparable from serving other people and community, working for family and society, and devotion to health, happiness, peace, and freedom.

Macrobiotics is not the limited philosophy of one time or place, one country or people. It is universal in its scope and eternal in its duration. It encourages the

East to learn from the West, and the West to learn from the East. Both the North and the South have much to teach each another. All antagonisms are seen as complementary: analysis and synthesis, reason and intuition, traditional and modern, spiritual and material. Macrobiotics recognizes that our understanding and practice are not fixed but constantly growing and developing. Following a pattern of general dietary decline over many centuries, it may take humanity possibly several hundred years to fully recover its health and develop the theoretical side of macrobiotics relating to technology, communications, new energy sources, and space travel, as well as reorient society in a more holistic direction.

This small book introduces the dietary aspect of macrobiotics, a first step in our endless journey to the infinite realization of our infinite dream. The principles underlying the dietary approach presented in this work have been applied widely throughout history by all major cultures. For almost a generation now, hundreds of thousands of modern individuals and families in the United States, Canada, South and Central America, Europe, the Middle East, Asia, and Australia have followed this way of life and prepared their daily food based on macrobiotic principles. This food is nutritious, healthful, delicious, and satisfying, and it has contributed to fundamental improvements in the lives of countless individuals, families, and communities. It has brought improved health and longevity, freedom from degenerative disease and the fear of disease, more peaceful and loving relationships, and deeper appreciation of God, nature, and the universe.

Despite the steady growth of macrobiotics in the post-World War II era, its influence is still small compared to the refined and artificial modern way of eating that has spread rapidly around the world. Macrobiotics is still unknown in many towns, cities, regions, and states. Only recently, for example, has macrobiotic literature become available in East Germany, Rumania, Yugoslavia, Czechoslovakia, and other parts of Eastern Europe, and macrobiotic material is beginning to be translated into Russian, Arabic, and Hebrew.

Because of a lack of information or basic understanding, the diet has been often misunderstood. The macrobiotic approach is really very broad and universal. It satisfies both vegetarians and nonvegetarians, can be easily adjusted for those with different levels of activity, conditions of health, or metabolic requirements, and is readily modified for different climates, ages, sexes, and individual preferences and tastes.

The macrobiotic diet is based on the actual practice and common sense understanding of many cultures and peoples. While we present some recent scientific and medical findings in this book, it is not quantitative or statistical in its approach. (To this end, we have not footnoted references in the text but provided a scientific bibliography at the end of the book.) The macrobiotic dietary approach is based on whole foods and a holistic understanding of human beings and the environment, and of mind and body. There are no calories to count, no nutrients to weigh, no micronutrients to measure. No foods are entirely prohibited, and no individual food items are recommended exclusively as the answer to all our needs. The guidelines are based on principles of balance and moderation, harmony and variety. They are easy to understand and easy to follow. I hope that any insufficient explanations will be corrected, added to, and revised in successive generations by those who share the same dream.

I am deeply grateful to my wife, Aveline, and to our family for their love and devotion; to Alex Jack, our coauthor, for his help in writing and editing this book; and to our associates and friends around the world who have contributed to the growth and development of contemporary macrobiotics, including the staffs of the Kushi Foundation, the Kushi Institute, the East West Foundation, the *East West Journal*, and other associated educational centers. I am especially thankful to Olivia Oredson, one of our senior teachers, for her editorial help in the early writing stage of this project and to Florence Nakamura and Donna Cowan for secretarial assistance. My son Lawrence, who is an epidemiologist in the field of heart disease and cancer research, reviewed the nutritional chapter in this book, for which I am grateful. I further extend my appreciation to Japan Publications, Inc., especially its president, Iwao Yoshizaki, and New York representative, Yoshiro Fujiwara, for their thoughtfulness and hard work through the years on this and other manuscripts, as well as distributors of this and other macrobiotic publications.

I sincerely hope that this book will help people recover a healthy way of life, contribute to reversing the modern trends toward biological degeneration and nuclear annihilation, and lead to the eventual realization of one peaceful world.

MICHIO KUSHI
January 1, 1985
Becket, Massachusetts

Contents

Part 1

The Meaning of
the Macrobiotic Diet

The Biological Regeneration of Humanity

Biological Degeneration

The problem facing us today under present civilization is the possible extinction of humanity. Because of the vast scale of this issue, which governs and influences our daily life, it is difficult to comprehend the entire scope of the problem. We do not see clearly how the tide of human destiny is proceeding in the direction of possible human extinction, shaping our lives and consciousness.

There are two major ways the end of civilization and our species could come about. The first is through the degeneration of humanity's physical, psychological, and spiritual quality. This kind of crisis—characterized by epidemic rates of heart disease, cancer, mental illness, and loss of reproductive and immune ability—has been spreading across the world regardless of differences in social and economic system, race and culture, beliefs and customs, age and intellect. Nearly every family and every person in the modern world is touched by one or more of these degenerative conditions. The second crisis is possible world destruction through thermonuclear war, which may arise at any time, annihilate the vast majority of the Earth's population, and leave the world uninhabitable in the future.

Other critical issues can be seen to arise from these two fundamental threats. These include the decomposition of the family, distrust among people, disputes among generations, an increase in criminal behavior, environmental pollution, world poverty and hunger, economic instability, decline of spiritual influence and ethical values, racial, religious, and cultural prejudice, and international conflicts.

However, the second problem of imminent world disaster through nuclear war arising out of social, economic, and political disorder is a global symptom and an inevitable result of the first problem: the underlying biological, psychological, and spiritual degeneration of humanity. As we lose our health and consciousness, as a society we become more rigid in our thinking, more fearful in our responses, and more reckless and extreme in our actions. To reverse the international arms race and create one peaceful world, we must recover our health and judgment. A peaceful mind will naturally prevail among healthy people, generating the spirit of parenthood, brotherhood, and sisterhood necessary to turn away from global war.

What then is the solution? How do we prevent or halt the march toward biological, psychological, and spiritual degeneration and reestablish a healthy, peaceful, happy humanity? Various educational, legal, moral, and religious steps have been urged. Unfortunately, modern education's capacity to contribute to strengthening human understanding has declined as its orientation has shifted to technical and professional training. Similarly, the legal and economic structures of modern society have lost their power to maintain the integrity of the human spirit. Religious and moral influences, which also have been institutionalized, have lost their ability to guide our future development. Modern science and medicine, because of their mechanistic and symptomatic approach to illness, have lost the ability to prevent and relieve physical and psychological disorders. Table 1 summarizes the extent of the degenerative changes we now face.

If biological degeneration—and therefore social decline—proceed at the present rate, humankind will inevitably face total collapse within the next fifty years. This collapse will include economic systems overburdened by rising expenditures for physical and mental health, disabled workers, and a decline in productivity and efficiency of the remaining workforce. Paralysis of political systems will arise from disorders with which a deluded majority or a fanatical minority constantly suffers, while uncontrollable social chaos may result from increasing environmental destruction, accelerated industrialization, and sense of futurelessness living in the

Table 1 Biological and Social Decline

The following figures give a statistical profile of the current biological and social decline of modern society, as represented by the United States. They are derived from the most recent reports of the American Heart Association, the American Cancer Society, and other national medical and public health organizations. The U.S. population is about 225 million.

Cardiovascular Disease	Heart attacks, stroke, and other circulatory disorders are the primary cause of death in modern society, taking 1 in every 2 lives. This has climbed from about 1 death in 9 due to heart and blood vessel disease in 1920. Today 37 million people have high blood pressure, a major risk factor. Each year about 1.5 million Americans have a heart attack, and 550,000 of them will die. Another half million will suffer a stroke, about one-third of which are fatal. Surgically, 1.6 million circulatory operations and procedures are performed each year in the U.S., including 159,000 bypass grafts, 177,000 pacemaker operations, and 414,000 cardiac catheterizations.
Cancer	The second leading cause of death in modern society, cancer claims about 440,000 Americans each year. In addition, 850,000 new cases will develop along with another 400,000 cases of usually nonfatal skin cancer. At the turn of the century, the cancer rate was about 1 in 25 persons. By 1950 it had risen to about 1 in 8, and today it will affect

about 1 in every 3 Americans now living. Lung cancer is rising the most rapidly, while breast cancer will develop in 1 of every 11 women. About 1.5 million biopsies are performed each year.

Arthritis

Fifty million Americans (about 1 in 4) are affected by arthritis. This includes 7.3 million crippling cases, mostly rheumatoid arthritis. Osteo-arthritis, or degenerative joint disease, affects 97 percent of all people over 60. About 250,000 children also suffer from some form of this disease.

Osteoporosis

About 25 percent of all women over 60 will break a bone, due primarily to the degenerative thinning of the bones, which makes them more susceptible to fracture. Older men are also affected.

Mental Illness

At any given time, 29 million Americans—nearly 1 in 5 adults—suffer psychiatric disorders ranging from mildly disabling anxiety to severe schizophrenia. About 5 million of these people seek medical treatment every six months.

Alzheimer's Disease

This degenerative disease of the brain cells affects as estimated 1 million persons, usually between the ages of 40 and 70. There is no current medical treatment.

AIDS

Acquired Immune Deficiency Syndrome (AIDS) has stricken several thousand persons in the last five years and is doubling every six months. It originally affected primarily male homosexuals, intravenous drug users, hemophiliacs, and persons from certain tropical climates. However, now it is beginning to turn up in women, heterosexual men, and other groupings. There is no current medical treatment.

Drug Abuse

From 1970 to 1980, there was an estimated 50 percent increase in illegal drug use and a 250 percent increase in prescriptive drugs such as tranquilizers, sedatives, and stimulants. Medical surveys indicate that about 40 percent of men and 60 percent of women report having used one or more medications in the 48 hours before the survey.

Alcohol Abuse

An estimated 14 million Americans are alcoholics, about 1 in 10 adults. Alcohol abuse is a growing problem among young persons as well.

Diabetes

Eleven million Americans currently have diabetes, about 1 in 20.

Birth Defects

12.7 million Americans have birth defects. In the last 25 years, the number of children reported born with physical abnormalities, mental retardation, or learning defects has doubled, jumping from 70,000 in the late 1950s to 140,000 in 1983, including about 25,000 babies born each year with congenital heart defects. This represents a jump from 2 percent of babies born with defects to 4 percent.

Hearing Loss

Severe hearing loss in infants appears to have increased dramatically in the early 1980s. The number of cases of profound hearing impairment reported in babies under 18 months rose almost five times between 1982 and 1983.

Disability

Five million Americans are incapacitated, requiring help in one or more basic activities such as walking, going outside, bathing, dressing, using the toilet, getting in or out of bed, or eating.

Epilepsy

2.1 million Americans have epilepsy, about 1 in 100.

Parkinson's Disease

About 1.5 million Americans have this disorder, about 1 in 150.

Cerebral Palsy	An estimated 750,000 Americans have this disorder, about 1 in 300.
Multiple Sclerosis	About half a million Americans have this disorder, about 1 in 450.
Sexually Transmitted Diseases	An estimated 30 million Americans have herpes or other new S.T.D. The number is expected to increase geometrically, with no effective medical prevention and relief at the present time. Syphilis, gonorrhea, and other older venereal diseases affect slightly over 1 million people.
Reproductive Disorders	One out of every 5 American couples is infertile. Sperm count in men has dropped 30 to 35 percent since 1920. More than 20 percent of sexually active males are estimated to be sterile. An estimated 40 percent of women have Premenstrual Syndrome (PMS), including 3 percent with severe cases. Forty percent of women have fibroid tumors. Annually there are about 4.2 million operations on female genital organs, including about 700,000 hysterectomies, so that at least half the women over age 60 have had their wombs or ovaries removed. About 1 in 5 babies is now delivered by Cesarean section.
Sterilization	Eighteen percent of couples of childbearing age avoid pregnancy through voluntary sterilization of either partner, making it the most popular form of birth control. Between 1965 and 1982, female sterilization rose from 7 to 26 percent, while male sterilization rose from 5 to 15 percent.
Surgery	In 1981, 25.6 million medical operations were performed, a 62 percent increase over the previous decade.
Abortion	Between 1974 and 1984, the number of legal abortions doubled. Currently 1.5 million abortions are performed each year, about 1 for every 3 births.
Kidney Dialysis	Between 1972 and 1982 the number of kidney dialysis patients rose from 10,300 to 82,000.
Transplants	Each year about 6,000 kidney transplants are performed, 200 pancreas transplants, 175 heart transplants, and 165 liver transplants.
Hospitalization	More than 70 percent of the population die in modern hospitals. In contrast, at the turn of the century, most people died at home.
Divorce	At the turn of the century, 1 in 12 marriages ended in divorce. By 1940 the rate had increased to 1 in 6. In 1970 it was 1 in 3, and in the early 1980s it was 1 in 2.
Family Violence	An average of 456,000 cases of family violence are reported each year, though many additional cases are believed to be unreported. About half of these involve spouses or ex-spouses and the others concern abuse of parents, children, siblings, or other relatives.
School Violence	In a typical month, 282,000 secondary students are physically attacked, 112,000 robbed, and 2.4 million report thefts at school.
Accidents	About 90,000 people die accidentally each year, and 8.8 million receive disabling injuries. An estimated 84 percent of these accidents involve human error.
Crime	Twenty-three million households are touched by crime each year, representing about 27 percent of all households. About one-third of these households experience violent or frightening crimes such as rape, robbery, burglary, or assault by strangers.
Pet Degeneration	An estimated 30 percent of all dogs, including up to 75 percent of older dogs, suffer from heart disease. Cancer in pets is also epidemic.

nuclear age. The family and social system will further deteriorate through the inability of humans to produce healthy offspring by natural means.

If the trend toward degeneration remains unchecked, almost the entire population of the modern world will lose one or more organs, glands, or other body parts through medical operations before the end of the century. Many will attempt to relieve their degenerative condition by turning to artificial organs and functions monitored by mechanical controls such as artificial heart implants, kidney dialysis, or hormonal controls with chemical and electronic intervention. Toward the end of this century and into the early part of the next century, psychological artificialization will begin to develop in parallel with this physical artificialization and will threaten to control human thought processes as well as bodily functions. Such control has already begun in mental and correctional institutions with the use of mood- and behavior-altering drugs and is now being extended to schools, hospitals, companies, and even families and private lives. The use of sleeping pills, birth control pills, stimulants, tranquilizers, and many other synthetic controls has become widespread. In the decades ahead this tendency will spread far more extensively through various chemical, mechanical, electrical, and magnetic means and become an even greater part of everyday life.

Following these changes, bionization—the artificialization of physical structures and functions—and psychonization—the artificialization of mental and spiritual processes—will begin. Erasure of memory and the input of artificial memory will commence. Biocomputers that can interact directly with the human mind, electromagnetic devices, synthesized chemical compounds, and other advances will make possible adjustment and reorientation of human thought. It will become possible to change human views of life by replacing them with artificial views, programming basic concepts such as health, love, peace, justice, life, death, and God. If this happens, *homo sapiens* will lose its natural human quality and become an artificially controlled, mechanical species.

Ironically, modern science and technology have already begun the mass production of lifelike artificial devices similar to natural human beings: robots. While human degeneration and artificialization rapidly spreads, the robot will be developed with more refined qualities of mechanization, controlled by more advanced computers and becoming more "human" in appearance and function. As years pass, this new species will drive away the natural human species more and more from all working domains, beginning from simple, repetitive labors to highly intellectual work, and eventually take over the most responsible positions of governing entire human societies.

During this period of transition, as natural human abilities are replaced by artificial ones, fierce competition will arise between robots and humans and between the semi-humans or semi-robots that may arise from their union as the result of advances in recombinant DNA research and other biogenetic techniques. The competition will inevitably end with victory of the new species because of its perfected artificial mechanical structures and functions in comparison with semi-artificialized human bodies and impaired human judgment. Even if the world escapes annihilation from nuclear weapons, the end of natural *homo sapiens* could come at the early part of the next century if this trend toward biological degeneration and artificialization continues.

What is the cause of biological degeneration that has brought us to the edge of human extinction? The cause involves various physical, psychological, social, and spiritual factors as well as changes in environment—water, soil, and air quality— brought about by the rapid advance of industrialization around the world. However, though influenced by various social and environmental factors, the decline of modern humanity must be directly related to a change of immediate biological origin. The quality of our health and judgment, our thinking and behavior, depends upon the quality of our organs and tissues, our blood and cells, and our health and vitality depend largely on dietary patterns.

Various social changes have taken place during the pageant of human history from Aegean and Vedic times to the present. Political and economic systems have come and gone, technology and the sciences have advanced, culture and the arts have experienced many cycles. However, the greatest change during the last several thousand years has been in our way of eating. Changes in diet in each distinctive historical epoch, especially from the late nineteenth century to the present, have caused far-reaching social change. We are what we eat. Change of what we eat changes our physical, psychological, and spiritual conditions. Change of body, mind, and spirit results in the change of social and cultural expressions as well as personal health and development. A change of food precedes a change of human history. In the past, changes in natural environmental conditions primarily caused changes in the way people ate. However, since the late nineteenth century, change in food quality has arisen largely as a result of technological intervention into the processes of farming, cooking, and natural food preparation.

The change of dietary pattern that has occurred during this recent period up to the present includes the following characteristics:

1. *Loss of principal food:* Whole cereal grains, the traditional Staff of Life in all previous civilizations, have rapidly declined as the principal food in proportion to other categories of foods. This period has also entailed the refinement of whole grains into polished grains as well as the mass production of refined flours.

2. *Increased consumption of animal-quality food:* Meat, poultry, egg, and dairy food intake has substantially risen, replacing whole grains, noodles, pasta, flour, and other grain products as the center of the modern meal. The quality of animal foods, moreover, has deteriorated as a result of the artificial quality of the feed given to animals and the processing of animal foods, including the use of chemicals, hormones, and other synthetic ingredients.

3. *Increased consumption of sugar and sugar-treated products:* White sugar, brown sugar, molasses, dextrose, and other refined sweeteners have been consumed in record amounts, incorporated into many cooked, canned, and bottled foods, including confections and soft drinks, together with artifi-

cially processed sweeteners, either chemically synthesized such as saccharin and nutrasweet or imported from totally different climatic regions.

4. *Change in vegetable consumption:* The modern era has given rise to the mass production of certain limited vegetables such as potato and tomato as the daily use of other kinds of vegetables has declined. Widespread adoption of chemical farming, as well as canning, freezing, and artificial preservation techniques to accommodate longtime storage and distant transport, have resulted in a deterioration in the quality of most vegetables.

5. *Change in fruit consumption:* Wild and naturally cultivated fruits have been replaced by uniform, hybrid species that have been chemically cultivated and sprayed. Consumption of fruits treated with sugar, preservatives, and other additives, as well as canned and frozen fruits, has increased, while that of fresh and naturally dried fruits has declined. Meanwhile, the modern juice industry has been born, emphasizing frozen concentrates and other highly processed products, as well as sugared and artificially colored liquids containing no fruit at all.

6. *Change in legume use:* Traditionally, human beings have received most of their protein from beans and bean products in combination with grains and vegetables. However, today, beans and legumes are raised principally for feeding to livestock rather than utilized for direct human consumption.

7. *Emergence of nonessential food:* The modern supermarket, drive-in restaurant, and vending machine have given rise to the "junk food" meal. Wholesome foods such as whole grains, beans, and vegetables have disappeared from many daily menus altogether in favor of quick, ready-made foods, soft drinks, candy bars, ice cream, coffee, and other excessively fatty, oily, sugary, salty, or spicy foods and beverages that provide a burst of energy or stimulate the senses but provide little nutrition.

8. *Change in farming practices:* Since the Neolithic Era, humanity has cultivated the soil with natural, organic methods of farming. With the rise of mechanical agriculture, chemical fertilizers, pesticides, and other sprays, the quality of food crops as well as livestock products has dramatically altered during the last century.

9. *Change in salt quality:* In recent decades naturally unrefined sea salt has been replaced with artificially refined salt from which nearly all the mineral compounds other than sodium chloride and trace minerals have been removed. As a result of this change, together with the lack of other natural foods including whole grains and vegetables which also supply minerals, a deficiency in mineral balance is now prevalent.

10. *Rise of vitamin consumption:* To furnish some of the nutrients removed from refined grain, white flour, and table salt, as well as those lacking in chemically grown fruits and vegetables, the modern food industry has created synthetic vitamins, minerals, and other food supplements. In the past, human beings received all of these items as part of a balanced whole foods diet.

In brief, as commercialization has become the driving force for the production, processing, and distribution of food, the modern food system has lost the capacity to sustain human health and ensure the future of the human species. Ironically, modern mechanical methods of agriculture, mass production, and artificial processing of food require the input of far more energy to produce food than traditional methods and are thus far less economical. The necessity of machinery, equipment, fuels, artificial fertilizers and pesticides, transportation, chemicals, canning, freezing, packaging, labeling, and advertising all drive up the cost of modern food. To gain one unit of food energy, the modern food and agricultural industry must invest from three to thirty times more energy.

This extreme overinvestment of energy for less energy harvest is totally against the principle of economy. Needless to say, this wasted energy comes largely from natural resources: various types of fuel materials such as gas, petroleum, radio-active elements, as well as mineral ores for equipment and machinery. Thus the modern economy is carrying on a constant deficit of energies, which in combination with other energy uses is contributing to environmental destruction and will eventually exhaust natural resources within a short period, possibly before the middle of the next century by most estimates. To avoid such a crisis, we must either develop new renewable sources of energy or revolutionize current methods of food production and processing toward more energy-saving and natural organic methods. This would also require drastic reduction in consumption of livestock and animal by-products such as dairy food and shifting the sources of animal protein and fat to more vegetable-quality protein and fat from beans, bean products, fish and seafood.

Nutritionally, the changes in modern dietary patterns can be summarized as follows:

1. A drastic increase of simple carbohydrates such as those found in sugar, fruit, milk and other dairy products and a decrease of complex carbohydrate intake as found in whole grains, beans, and their products.
2. A drastic increase of animal protein from sources such as meat, poultry, eggs, and dairy food and a decrease of vegetable protein such as from whole grains, beans, and their products.
3. A drastic increase of saturated fats represented mainly by various animal-quality foods and decrease of unsaturated fats represented mainly by vegetable-quality oils.
4. A drastic increase of nonfibrous products such as various foods of fatty, greasy, oily, creamy, or floury substances and a drastic decrease of fiber foods such as whole grains, beans, and fresh vegetables.
5. A drastic increase of synthetic chemicals in the form of fertilizers, insecticides, preservatives, emulsifiers, stabilizers, and artificial colorings and decrease of natural quality including natural textures, colors, tastes, and odors.
6. A drastic increase of artificial additives such as vitamins, minerals, hormones, and other supplements as seen in the rise of the vitamin industry

and decrease of whole foods containing these nutrients as natural organic substances.

Table 2 shows a change in food patterns in the United States since 1910. A similar pattern is common to many industrial countries and is now beginning to emerge in the developing world with the spread of the modern diet.

Table 2   Food Changes in 1910–1976

(Per capita annual consumption in pounds unless otherwise noted.)

Food	1910	1976	Change (%)
Eggs	305 whole	276 whole	−10
Meat	136.2	165.2	+21
Beef	55.5	95.4	+72
Poultry	18.0	52.9	+194
Fish	11.4	13.7	+20
Canned tuna	0.2	3.1 (1974)	+1,300
Grains	294.0	144.0	−51
Wheat	214.0	112.0	−48
Corn	51.1	7.7	−85
Rice	7.2	7.2	none
Rye	3.6	0.8	−78
Barley	3.5	1.2	−66
Oats	3.5	3.5	none
Buckwheat	2.1	0.05	−98
Beans, peas	13.0	7.0	−46
Fresh vegetables	188.0	144.5	−23
Fresh cabbage	23.2 (1920)	8.3 (1965)	−64
Sweet potato	22.5	4.4	−80
Fresh potato	80.4	48.3	−40
Frozen potato	6.6 (1960)	36.8	+457
Tomato products	5.0 (1920)	22.4	+348
Canned vegetables	12.6 (1920)	53.0	+320
Frozen vegetables	0.57 (1940)	9.9	+1,650
Fresh fruit	123.0	82.0	−33
Processed fruit	20.5	134.6	+556
Grapefruit	1.0	9.0	+800
Frozen citrus	1.0 (1948)	117.0	+11,600
Frozen foods	3.1 (1940)	88.8	+2,764
Dairy	320.2	354.3	+11
Whole milk	29.3 gal.	21.5 gal.	−27
Low fat milk	6.8 gal.	10.6 gal.	+56
Cheese	4.9	20.7	+322
Ice cream	1.9	18.1	+852
Frozen dairy	3.4	50.2	+1,376
Yogurt	0.5 (1967)	2.0	+300
Margarine	1.5	12.5	+733
Sweeteners	89.0	134.6	+51
Corn syrup	3.8	32.7	+761

Food	1910	1976	Change (%)
Sugar	73.7 (1909)	94.8	+29
Soft drinks	1.1 gal.	30.8 gal.	+2,638
Saccharine	2.0 (1960)	8.0	+300
Tea	1.0	0.8	−20
Coffee	9.2	12.8	+39
Alcohol	2.69 gal.	2.69 gal.	none
Food colors	0.03 oz. (1940)	0.34 oz. (1977)	+995
Total food	4.4 per day	4.1 per day	−9
Calories	3,490 per day	3,380 per day	−3
Protein	102 gms.	103 gms.	+1
Fat	124 gms.	159 gms.	+28
Carbohydrate	495 gms.	390 gms.	−21

Sources: U.S. Department of Agriculture statistics summarized in *The Changing American Diet*, published by the Center for Science in the Public Interest and adapted for this chart. Figures do not measure quality, whether organically grown, or naturally processed. For example, the USDA makes no distinction between whole wheat or white refined bread (included in Grain and Wheat categories).

The Biological Revolution of Humanity

In order to save humanity's natural physical, psychological, and spiritual health, it is apparent that we need to change the orientation of our modern civilization. This is biological revolution in a large sense: to preserve, maintain, and develop the human species. This biological revolution does not require any violence, treaties, power politics, or ideological battles. This biological revolution is the first revolution of its kind in history which we—humanity as a whole—has created. It is the most fundamental, most universal, most peaceful revolution. This is a revolution to be carried and spread all over the surface of the Earth wherever the human species dwells. It is far more important than any other movement, whether it be political, economic, religious, psychological, social, cultural, artistic, or humanitarian, because this revolution directly concerns the survival and prosperity of the human species far beyond differences of nationality, religious belief, racial origin, cultural tradition, and ideological pursuation, as well as all difference of modern political, economic, and social systems.

The biological revolution sharply contrasts with recent scientific and medical advances in developing the bionic man and bionic woman. Some examples of bionization include the following:

1. Removal of tonsils, adenoids, glands, and appendixes as preventive measures.
2. Vaccine injections or medications for immunizing against certain diseases

such as smallpox and measles.

3. Replacement of teeth, in part or whole, with artificial teeth of metal, ceramic, or other material.

4. Replacement of degenerated natural hearts, valves, arteries, and other circulatory vessels with artificial hearts and parts made from plastic, metal, or animal organs.

5. Implantation of artificial pancreases to monitor sugar levels and provide insulin as needed in the case of diabetes.

6. Use of pills and medications to control thyroid hormones and/or the removal of the thyroid in whole or part.

7. Removal of the uterus and/or ovaries to prevent fibroid tumors, uterine and ovarian cancer, or other disorders in the female reproductive organs.

8. Periodic supply of chemicals such as estrogens and other hormones to control the menstrual cycle and/or to induce fertility or infertility.

9. Vasectomy, tubal ligation, and other operations to temporarily or permanently block the natural ability of fertilization or conception.

10. Replacement of eye lenses or eyeballs in cases of cataracts, glaucoma, and other serious sight impairment.

11. Implantation of electrodes in the inner ear in order to help the totally or partially deaf to hear some sounds, together with monitoring the individual's own voice level mechanically.

12. Implantation of electrodes in the brain to help some blind to see rough patterns of images.

13. Removal of various lymph glands from the armpit, chest, or groin areas, with the objective of preventing the spread of cancer through the lymphatic system.

14. Removal of testicles or ovaries and giving hormonal substances to supersede the effects of natural hormones, as in the cases of prostate, ovarian, and breast cancer.

15. Skin grafts from other parts of the body with supplemental skin-equivalent tissues to replace burned or discolored skin.

16. Replacement of feet and hands, legs and arms, with artificial ones in order to save other parts of the body from spreading infections or degeneration as in the case of cancer.

17. Periodical cleaning of blood by dialysis in persons with removed or nonfunctional kidneys.

18. Replacement of paralyzed arms with artificial arms which are devised to respond to spoken commands to handle objects.

19. Removal of a part or all of certain organs such as a part of the liver, part or all of the stomach, part or all of the esophagus, the larynx, vocal cords, thyroid glands, a part or all of the spleen, a part or all of either lung, a part of the colon or small intestine, a part or all of the prostate gland, as well as partial removal of certain bones such as those in the rib cage, cervical area, certain vertebrae, and many other parts of the body.

20. Prescribing medications and chemical compounds to monitor, adjust, and control emotional and intellectual thinking as in the case of tranquilizers, stimulants, and sedatives.
21. Prophylactic removal of one or both breasts in the case of healthy women who are said to be in a high-risk category for breast cancer.
22. Removal of part of the brain, with the supplement of chemicals to monitor mental processes and psychological activities.
23. Creation of test-tube babies, surrogate mothers, sperm bank fathers, embryo transfer pregnancies, and other artificial methods of giving birth.

All of these methods of bionizing the natural human body and its physical and mental functions have been already introduced. Further methods, involving direct intervention into DNA, are on the drawing board and may be introduced experimentally and clinically in the late 1980s and 1990s.

The fundamental reason we resort to these artificial methods of bionization is to balance modern physical and psychological disorders. Unfortunately, modern medical science is not oriented to deal with the fundamental causes of disease and disability, which are largely dependent upon our daily way of life including our dietary practice. Modern medicine is directed toward the relief of outward symptoms and emergency life-saving methods. In specific areas, these advances are undeniably of value such as in the treatment of infectious diseases and in lowering the incidence of infant mortality. However, this tendency—especially toward chronic disease—contrasts sharply with traditional medicine, such as that taught by Hippocrates and other Western philosophers and by traditional Oriental medical practitioners, which was oriented toward the prevention of illness and fundamentally curing disease by correcting the underlying cause.

We need to spread biological revolution to make the connection between cause and ailment and to eliminate the causative factors from our daily life that give rise to degeneration and the mistaken solution of artificialization and bionic reconditioning. We need to reorient our daily way of life including day to day dietary patterns, physical exercise, consciousness and way of thinking, human relations with other people, and respect for the natural environment.

Biological revolution is education to change diet and life-style to harmonize with the natural order and thereby safeguard the integrity of humanity for endless generations to come. Such education begins in every home by individual family and community members. This revolution does not begin with any political party, social organization, or ideological platform. It begins from kitchens and pantries, gardens and backyards, where the physical source of our daily life—daily food—is grown and prepared.

In this biological revolution, woman's participation is essential. More so than man, she is the one who produces healthy children through the period of pregnancy before birth and that of breastfeeding after delivery. She is the biological center of the family, and this peaceful revolution of humanity is carried on and realized largely by her initiative and around her awareness and practice. Of course, parenting is also the responsibility of the man, and every one, male or female, is encouraged to learn how to cook, take care of children, and contribute to the housekeeping.

To prevent the extinction of the natural human race and to recover natural pregnancy and delivery, the woman's participation is of utmost importance in the biological revolution. The loss of natural reproductive ability through love and care between woman and man indicates loss of family, followed by loss of physical, emotional, and spiritual unity between them—or marriage. Living together, as a substitute for marriage, will generally become only a means for sensory, emotional, economical, and social convenience. In such circumstances, the natural development of kinship between children and parents and between brothers and sisters, as well as ancestors, offspring, and relatives, will eventually disappear. The recovery of our natural human health and consciousness will also secure the spiritual heritage of humanity. Health and happiness are our natural birthright on this planet. From them are directly derived the spirit of family love, the unity we feel with the natural world, and the trust and vision necessary to build a peaceful world community.

Recovery from Degeneration and the Realization of One Peaceful World

This universal revolution involving the biological reconstruction of humanity is not a medical revolution nor even a nutritional one, though it shall begin from the recovery of proper dietary practice and protection from degenerative disease. The biological revolution has a deeper and wider meaning of changing the entire orientation of modern civilization: to realize one peaceful world and to secure the future of the human species with maximum health, optimal mental and psychological well-being, and the highest spirit.

The biological and spiritual reconstruction of humanity begins with centering the modern diet and returning to a way of eating more in harmony with the environment and human heritage over the last several thousand years. Since the beginning of the Industrial Revolution, the importance of daily food has diminished, and very few people today really understand that diet is the crucial factor in determining and shaping physical health, psychological character, and social behavior. Today the overwhelming majority of scientists, physicians, educators, religious and spiritual leaders, historians, journalists, social workers, business executives, and government leaders still have little awareness of the effects of the foods they eat on personal or social health.

Future generations will probably find it unbelievable that the modern theory of evolution did not see that the dietary pattern of certain species or individuals in relation to environmental conditions was a chief determinant of major characteristics of that species or individual, as well as an essential factor in genetic characteristics or what we call heredity. It is unbelievable that modern psychologists

have overlooked dietary habits in relation to environmental stimuli as basic deter-
minants of psychological and mental tendencies. It is unbelievable that modern
social scientists have not seen that society's dietary patterns in relation to changing
natural climatic conditions are a major factor in the life of the individual, the
family, community and business institutions, and society as a whole. It is unbelievable that modern political scientists and economists do not see that food and
agricultural quality is the primary factor underlying political and economic trends,
including patterns of world hunger and plenty, cycles of war and peace, and the
health and stability of world leaders. It is unbelievable that modern medical
scientists and technologists are not aware of the importance of diet in the prevention and relief of physical and mental disorders.

Because of the lack of understanding regarding the relationship between dietary
patterns and physical, psychological, social, and spiritual affairs, our modern
world has entered into confusion and disorder on a vast scale. Within the capi-
talist, communist, and nonaligned blocs of nations, no viable solution has been
discovered for the possible extinction of humanity through internal biological
degeneration and the possible annihilation of humankind through external
aggression.

Needless to say, there are many factors other than dietary habits which influence
human destiny, but among all of them, dietary habits in relation to natural climatic conditions are the primary factor, directing, motivating, and reciprocally
interacting with other factors. Accordingly, without correcting individual dietary
habits, personal health and happiness will not be achieved, and without correcting
society's dietary habits global peace and harmony will not be realized.

Principles of Macrobiotic Diet

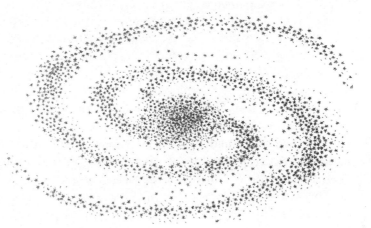

The Order of the Universe

The infinite universe is without beginning and without end. It is spaceless and timeless. However, because it is moving in all dimensions at infinite speed it creates phenomena that are infinitesimal and ephemeral. These manifestations have a beginning and an end, a front and a back, measure and duration, and may be viewed as forms appearing and disappearing in an ocean of nonbeing.

The infinite universe, though itself invisible and beyond the apprehension of the senses, differentiates into two antagonistic and complemental tendencies of centrifugality and centripetality or expansion and contraction, time and space, beginning and end, yin and yang. From the intersection of these two forces, numerous spirals are produced in every dimension.

All phenomena are spirallic in nature, regardless of whether they are visible or invisible, spiritual or physical, energetic or materialistic. Many of the spirals arising in the infinite ocean of existence appear manifest to our eyes. The physical universe, stretching over 10 billion light years in every direction and itself spirallic in structure, contains billions of spiral galaxies, some hundreds of thousands of light years in diameter, which periodically appear and disappear. In turn, these galaxies contain hundreds of millions of spirallic solar systems.

In each spirallic solar system, various planets, together with millions of comets, are spiralling around the spirallic center called the sun. Each planet receives a charge of incoming centripetal force toward its center—a spirallic energy we call gravity. Meanwhile, as a result of turning on its axis, an outgoing centrifugal force is generated toward the periphery. Together these two forces combine to keep the planet in orbit about the sun.

On Earth, a small planet within this solar system belonging to the spiral galaxy called the Milky Way, centripetal inward coming force and centrifugal outward going force produce unaccountable phenomena that appear and disappear, changing constantly. These planetary phenomena include invisibly minute spirals such as electrons, protons, and other subatomic particles; various kinds of elements that combine to form organic and inorganic compounds; numerous kinds of botanical and zoological life; and human beings which appeared during the most recent era of biological evolution on the planet.

As all life exists within worlds of multiple spirals, human life is also spirallically constituted and governed. Not only individual human lives but also human civilizations are subject to the laws of spirallic motion and change. The two antagonistic and complementary forces govern the development of human affairs, underlying patterns of growth and decay, health and sickness, peace and war.

The laws of the inifinite universe have been the subject of study since the beginning of human culture. The principles of spirallic motion and change have been written up, codified, symbolized, depicted, and expressed in many other ways by all traditional human societies and civilizations, with varying degrees of wisdom and understanding. In the Far East, the two primary universal antagonistic and complementary forces were known as yin and yang. In Bible lands they were called movement and rest. Modern science sometimes refers to their electromagnetic charge as plus and minus. In the appendix to this book is a summary of the laws and principles of spirallic motion and change.

One of the principal laws is the law of harmony. According to this law, yin and yang are always balancing in different dimensions to maintain harmony at all times during every step of the changing process. Thus each being is constantly realizing a harmony within itself as well as harmony with external conditions. Harmony is continually being made between past and present, and the future. Each being is continually achieving harmony with other beings, with groups of beings, with the environment, and with the universe itself. The two antagonistic and complementary forces do not act as destructive forces against each other, but they act as opposite factors to maintain balance. Opposite energies attract each other and similar energies repel each other in order to achieve harmony always as a whole.

Another law summarizes the principles of cause and effect. In the process of endless change, yin and yang intersect in serial motion. Upward motion, for example, causes downward motion as the next step; downward motion causes upward motion in the succeeding phase. Faster motion causes slower motion as the next step; the slower motion is succeeded by faster motion. The rate of change varies, furthermore, according to whether the spiral is predominantly centripetal or centrifugal and whether we are at the beginning, middle, or end of the spiral. Meanwhile, there are no independent manifestations that rise separately out of time—unconnected with the past—or out of space—unconnected with the environment in which we live. Therefore, there are no mutations and accidents in the modern sense occurring in the universe. Everything has its cause, and everything becomes the cause for the next process in its change. Therefore, all phenomena are related to each other, and all are connected to each other in the process of change, in time and in space.

Isolation, separation, randomlessness, and meaninglessness exist only in deluded imagination. In reality, there are no separate and autonomous manifestations. The infinite universe is always in perfect harmony. Though we live in the relative world, we are governed by the absolute world. Human destiny is subject to the universal destiny of the cosmos, though the dimensions of time and space differ from each other. According to the law of unity, all phenomena appear differently yet all phenomena arise from the same origin and return to the same source. All beings move differently, yet all beings are governed by the same universal laws of change. The infinite universe, or what we may call God, is our common origin and destiny. From an absolute viewpoint, everything is one. Matter equals non-matter, and nonmatter equals matter. The manifest equals the unmanifest, and the unmanifest equals the manifest. The visible equals the invisible, and the invisible equals the visible. Body equals spirit, and spirit equals body. One equals infinity, and infinity equals one. This dualistic, paradoxical, yet monistic order is the spirallic constitution of the universe. The dialectical harmony of complementary opposite energies—time and space, life and death, day and night, summer and winter, health and sickness, and countless other phenomena—is the order of the infinite universe. There is a purpose and a meaning to this everchanging process, and beyond all appearances everything is always in harmony with endless oneness.

The Order of the Universe, described in these laws is permanent, invincible, and unchanging. These universal principles, though expressed slightly differently here and there, have been known under various names and forms by all traditional human cultures. Today, the laws of spirallic motion and change are occasionally approached by modern poets and philosophers, artists and scientists. However, generally they have completely been forgotten in modern times or have been expressed in very limited and fragmented form. The Order of the Universe is really very simple. Most children readily understand it, and it is apprehended by the adult mind through more intuitive natural and aesthetic comprehension. This capacity is nothing but primary common sense, the birthright of everyone who is living in harmony with nature and their environment.

Modern theories, assumptions, hypotheses, and laws of a psychological, physical, social, and intellectual nature are usually partial or at variance with this traditional understanding. Because they are not based on a comprehensive view of universal order, modern technologies including those responsible for health and human services, medical care, and freedom from violence and aggressive behavior are unable to safeguard humanity's health and happiness. On the contrary, through an unnatural food and agricultural system and an uncontrollable nuclear armaments race, modern civilization is threatening to destroy human life altogether on this planet.

From the point of view of universal justice, if these trends continue, biological degeneration and/or nuclear war can be seen as the universe's way of making evolutionary balance with a species that refuses to respect the laws of nature.

However, such a tragic destiny is not inevitable. We have a choice. Applying the universal principles of change described above to problems of human life and its development, we can make the following judgments:

1. Humanity as a whole is constantly changing, as is every individual.
2. All of the facets of human life are constantly changing and evolving, including the physical, psychological, spiritual, and social dimensions, as well as the relationship between human beings and their environment.
3. All physical and psychological changes that human beings experience, as well as all other aspects of life, change according to orderly laws and principles. Yin and yang—the laws of harmony and relativity—govern all bodily and mental functions including digestion and elimination, inhalation and exhalation, extension and constriction in muscular motion, expansion and contraction of internal organs, antagonistic and complementary functions between the orthosympathetic and parasympathetic nerves, harmonious balance between hormones, balance between red and white blood cells in the circulatory system, smooth coordination between right and left hemispheres of the brain, balance between salt and water retention in the kidneys, and many other similar relationships.
4. All human functions and movements are proceeding in relative harmony between the internal environment (body, organs, thoughts, emotions) and the external environment (natural and social conditions).
5. All physical and psychological manifestations arising in human beings, including symptoms of disease, do not occur accidentally but arise as the result of certain causes.
6. Human behavior and consciousness, including symptoms of disease, are conditioned by outward causes. Humanity's internal condition mirrors the external environment and, in turn, reciprocally influences that environment for better or worse. The primary factors absorbed from the environment are:
   - Food to eat
   - Liquid to drink
   - Air to breathe
   - Vibrations to hear
   - Light waves to see
   - Atmospheric impulses and other external stimulants to sense for reaction
   - Cosmic rays, waves, and invisible forces to influence thought and consciousness
7. Each of these causative forces is composed of antagonistic and complementary factors. For example:
   - *In food and liquid*, yin and yang manifest as vegetable quality versus animal quality, protein versus carbohydrates, complex molecular structure versus simple molecular structure, unsaturated fat versus saturated fat, potassium versus sodium, high fiber versus low fiber, liquid form

versus solid form, vitamin C versus vitamin D or B_{12}, and numerous other antagonistic and complementary factors.

- *In the air*, yin and yang manifest as oxygen versus carbon, oxygen versus carbon dioxide, nitrogen versus hydrogen, wet versus dry, high humidity versus low humidity, low pressure versus high pressure, low temperature versus high temperature, negative ions versus positive ions, and other numerous antagonistic and complementary factors.
- *In vibrations, waves, and rays*, yin and yang manifest as low frequency versus high frequency, low speed versus high speed, long waves versus short waves, ultraviolet versus infrared, sensory detectable waves versus sensory undetectable waves, electromagnetic waves versus nonelectromagnetic waves, negatively charged waves versus positively charged waves, waves from a short distance versus waves from long distances, and other numerous antagonistic and complementary factors.
- *In stimuli and impulses*, yin and yang manifest as light pressure versus heavy pressure, dull pain versus sharp pain, cold sensation versus hot sensation, unpleasant sensation versus pleasurable sensation, stimulants that create ascending energy versus stimulants that create descending energy, dispersing energy versus gathering energy, and other numerous antagonistic and complementary factors.

8. Various combinations of these causative factors produce various differences in the internal physical condition, as well as psychological variations. These physical and psychological differences give rise to different expressions in daily thought, action, and behavior, as well as various conditions including health and sickness, orderliness and disorderliness, life and death.

9. When these causative factors are observed in proper harmony, the individual realizes and maintains physical health and psychological well-being. When they are observed chaotically, the individual experiences physical and psychological disorder.

10. Among the causative factors, food and drink are the two primary factors that the individual can control and manage, while other factors—such as air quality, atmospheric conditions, external vibrations, stimulations and impulses, cosmic rays and waves—are less manageable or practically impossible to control.

11. Food and liquid, as a part of the organic and inorganic life of this planet, synthesize the fundamental forces and energies of the universe and are themselves the culmination of preceding biological evolution. By observing food and liquid intake in proper balance, the individual is able to maximize his or her adaptation to the environment, realize physical health, psychological well-being, and continued mental and spiritual development.

12. By observing a proper diet, the individual maintains a healthy and orderly condition in harmony with the natural and social environment. Food and drink largely determine the internal quality of the individual's blood and lymph, the quality of cells, tissues, and organs, the quality of digestive,

circulatory, nervous, and reproductive systems, the quality of thought and consciousness, the quality of behavior, the quality of human relations, the quality of society, the quality of human interaction with the natural environment, and the quality of the human spirit to be passed on to future generations. Diet is the primary means by which the individual controls his or her destiny and produces all human social activity, including culture and civilization.

Dietary Order According to Yin and Yang

Food is the mode of evolution, the way one species transforms into another. To eat is to take in the whole environment: sunlight, soil, water, and air. The classification of foods into categories of yin and yang is essential for the development of a balanced diet. Different factors in the growth and structure of foods indicate whether the food is predominantly yin or yang:

YIN Energy Creates:	*YANG Energy Creates:*
Growth in a hot climate	Growth in a cold climate
More rapid growth	Slower growth
Foods containing more water	Drier foods
Fruits and leaves, which are more nurtured by expanding energies	Stems, roots, and seeds, which are more nurtured by contracting energies
Growth upward high above the ground	Growth downward below ground
Sour, bitter, sharply sweet, hot, and aromatic foods	Salty, plainly sweet, and pungent foods

To classify foods we must see the predominant factors, since all foods have both yin and yang qualities (see Table 3). One of the most accurate methods of classification is to observe the cycle of growth in food plants. During the winter, the climate is colder (more yin); at this time of year the vegetal energy together with the atmospheric energy descend into the root system. Leaves wither and die as the sap descends to the roots and the vitality of the plant becomes more condensed. Plants used for food and grown in the late autumn and winter are drier and more concentrated. They can be kept for a longer time without spoiling. Examples of these plants are carrots, parsnips, turnips, and cabbages. During the spring and early summer, the vegetal energy together with the atmospheric energy ascend and new greens appear as the weather becomes hotter (more yang). These plants are more yin in nature. Summer vegetables are more watery and perish more quickly. They provide a cooling effect, which is needed in warm months. In late summer, the vegetal energy has reached its zenith and many fruits become ripe. They are very watery and sweet and develop higher above the ground.

Table 3   Examples of Yin and Yang

	YIN ▽*	YANG △*
Attribute	Centrifugal force	Centripetal force
Tendency	Expansion	Contraction
Function	Diffusion	Fusion
	Dispersion	Assimilation
	Separation	Gathering
	Decomposition	Organization
Movement	More inactive, slower	More active, faster
Vibration	Shorter wave and higher frequency	Longer wave and lower frequency
Direction	Ascent and vertical	Descent and horizontal
Position	More outward and peripheral	More inward and central
Weight	Lighter	Heavier
Temperature	Colder	Hotter
Light	Darker	Brighter
Humidity	Wetter	Drier
Density	Thinner	Thicker
Size	Larger	Smaller
Shape	More expansive and fragile	More contractive and harder
Form	Longer	Shorter
Texture	Softer	Harder
Atomic particle	Electron	Proton
Elements	N, O, P, Ca, etc.	H, C, Na, As, Mg, etc.
Environment	Vibration . . . Air . . . Water . . . Earth	
Climatic effects	Tropical climate	Colder climate
Biological	More vegetable quality	More animal quality
Sex	Female	Male
Organ structure	More hollow and expansive	More compacted and condensed
Nerves	More peripheral, orthosympathetic	More central, parasympathetic
Attitude, emotion	More gentle, negative, defensive	More active, positive, aggressive
Work	More psychological and mental	More physical and social
Consciousness	More universal	More specific
Mental function	Dealing more with the future	Dealing more with the past
Culture	More spiritually oriented	More materially oriented
Dimension	Space	Time

* For convenience, the symbols ▽ for Yin, and △ for Yang are used.

This yearly cycle shows the alternation between predominating yin and yang energies as the seasons turn. This same cycle can be applied to the part of the world in which a food originates. Foods that find their origin in hot tropical climates where the vegetation is lush and abundant are more yin, while foods originating in northern or colder climates are more yang. We can also generally classify plants according to color, although there are often exceptions, from the more yin colors—violet, indigo, green, and white—through the more yang colors—yellow, brown, and red. In addition, we should also consider the ratio of various chemical components such as sodium, which is yang or contractive, to potassium, which is yin or expansive, in determining the yin/yang qualities of various foods.

In the practice of daily diet, we need to exercise proper selection of the kinds, quality, and volume of both vegetable and animal food. With some minor exceptions, most vegetable food is more yin than animal food because of the following factors:

1. Vegetable species are fixed or stationary, growing in one place, while animal species are independently mobile, able to cover a large space by their activity.
2. Vegetable species universally manifest their structure in an expanding form, the major portion growing from the ground upward toward the sky or spreading over the ground laterally. On the other hand, animal species generally form compact and separate unities. Vegetables have more expanded forms, such as branches and leaves, growing outward while animal bodies are formed in a more inward direction with compact organs and cells.
3. The body temperatures of plants are cooler than some species of animals and generally they inhale carbon dioxide and exhale oxygen. Animal species generally inhale oxygen and exhale carbon dioxide. Plants are mainly represented by the color green, chlorophyll, while animals are manifested in the color red, hemoglobin. Their chemical structures resemble each other, yet their nuclei are, respectively, magnesium in the case of chlorophyll and iron in the case of hemoglobin.

Although plant species are more yin than animal species, there are different degrees even among the same species, and we can distinguish which plants are relatively more yin and which are more yang. For example, fruits are more yin than vegetables or grains because they are generally more expanded in shape and size, more watery, and sweeter tasting. However, among fruits, the smaller, harder ones such as apples are more yang than oranges or grapefruits, which are larger, softer, and thus more yin. In turn, certain types of apples that are smaller, drier, and more bitter to the taste, such as crab apples, are more yang than larger, more juicy, and sweeter tasting varieties such as red delicious. Furthermore, crab apples that come from trees growing in stony soil and in a sunny environment are usually more yang than those growing in soft soil or in the shade. Even apples from the same tree may differ in their energy and nutrients depending upon the side of the tree they grow on, the height on the tree at which they grow, and the time of season and even time of day at which they fall or are picked.

Thus we are able to classify, from yin to yang or yang to yin, the entire scope of food and drink as well as classify within each category. In the beginning, the simplest division is made among foods that are excessively yang and excessively yin and should be avoided or reduced whenever possible and between foods of more central balance that are suitable for regular consumption.

These categories are summarized below. Note that in the strong yang column, items are categorized from most contractive (refined salt and eggs) to least contractive (fish and seafood), which are thus more suitable for occasional consumption if desired. In the strong yin column, items are listed from least expansive (white rice and white flour) to most expansive (drugs and many medications), so that when traveling or eating out we occasionally find ourselves in a position of selecting polished grains as the least objectionable of the highly processed foodstuffs available. Foods in the center column are generally listed from those of most central balance (whole cereal grains, beans, vegetables, and sea vegetables) that are eaten regularly to those of lesser balance (fruits and natural sweeteners) that are eaten only occasionally and in moderate volume.

Strong Yang Foods
Refined salt
Eggs
Meat
Cheese
Poultry
Fish
Seafood

More Balanced Foods
Whole cereal grains
Beans and bean products
Root, round, and leafy green vegetables
Sea vegetables
Unrefined sea salt, vegetable oil, and other seasonings (if moderately used)
Spring water and well water
Nonaromatic, nonstimulant teas and beverages
Seeds and nuts
Temperate-climate fruit
Rice syrup, barley malt, and other grain-based natural sweeteners
  (if moderately used)

Strong Yin Foods
White rice, white flour
Frozen and canned foods
Tropical fruits and vegetables
Milk, cream, yogurt, and ice cream
Refined oils
Spices (pepper, curry, nutmeg, etc.)
Aromatic and stimulant beverages (coffee, black tea, mint tea, etc.)
Honey, sugar, and refined sweeteners

Alcohol
Foods containing chemicals, preservatives, dyes, pesticides
Drugs (marijuana, cocaine, etc., with some exceptions)
Medications (tranquilizers, antibiotics, etc., with some exceptions)

Since we need to maintain a continually dynamic balance and harmony between yin and yang in order to adapt to our immediate environment, when we eat foods from one extreme, we are naturally attracted to the other. For example, a diet consisting of large quantities of meats, eggs, and other animal foods, which are very yang, requires a correspondingly large intake of foods in the extreme yin category such as tropical fruits, sugar, alcohol, spices, and in some cases, drugs and medications. However, a diet based on such extremes is very difficult to balance, and often results in sickness, which is nothing but imbalance caused by excess of one of the two factors, or both.

After the transition from the old way of eating to the new is accomplished, our use of yin and yang can become more refined and intuitive. Within the category of balanced foods, we may wish to make a distinction among the relatively good-quality yang foods such as grains, unrefined sea salt, *miso*, *tamari* soy sauce, sea vegetables, and root vegetables such as burdock, carrots, and onions and good-quality yin foods such as beans, leafy green vegetables, unrefined vegetable oil, temperate-climate fruit, and natural sweeteners. Over time, as our cooking improves and we become accustomed to the effects of these foods on our bodies and minds, we can begin to balance them according to these relative qualities, as well as taking into account the climate in which we live, the season of the year, the daily weather, the age and sex of family members, and their level of activity, health, and personal needs.

As a general rule, for example, when we plan our menus in the warmer season of the year or in a warmer environment, it is safer to balance these yang climatic factors with slightly more foods from the yin category. Conversely, when selecting foods in the colder season of the year or in colder regions, we can offset these yin environmental factors with a diet slightly higher in food from the yang category. Food can also be made more yang by increasing the length of cooking as well as by increasing other factors such as heat, pressure, and salt or other seasoning. Conversely, food dishes can be made more yin by decreasing cooking time or serving them raw as well as reducing heat, pressure, and salt or other seasoning.

Yin and yang constitute a compass to help guide us through life, including the selection and preparation of daily foods. However, there is a danger of using this tool too conceptually. As we have seen, yin and yang are very relative concepts, and nothing is exclusively one or the other but always a combination of both and subject to constant change. In planning our diet, therefore, we need to keep in mind the balance of the whole, as well as the quality of individual foods we select. As we return to a condition of more sound physical and psychological health, we find that our bodies and minds intuitively respond to the environment according to these universal principles. The judgment according to yin and yang is nothing but the native, intuitive judgment of common sense.

Dietary Order According to Biological Evolution

Nature is continually transforming one species into another. A great food chain extends from bacteria and enzymes to sea invertebrates and vertebrates, amphibians, reptiles, birds, mammals, and human beings. Complementary to this line of animal evolution is a line of plant development ranging from bacteria and enzymes to sea moss and sea vegetables, primitive land vegetables, ancient vegetables, modern vegetables, fruits and nuts, and whole cereal grains. Whole grains evolved parallel with human beings and therefore should form the major portion of our diet, just as nuts and fruits developed with chimpanzees and apes and formed the staple of their diet and as giant ferns and other primitive plant life evolved in an earlier epoch in conjunction with the dinosaurs. The remainder of our food as human beings may be selected from earlier evolutionary varieties of plants and animals, including land and sea vegetables, fresh fruit, seeds and nuts, fish and seafood, and soup containing fermented enzymes and bacteria representing the most primordial form of life and the ancient sea.

In traditional societies, this way of eating is reflected in the natural development of infants and children. After conception, the human embryo develops from a single-celled fertilized egg into a multicellular infant and is nourished entirely on its mother's blood, analogous to the ancient ocean in which biological life began. At birth, mother's milk is the principal food, and as children begin to stand, whole grains and vegetables become their staple fare, with a smaller portion of other supplemental foods.

The exact proportion of plant food to animal food, with the latter being eaten primarily as a condiment or dietary supplement, also reflects humanity's traditional understanding of nature's delicate balance. The ratio approximated seven parts vegetable food to about one part animal food, with the exception of unusual or extreme climatic regions or natural environments such as in the polar zones and in the high mountains. Modern geologists and biologists have found approximately the similar proportion in the evolutionary period of water life, roughly 2.8 billion years, compared to the period of land life, approximately 0.4 billion years. The structure of the human teeth offers another biological clue to humanity's natural way of eating. The thirty-two teeth include twenty molars and premolars for grinding grains, legumes, and seeds; eight incisors for cutting vegetables; and four canines for tearing animal and seafood. Expressed as a ratio of teeth designed for plant use and for animal use, the proportion of twenty-eight to four also comes to 7:1. Other examples of comparative anatomy, such as the length of the intestines, show that the human constitution is suited primarily to the consumption of vegetable-quality food. If animal food is eaten in the human diet, it is ideally selected from among species most distant in the evolutionary order, especially fish and primitive sea life.

With the rise of the Darwinian theory of the survival of the fittest, there developed a modern notion that primitive human societies lived primarily on animal-quality food killed in the hunt. However, recent studies of Paleolithic cultures, as well as dietary investigation of the hunter-gatherer tribes remaining on the planet today, have shown that they consumed primarily vegetable-quality food, including undomesticated grains, wild plants and grasses, tubers, berries, and roots. Fish and animal life, comprising about 5 to 25 percent of food intake, was taken only when necessary and consumed in small amounts. Summarizing the new view of the early diet, the *New York Times* reported in its science section:

"Recent investigations into the dietary habits of prehistoric peoples and their primate predecessors suggest that heavy meat-eating by modern affluent societies may be exceeding the biological capacities evolution built into the human body. The result may be a host of diet-related health problems, such as diabetes, obesity, high blood pressure, coronary heart disease, and some cancers.

"The studies challenge the notion that human beings evolved as aggressive hunting animals who depended primarily upon meat for survival. The new view—coming from findings in such fields as archaeology, anthropology, primatology, and comparative anatomy—instead portrays early humans and their forebears more as herbivores than carnivores. According to these studies, the prehistoric table for at least the last million and a half years was probably set with three times more plant than animal foods, the reverse of what the average American currently eats."

Dietary Order According to Traditional Practice

Generally speaking, if we continue to live in a certain place throughout our lifetime or a large part of our life, we should follow the dietary practices that have been traditionally observed by the majority of people in that particular place. Like most traditional cultures throughout the world, the people of Hunza in Pakistan, the people of Vilcabamba in Ecquador, and the native Inuit people of the Arctic, have maintained certain patterns of eating that have enabled them to enjoy health and longevity down through the centuries. In fact, the word *macrobiotic* meaning "Great Life" or "Long Life" originated in ancient Greece and was used by classical writers to refer to persons who enjoyed unusual health and exceeding old age, such as the Biblical patriarchs, the Chinese sages, and the centenarians of Ethiopia.

However, if long-lived traditional societies begin to adopt foods from another climate zone or use manufactured food they inevitably lose their adaptability to their environment. This is happening in many cases today with the spread of sugar, white flour, soft drinks, hamburgers, and other highly processed foodstuffs.

The traditional way of eating has been developed through the centuries by the accumulated experience of many generations. In many parts of the world there developed religious and ceremonial customs dedicated to certain kinds of energy that food embodied, which their ancestors experienced through the long period of history as the foundation of their cultural and social life. Shintoism in Japan, for example, enshrined the spirit of rice and other grains. North and South American Indians developed an elaborate mythology of gods and goddesses relating to maize. The early Jewish and Christian people respected unleavened bread as a holy means to commune with God. The Greeks and Romans worshipped Demeter and Ceres, the goddesses of grains and the harvest. Through rituals and pageants such as these, ancient peoples handed down their understanding to offspring, teaching them about the way of eating in harmony with their environment and the unity of mind, body, and soul. In many cases, such traditions included special types of dishes and special types of cooking. Proverbs and parables were also left by early societies to tell future generations the importance of certain ways of eating in that environment.

Therefore, wherever we go and live we should respect and integrate into our own dietary practice the way of eating traditionally developed in that locality over many centuries. Of course, over the millennia, traditional cultures went through many cycles of growth and decay so that customs prevailing today are not necessarily those observed during more harmonious times. Moreover, today as modern world citizens, we are building a peaceful, planetary commonwealth that is synthesizing various traditions and values from East and West, and North and South. As a result, our understanding and practice is broader and more universal than that of those who have come before, just as those who come after us will build and improve upon what they have inherited from our era.

Dietary Order According to Natural Environment

From ancient times, each civilization developed a way of eating in harmony with its natural environment. Bound together by common food, mythology, and language, primitive societies learned to adjust to their unique surroundings and to maintain a balance with nature. Degenerative disease was almost unknown, and these early cultures often lasted for a hundred generations or more.

With the introduction of farming in Neolithic times, domesticated grains replace wild cereal grasses and foraged plants as principal fare. The Staff of Life, celebrated in ancient teachings, differed with each culture according to geography and climate. In the Orient it was largely rice and millet. In the Middle East it was mostly barley and wheat. In Europe it was mostly oats and rye, in Russia buckwheat, in Africa sorghum, and in the Americas maize or Indian corn. Staple food was supplemented with beans and legumes, seeds and nuts, garden and wild vegetables, sea vegetables, seasonal fruits, and small supplementary amounts of fish, poultry, meat, or other products of animals mainly living naturally.

Even today, cooked whole grains and beans continue to form the basic nourishment in regions where the modern way of life has not fully penetrated. Thus corn tortillas and black beans form the daily diet in rural and low-income urban areas of Mexico and parts of Central America. Rice and soybean products make up

Figure 1 World Climates

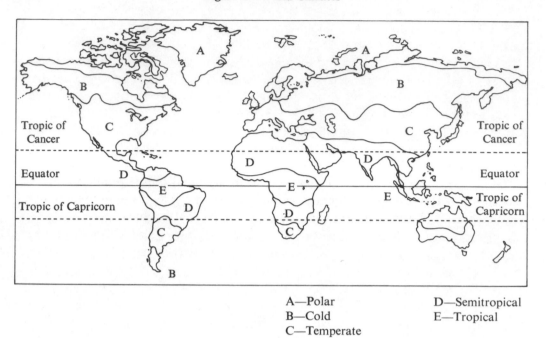

A—Polar   D—Semitropical
B—Cold   E—Tropical
C—Temperate

the staple fare outside the major cities in China, Southeast Asia, and Indonesia. Whole wheat chapatti bread and lentils provide sustenance in India, Pakistan, and Afghanistan. Bulgur, tahini, hummus, and falafel—made from wheat and various beans and seeds—are eaten throughout North Africa and the Middle East.

The two exceptions to this pattern of eating, which extends across the temperate zones of the world, are in the polar regions and in the tropics (see Figure 1). In the northern latitudes, where the growing season is short, a balanced diet evolved over the millennia higher in animal and seafood. In cold regions, while these animal foods were often consumed fresh and raw, cooking of vegetable-quality foods was longer than in warm climates, and salt was used more in cooking and in preserving foods for use throughout the year. In the southern tropical latitudes, where animal food rapidly spoils, people tended to adopt a more completely vegetarian diet higher in fruits, spices, and liquids. In these hotter regions, cooking was lighter and raw foods were consumed more frequently. These types of foods helped to protect against the hot and humid climate as well as, in the case of spices, activate and energize.

The different ways of eating in the polar, temperate, and the equatorial regions are a good example of the dynamic balance of yin and yang. At the poles, the Earth's features are more still. There are barren stretches of snow and ice, long periods of intense cold, and abundant darkness. We may classify the polar and semipolar environment as yin. In the tropics, the landscape teems with life, the weather is hot and humid, and the days are bright and sunny. We may classify the more active tropical and semitropical environment as yang. In-between these two extremes, our four-season temperate climate displays moderate fertility, medium temperature, and days and nights of more balanced fluctuation.

As we saw earlier, yin and yang never exist in isolation. They are always found together in different proportions, and at their extremes they produce their opposites. The further north we go into a cold yin environment, the forms of life become more yang—smaller, harder, and stronger. The further south we go into a hot yang environment, the flora and fauna become more yin—larger, softer, and more delicate. In the temperate zones, the size and shape of plants and animals are more balanced. Thus cranberries and currants grow naturally in colder climates, apples and pears grow in temperate climates, and mangoes and coconuts grow in hot climates.

Of course, these three divisions are the most basic and there are many subdivisions. Within the same climatic region, people who live in the high mountains naturally eat differently from people who live in the lower plains. People who live far inland naturally differ in their way of eating from those along coastal regions or by major waterways. Even within the same local environment, different soil conditions, varying temperatures, and levels of precipitation can give rise to unique strains and varieties of life (see Tables 4 and 5).

To return to the list of strong yang, strong yin, and more balanced foods earlier in this chapter, a number of interesting environmental relationships emerge from studying this order. The foods in the strong yang column are primarily animal foods and are naturally eaten in higher proportions in the colder regions of the world. The foods in the strong yin column are mostly vegetable-quality foods and are primarily native to the tropics. Those in the middle column are common to temperate zones.

Table 4   Yin and Yang in the Animal Kingdom

	Yin (▽) Centrifugal	Yang (△) Centripetal
Environment:	Warmer and more tropical; also, in warm current	Colder and more polar; also in cold current
Air humidity:	More humid	More dry
Species:	Generally more ancient	Generally more modern
Size:	Larger, more expanded	Smaller, more compacted
Activity:	Slower moving and more inactive	Faster moving and more active
Body temperature:	Colder	Warmer
Texture:	Softer, more watery and oily	Harder and drier
Color of flesh:	Transparent——white——brown——pink——red——black	
Odor:	More odor	Less odor
Taste:	Putrid——sour——sweet——salty——bitter	
Chemical components:	Less sodium (Na) and other yang elements	More sodium (Na) and other yang elements
Nutritional components:	Fat.....................Protein.....................Minerals	
Cooking time:	Shorter	Longer

Table 5 Yin and Yang in the Vegetable Kingdom

	Yin (▽) Centrifugal	Yang (△) Centripetal
Environment:	Warmer, more tropical	Colder, more polar
Season:	Grows more in spring and summer	Grows more in autumn and winter
Soil:	More watery and sedimentary	More dry and volcanic
Growing direction:	Vertically growing upward; expanding horizontally underground	Vertically growing downward; expanding horizontally above the ground
Growing speed:	Growing faster	Growing slower
Size:	Larger, more expanded	Smaller, more compacted
Hight:	Taller	Shorter
Texture:	Softer	Harder
Water content:	More juicy and watery	More dry
Color:	Purple——blue——green——yellow——brown——orange——red	
Odor:	Stronger smell	Less smell
Taste:	Spicy——sour——sweet——salty——bitter	
Chemical components:	More K and other yin elements Less Na and other yang elements	Less K and other yin elements More Na and other yang elements
Nutritional components:	Fat——protein——carbohydrate——mineral	
Cooking time:	Faster cooking	Slower cooking

From this list we see that the modern diet combines foods mostly from the strong yang category and the strong yin category. Historically most of these foods originated in either colder northern climates or in hotter southern climates, even though they are now produced in temperate zones owing to advances in transplanting, hybridization, refrigeration, and artificial methods of preservation. In their original habitats, some of these foods are part of a balanced natural diet, for example, curry and spices in India, coconuts in the Pacific Isles, and meat and dairy food in Siberia and Alaska. However, when consumed on a regular basis in a four-season climate, strong yin and strong yang foods are unnatural. Today most Americans, Europeans, Soviets, and Japanese eat large amounts of meat and dairy products suited to a colder, semipolar climate, fruits and vegetables native to the tropics, refined sugar from the tropics, and cola beverages, coffee, and other stimulants prepared from tropical ingredients. This way of eating in a temperate environment violates the ecological order and sooner or later leads to serious physical and psychological imbalance.

Standard Macrobiotic Diet

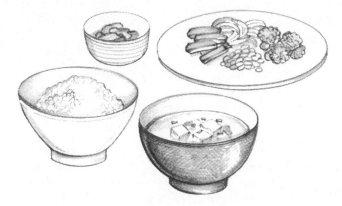

General Guidelines

Macrobiotic "standard" diet varies according to different environmental conditions, especially climate, season, temperature, and atmosphere. It also varies according to personal differences in age, sex, activity, and cultural background as well as individual condition of health and personal needs.

For example, people living in polar regions have to depend heavily on fresh or naturally processed animal meat and fat including whales, caribou, and muskrat, with a relatively smaller percentage of vegetable-quality food, as seen historically in the traditional dietary practice of the Inuit and other arctic populations. Their macrobiotic "standard" diet consists of much more animal food than in temperate or tropical regions. As another example, people living in the middle region of the Soviet Union have heavily depended upon the consumption of buckwheat groats—kasha—as their principal food for many centuries, and this hardy cereal grass is climatically proper in accordance with the macrobiotic view. Conversely, people living in more equatorial areas have culturally depended upon corn or maize, as seen in the history of the native peoples of Central and South America.

People who for generations have lived in the high mountains where the geographical, geological, and climatic conditions make unavailable cereal grains and vegetables usually grown on the plains depend more upon seeds, roots, bark, and other wild grasses as well as mountain grains and wild birds and animals. All the above different patterns of eating have been practiced for thousands of years and can be considered as the macrobiotic "standard" diet for these particular people and regions. However, minor modifications may be needed from the perspective of modern nutrition in the combinations of foods served at the meal and the ways of preparation.

The "Standard Macrobiotic Diet" outlined in this book deals with the majority of the world population living in a temperate four-season climate zone, generally including most of North America, Europe, the Soviet Union, China, Japan, and the major part of Asia, and parts of Latin America and Australia. People in this climatic region—except for certain distinctive areas such as the high mountains, deserts, islands, or swamps, where different dietary patterns are required—have developed modern industrial societies and their way of life, especially patterns of health and sickness and of peace and war, are crucial to the destiny of humanity as a whole.

In this broad geographical area, rapid physical and psychological degeneration is spreading because of chaotic dietary patterns observed individually and collectively in the family and in the community. It is essential for the well-being of the entire planet that a clear understanding of proper dietary patterns be reestablished in the temperate region. The following principles provide a compass for reorienting our direction to one more in harmony with the natural Order of the Universe:

1. *Distinction of principal food from supplemental food:* Consumption of whole cereal grains and their products as the main daily food provides a natural balance of energy and nutrition, leading to centered thinking and behavior and the maintenance of human health, family unity, and community harmony. All other foods, including soup, beans, vegetables, sea vegetables, fruit, fish and seafood, other animal food, seeds and nuts, condiments, and seasonings, are supplemental. Principal food—such as brown rice, whole wheat berries, barley, millet, and other grains—is to be consumed at every meal while the supplemental foods may vary daily, seasonally, and regionally, as well as according to family tradition. Principal food preserves and develops our fundamental characteristics as human beings and creates our physical, psychological, and spiritual foundation and qualities. Without principal food in the past, human civilization would not have developed, and without principal food today and in the future it will degenerate, disappear, and be replaced by an artificial society.

2. *Distinction of supplementary foods in accordance with their importance and frequency of consumption:* The volume, proportion, combination, and style of preparing supplemental foods, such as soup, vegetables, beans and bean products, and sea vegetables, will vary according to climate, season, and other environmental factors as well as personal condition and needs. Supplemental foods, depending upon how they are used, either emphasize or deemphasize certain physical, psychological, and spiritual qualities. On account of different soil conditions, geological features, weather patterns, and other environmental factors, the kinds and combinations of supplemental foods consumed differ widely and contribute to different cultural, familial, and personal expressions. Such diversity in thought, customs, behavior, and language springs directly from the land and its products. This wonderful facet of our human heritage is imperiled by the modern food system and its homogenous, uniform diet.

3. *Distinction of pleasure foods in accordance with individual sensory and emotional satisfaction, social occasions, cultural flavor, fashionable trend, and other*

factors: Party and snack foods such as good-quality hors d'oeuvres, canapés, *tempura* and deep-fried foods, other rich-tasting main courses, sauces, and stews; sweetbreads and pastries; desserts; fruit; juice; beer, wine, *saké*, and other mild alcoholic beverages; and similar items may be used occasionally for variety and enjoyment but are not regular foods for everyday consumption. Pleasure foods are unnecessary for maintaining and developing human physical, psychological, social, and spiritual qualities. But they do influence individual emotional and social behavior, depending upon the volume and frequency of their usage. In moderation, they may be enjoyed by those in usual good health. In modern society, however, pleasure foods have become staple daily fare for many individuals and families, with devastating results to their health and consciousness.

Besides the above three categories of foods, there is a fourth category: medicinal use of food substances. Relief from ailments and disease can usually be achieved by temporary use of certain food substances, singly or in combination with other ingredients, and prepared in various ways. Medicinal foodstuffs sometimes include strong foods, beverages, or herbs not recommended for either regular or occasional use in the ordinary daily diet. The use of medicinal foods is symptomatic, rather than fundamental, and should preferably be observed under the guidance of an experienced macrobiotic family member or counselor. Medicinal preparations are not considered part of the Standard Macrobiotic Diet and will be discussed separately in a later chapter.

Based on these principles, the following macrobiotic dietary guidelines have been formulated for temperate regions of the world (see Figure 2). These guidelines also take into account harmony with evolutionary order, universal dietary traditions in East and West and in North and South, the changing seasons, and individual conditions and needs. They have been further modified with a view to enjoying, within moderation, the benefits and conveniences of modern civilization.

1. *Whole Cereal Grains:* The principal food of each meal is whole cereal grain, comprising from 50 to 60 percent of the total volume of the meal. Whole grains include brown rice, whole wheat berries, barley, millet, and rye, as well as corn, buckwheat, and other botanically similar plants. From time to time, whole grain products, such as cracked wheat, rolled oats, noodles, pasta, bread, baked goods, and other flour products, may be served as part of this volume of principal food. However, their energy and nutrients are substantially less than grain consumed in whole form, which ideally constitutes the center of each meal.

2. *Soup:* One to two small bowls of soup, making up about 5 to 10 percent of daily food intake, are consumed each day. The soup broth is made frequently with miso or tamari soy sauce, which are prepared from naturally fermented soybeans, sea salt, and grains, to which several varieties of land and sea vegetables, especially *wakame* or *kombu*, and other vegetables such as carrots, onions, cabbage, Chinese cabbage, *daikon* greens and root, may be added during cooking. The taste of miso or tamari broth

Figure 2   The Standard Macrobiotic Diet

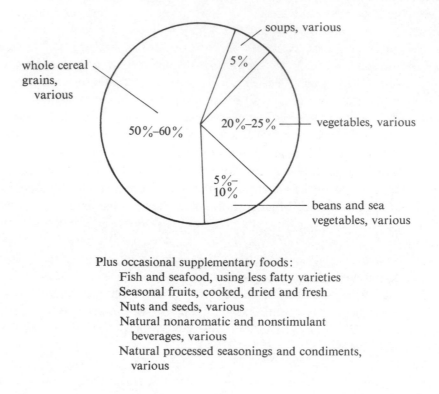

Plus occasional supplementary foods:
  Fish and seafood, using less fatty varieties
  Seasonal fruits, cooked, dried and fresh
  Nuts and seeds, various
  Natural nonaromatic and nonstimulant
    beverages, various
  Natural processed seasonings and condiments,
    various

soup should be mild, not too salty nor too bland. Soups made with grains, beans, vegetables, and occasionally a little fish or seafood may also be prepared frequently as part of this category.

3. *Vegetables:*   About 25 to 30 percent of daily food includes fresh vegetables prepared in a variety of ways, including steaming, various types of boiling, baking, sautéing, salads, marinades, and pickles. The vegetables include a variety of root vegetables (such as cabbage, carrots, burdock, and daikon radish), ground vegetables (such as onions, fall and winter squashes, and cucumbers), and leafy green vegetables (such as kale, collard greens, broccoli, daikon greens, turnip greens, mustard greens, and watercress). The selection will vary with the region, season, availability, personal health, and other factors. More than two-thirds of the vegetables are usually served cooked and up to one-third may be prepared in the form of fresh salad or pickles. Vegetables that historically originated in the tropics, such as tomato and potato, are avoided.

4. *Beans and Bean Products:*   A small portion, about 10 percent by volume, of daily food intake includes cooked beans or bean products such as *tofu*, *tempeh*, and *natto*. These foods may be prepared individually or be cooked together with grains, vegetables, or sea vegetables, as well as served in the form of soup. Though all dried and fresh beans are suitable for consump-

tion, the smaller varieties such as *azuki* beans, lentils, and chick-peas contain less fat and oil and are preferred for regular use.

5. *Sea Vegetables:* Sea vegetables, rich in minerals and vitamins, are eaten daily in small volume, about 5 percent or less. Common varieties including kombu, wakame, *nori*, dulse, *hijiki*, *arame*, and others may be included in soups, cooked with vegetables or beans, or prepared as a side dish. They are usually seasoned with a moderate amount of tamari soy sauce, sea salt, or brown rice vinegar.

6. *Animal Food:* A small volume of fish or seafood may be eaten a few times per week by those in usual good health. White-meat fish generally contain less fat than red-meat or blue-skin varieties. Currently, saltwater fish also usually contain fewer pollutants than freshwater types. To help detoxify the body from the effects of fish and seafood, a small volume of grated daikon, horseradish, ginger, or *wasabi* horseradish is usually consumed at the meal as a condiment. Other animal-quality food, including meat, poultry, eggs, and dairy food, are usually avoided, with the exception of infrequent cases when they may be recommended temporarily for medicinal purposes.

7. *Seeds and Nuts:* Seeds and nuts, lightly roasted and salted with sea salt or seasoned with tamari soy sauce, may be enjoyed as occasional snacks. It is preferable not to overconsume nuts and nut butters as they are difficult to digest and high in fats.

8. *Fruit:* Fruit is eaten by those in usual health a few times a week, preferably cooked or naturally dried, as a snack or dessert, provided the fruit grows in the local climate zone. Raw fruit can also be consumed in moderate volume during its growing season. Fruit juice is generally too concentrated for regular use, although occasional consumption in very hot weather is allowable as is cider in the autumn. Most temperate-climate fruits are suitable for occasional use such as apples, pears, peaches, apricots, grapes, berries, melons, and others. Tropical fruits such as grapefruit, pineapple, mango, and others are avoided.

9. *Desserts:* Dessert is eaten in moderate volume two or three times a week by those in good health and may be consist of cookies, pudding, cake, pie, and other sweet dishes. Naturally sweet foods such as apples, fall and winter squashes, azuki beans, chestnuts, or dried fruit can often be used in dessert recipes without additional sweetening. However, to provide a stronger sweet taste, a natural grain-based sweetener such as rice syrup, barley malt, or *amazaké* may be used. Sugar, honey, molasses, chocolate, carob, and other sweeteners that are refined, extremely strong, or of tropical origin are avoided. A delicious sea vegetable gelatin called *kanten* made with agar-agar and various cut-up fruit, nuts, or beans is very popular and served often.

10. *Seasoning, Thickeners, and Garnishes:* Naturally processed, mineral-rich sea salt and traditional, nonchemicalized miso and tamari soy sauce are used in seasoning to give a salty taste. Food should not have an overly

salty flavor, and seasonings should generally be added during cooking and not at the table, though occasionally personal adjustments may need to be made at the table in which case a moderate amount of seasoning may be added. Other commonly used seasonings include brown rice vinegar, sweet brown rice vinegar, *umeboshi* vinegar, umeboshi plums, and grated ginger-root. The frequent use of spices, herbs, and other stimulant or aromatic substances is generally avoided. For sauces, gravies, and thickening, *kuzu* root powder or arrowroot flour is preferred over other vegetable-quality starches. Sliced scallions, parsley sprigs, nori squares or strips, fresh grated gingerroot, and other ingredients are commonly used as garnishes to provide color, balance taste, stimulate the appetite, and facilitate digestion.

11. *Cooking Oil:*   For daily cooking, naturally processed, unrefined vegetable-quality oil is recommended. Dark sesame oil is used most commonly, though light sesame oil, corn oil, and mustard seed oil are also suitable. Less occasionally or for special occasions, other unrefined vegetable-quality oils such as safflower oil, olive oil, and walnut oil may be used. Generally fried rice, fried noodles, or sautéed vegetables are prepared several times a week using a moderate amount of oil. Occasionally, oil may also be used for preparing tempura, deep-frying grains, vegetables, fish, and seafood, or for use in salad dressings and sauces.

12. *Condiments:*   A small amount of condiments may be used on grains, beans, or vegetables at the table to provide variety, stimulate the appetite, and balance the various tastes of the meal. Regular condiments include *goma-shio* (roasted sesame salt), roasted sea vegetable powders, umeboshi plums, *tekka* root vegetable condiment, and many others.

13. *Pickles:*   A small volume of homemade pickles is eaten each day to aid in digestion of grains and vegetables. Traditionally fermented pickles are made with a variety of root and round vegetables such as daikon, turnips, cabbage, carrots, and cauliflower and are aged in sea salt, rice or wheat bran, tamari soy sauce, umeboshi plums or *shiso* leaves, or miso.

14. *Beverages:*   Spring water or well water is used for drinking, preparing tea and other beverages, and for general cooking. *Bancha* twig tea (also known as *kukicha*) is the most commonly served beverage, though roasted barley tea, roasted brown rice tea, and other grain-based teas or traditional, nonstimulant herbal teas are also used frequently. Grain coffee, umeboshi tea, *Mu* tea, dandelion tea, and other nonaromatic root and herbal teas are prepared occasionally. Less frequently, green tea, fruit juice, vegetable juice, soy milk, beer, wine, saké, and other grain, bean, vegetable, and herbal beverages are served. The consumption of black tea, coffee, herb teas that have stimulant or aromatic effects, distilled water, soft drinks, milk and dairy beverages, and hard liquor is usually limited or avoided.

In Part II, we shall examine in detail each of these categories of foods, describing further their daily use, historical background, quality considerations, varieties and types, methods of cooking and preparation, special dishes, and nutritional and health benefits.

Way of Life Suggestions

The recommendations that follow will help guide you to a more natural way of living.

1. Chew your food well, at least fifty times or more per mouthful.
2. Eat only when you are really hungry.
3. Eat in an orderly and relaxed manner. When you eat, sit with a good posture and take a moment, inwardly or outwardly, to express gratitude for your food. You may eat regularly two or three times per day, as much as you want, provided the proportion is generally correct and each mouthful is thoroughly chewed.
4. It is best to leave the table feeling satisfied but not full.
5. Drink a moderate volume, only when thirsty.
6. Avoid eating for three hours before sleeping as this causes stagnation in the intestines and throughout the body.
7. Wash your body as needed, but avoid long, hot baths or showers which deplete the body of minerals.
8. Scrub and massage your entire body with a hot, damp towel until the skin becomes red, every morning and/or night. At the very least, scrub your hands and feet, including each finger and toe, to stimulate the smooth flow of electromagnetic energy through the body.
9. Wear cotton clothing directly next to the skin, especially cotton under-garments. It is best to avoid wearing synthetic, woolen, or silk clothing directly on the skin as well as wearing excessive metallic jewelry or accessories on the fingers, wrists, or neck as these can interfere with the smooth flow of energy. Try to keep such ornaments simple and graceful.
10. For the deepest and most restful sleep, retire before midnight and rise early in the morning.
11. Be as active as possible in your daily life, including activities such as scrubbing floors, cleaning windows, washing clothes, etc. Systematic exercise programs such as yoga, Dō-in or shiatsu massage, martial arts, and sports can also be helpful.
12. If your condition permits, go outdoors in simple clothing. Try to walk barefoot on the beach, grass, or soil whenever possible, as this stimulates energy flow in the body.
13. Keep your home environment clean and orderly, especially the areas where food is prepared and served.
14. All daily living materials should be as natural as possible. Cotton for

sheets, towels, blankets, and pillowcases, incandescent lighting and natural wooden furnishings, and cotton or wool carpets all contribute toward a more natural atmosphere.

15. It is advisable to use a gas stove or wood stove for daily cooking rather than electric or microwave cooking devices.

16. Avoid or minimize the use of electric objects close to the body, including electric shavers, hair dryers, blankets, heating pads, toothbrushes, etc.

17. Keep large green plants in your home to freshen and enrich the oxygen content of the air. Open windows daily to permit fresh air to circulate, even in cold weather.

18. Use earthenware, cast iron, or stainless steel cookware rather than aluminum or teflon coated pots.

19. If you watch television, do so at a great distance, in order to minimize exposure to radiation. Color television is best avoided.

20. Avoid using chemically produced cosmetics and body care products. For care of teeth, use natural toothpaste, sea salt, *dentie* powder, or clay.

Along with these way of life recommendations, we also suggest the following daily reflections:

1. Develop your appreciation for nature. Every day, try to set aside several minutes to observe and marvel at the wonder and beauty of our natural surroundings. Appreciate the sky, mountains, sun, wind, rain, snow, and all natural phenomena. Regain your sense of wonder at the miracle of life.

2. Live each day happily without being preoccupied with your condition or health. Keep mentally and physically active, and maintain an optimistic and positive attitude.

3. Greet everyone you meet with gratitude. Begin with your friends and family, teachers and elders, children and juniors, and extend your gratitude to all people. Be friends with all animals, too.

4. Introduce the members of your family to your new diet and way of life and encourage them to begin and practice macrobiotics with you. Family support and participation is one of the most important aspects of good health.

5. See your daily life, your work, tasks, chores, and family relations, as an inseparable part of creating a healthy, peaceful planetary commonwealth. Help and pray for others who are sick or suffering and regard everyone as brothers and sisters sharing a common origin and destiny. Persevere endlessly toward realizing one peaceful world, which is the common dream of all humanity.

Nutritional Balance

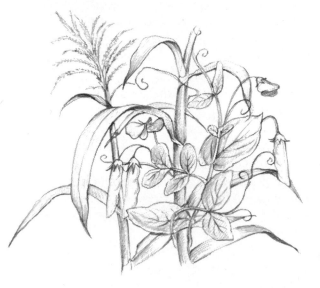

The macrobiotic way of eating is based upon native common sense and an intuitive understanding of the relation between humanity and the environment. It is governed by principles of balance and harmony dynamically achieved between antagonistic and complementary factors, or yin and yang. The macrobiotic way of life has been tested and experienced by billions of people over hundreds of centuries, in most parts of the world, under many names and forms. While all cultures and civilizations go through cycles of growth and decay, a traditional diet based on whole cereal grains remained the foundation of most societies until the advent of modern times. The Staff of Life protected populations from heart disease, cancer, mental illness, loss of reproductive capacity, loss of natural immunity, and the other degenerative diseases that are common today and that together lead to premature, unnatural death for about 99 percent of modern people.

Meanwhile, modern nutrition has made a valuable contribution to the symptomatic treatment of illnesses occasioned by the historic shift in our diet from whole foods and vegetables to refined and artificial foods. In traditional cultures, adoption of processed and chemicalized food has been accompanied by outbreaks of serious illness which modern nutritional science has helped stem. Deficiencies and imbalances in the standard American diet are also corrected to a limited extent by paying attention to calories, protein, vitamins, and other modern scientific categories of food composition.

However, as a whole, nutrition is a very young science, commencing only within the past two centuries. Modern scientific and nutritional studies are still immature and imperfect in many respects and will never reach a stage of perfection as long as they are based almost exclusively on analytical methods and overlook the dynamic relation of life and environment as an organic whole.

Modern nutritional science began in Germany in the nineteenth century and developed around the dietary practices of Prussian men who were considered to be among the healthiest at that time. This way of eating, high in animal protein, saturated fat, and sugar, became the standard for nutritional guidelines in the United States, Europe, and Japan. However, history has shown that the modern diet, and the science of nutrition on which it is based, is dangerously imbalanced and has contributed to the current epidemic of heart disease, cancer, and other degenerative disorders, as well as the consciousness and thinking that led to two devastating world wars.

Over the decades, recommended weight levels, caloric intake, and consumption of protein, fat, carbohydrate, vitamins, minerals, and other nutrients have been revised many times by dietitians and medical bodies, but the basic principles remain unchanged. Even today, many nutritionists still believe that animal-quality protein, sugar, enriched flour, polished rice, canned foods, foods containing chemical additives, and other highly processed substances are as healthy as, or even healthier than, whole natural foods.

Today some nutritionists are taking a more holistic approach to their field, challenging fundamental concepts such as the "basic four food groups" (including the emphasis on meat and dairy foods), and generally trying to harmonize the best of Western science with Eastern philosophy. In order to have a clear and practical understanding of this subject, we need to examine several issues raised by modern nutrition.

Meat and Dairy Products

Meat, poultry, eggs, milk, cheese, and other dairy foods are the backbone of the modern diet. Physiologically, they give the human organism an immediate burst of energy and strength. It was this raw power that allowed nomadic tribes of Indo-Europeans to overrun traditional grain- and vegetable-consuming cultures in ancient Greece, Italy, the Near East, and India. In the Americas, a heavy meat-centered diet enabled pioneers to level whole regions of the continent quickly and efficiently, though at high cost to native peoples and the environment.

While meat and other naturally processed animal-quality foods are part of the traditional diet in colder and polar regions of the world, their regular consumption in temperate and tropical climates can have adverse effects on human health. Meat begins to decompose as soon as it is killed, even with traditional preservatives such as salt or with refrigeration to retard spoilage. Meat is harder to digest than plant foods and continues to putrefy in the digestive tract, taking about 4 to $4\frac{1}{2}$ hours to be absorbed in the intestines versus 2 to $2\frac{1}{2}$ hours for grains and vegetables. Putrefaction produces toxins and amines that accumulate in the liver, kidneys, and large intestine, destroys bacterial culture, especially those that synthesize the vitamin B complexes, and causes degeneration of the villi of the small intestine where metabolized foodstuffs are absorbed into the blood. Saturated fatty acids, from meat and other animal products, accumulate in and around vital organs and blood vessels, often leading to cysts, tumors, and hardening of the arteries. Saturated fat also raises the amount of cholesterol in the blood, further contributing to the buildup of atherosclerotic plaque.

To compensate for eating meat, poultry, eggs, and other animal foods, the body requires more oxygen in the bloodstream. The breath rate rises after eating animal food, making it difficult to maintain a calm mind. Thinking in general becomes defensive, suspicious, rigid, and sometimes aggressive. A very narrow, analytical view is often the result.

Dairy food, which often accompanies meat consumption, contributes a soothing, stabilizing, and overall calming influence on a digestive and nervous system subjected to volatile red-meat elements. However, it can lead to illness in its own right or in combination with other factors.

Casein, the protein in cheese, milk, cream, butter, and other dairy foods, cannot be assimilated easily and begins to accumulate in an undigested state in the upper intestine, putrefying, producing toxins, and leading to a weakening of the gastric, intestinal, pancreatic, and biliary systems, as well as mucous deposits. The inability to digest milk or other dairy products is known as *lactose intolerance* and is found in about 50 to 90 percent of the world's population groups with the exception of those of Scandinavian origin and of some other European ancestries (see Table 6).

Dairy food affects all organs and systems. However, because it is a product of the mammary gland, it primarily affects the human glands and related structures, especially the reproductive organs. The most commonly affected are the breast, uterus, ovaries, prostate, thyroid, nasal cavities, pituitary gland, the cochlea in the ear, and the cerebral area surrounding the midbrain. Its adverse effects first appear as the accumulation of mucus and fat and then the formation of cysts, tumors, and finally cancer. Many people who eat dairy food have mucous accumulations in the nasal cavities and inner ear, resulting in hay fever and hearing difficulty. Accumulation of fatty deposits from dairy food consumption in the kidneys and also gallbladder leads to stones. The development of breast cysts, breast tumors, and finally breast cancer follows a similar pattern. Common problems from dairy also include vaginal discharges, ovarian cysts, fibrosis and uterine cancer, ovarian cancer, and prostate fat accumulation with cyst formation. Many diseases of the reproductive organs, including infertility, are associated with dairy consumption. In the case of the lungs, fat and mucous accumulation in the air sacs causes breathing difficulties. In combination with tobacco, dairy food can trap tars and other ingredients of tobacco smoke in the lungs, often leading to lung cancer.

Modern medical studies have begun to link milk and dairy food consumption with a wide variety of sicknesses including cramps and diarrhea, multiple forms of allergy, iron-deficiency anemia in infants and children, aggressive and anti-social behavior, atherosclerosis and heart attacks, arthritis, and several forms of cancer. Since more oxygen is needed to carry hemoglobin to cells enveloped with mucus,

Table 6 Lactose Intolerance

A majority of the world's population cannot digest milk or dairy products, a normally healthy condition known as lactose intolerance. Lactose is the sugar in dairy foods that is broken down in the intestinal tract by the enzyme lactase. After weaning, most individuals naturally lose lactase activity. However, over the centuries, Northern Europeans and their descendents have generally adapted to dairy food consumption and lactase activity continues past childhood. Lactose intolerance is one reason why developing peoples get sick from powdered milk, infant formula, and other dairy intake.

Population Group	Prevalence of Lactase Deficiency in Healthy Adults (%)
Filipinos	90
Japanese	85
Taiwanese	85
Thais	90
Indians	50
Peruvians	70
Greenland Inuit	80
U.S. Blacks	70
Bantus	90
Greek Cypriots	80
Arabs	78
Israeli Jews	58
Ashkenazi Jews	78
Finns	18
Danes	2
Swiss	7
U.S. Whites	8

Source: Frank A. Oski, M.D., and John D. Bell, *Don't Drink Your Milk*, Wyden Books, 1977.

Table 7 Comparison of Human Milk and Cow's Milk

The ratio of protein to fat and carbohydrate in mother's milk is about 1:7, which is the proper ratio of human width to height, while that of cow's milk is about 2:5 which is the ratio of cow's width and length. This is why people who eat dairy products tend to develop large bone structures and other bovine characteristics. Mother's milk also contains less protein, but it is soluble in water and easy to digest, while cow's milk protein is insoluble, coagulates (curdles) in the stomach and diarrhea occurs. The fat content is the same, but in human milk fat is more finely emulsified. The pH reaction means that with human milk, the blood's normal alkaline condition can be maintained without buffer action, whereas cow's milk requires minerals to offset the acidic reaction. In addition to more natural human qualities, breastfeeding creates psychological and spiritual unity between mother and child.

	Human Milk (%)	Cow's Milk (%)
Water	88.3	87.3
Salt-inorganic minerals	0.2	0.7
Protein	1.5	3.8
Fat	4.0	4.0
Carbohydrates	6.0	4.5
pH reaction	Alkaline	Acid

Source: *The Teachings of Michio Kushi*, 1971.

dairy food consumption contributes also to uneven thinking, dulled reactions, and emotional dependency. Some of these findings are reported in *Don't Drink Your Milk* by Frank A. Oski, M.D. and John D. Bell.

Human milk is the ideal food for human infants (see Table 7). The chief nutrients for which cow's milk and dairy foods are often eaten, such as calcium and iron, are found in proportionately greater amounts in vegetable-quality foods as shown in the tables in this chapter. If animal food is desired, fish and seafood may be taken occasionally. Marine products such as these contain unsaturated rather than saturated fat, and among them white-meat fish and slower-moving shellfish are less fatty than red-meat, blue-skin, or faster-moving varieties.

Calories

Present recommendations of caloric intake made by scientific and medical institutions tend to overestimate the volume of calories required by the average person. The modern method of calculating the calories required for various activities is based upon expenditure of energy as measured by discharge following activities rather than the actual amount of calories really required to carry on those activities. Guidelines based on such analytical examinations result in progressively higher recommendations of caloric intake needed in prosperous countries, where people are eating more rich and refined food, and progressively lower recommendations in countries where the people are eating more simply.

According to the macrobiotic view, one's natural appetite for whole, natural, properly cooked foods and one's regular bowel movements are more practical barometers for determining the necessary volume of food as well as required calories. Caloric requirements vary generally between 1,400 and 1,800 daily depending upon age, sex, and personal condition and need, if the Standard Macrobiotic Diet is generally practiced in a temperate region, with two or three meals consumed per day. In contrast, the average American consumes about 2,400 to 3,300 calories daily.

Furthermore, it is necessary to consider that some foods convert into calories with higher speed than other foods. For example, sugar processed from sugarcane produces calories rapidly, but the caloric discharge soon ceases, while glucose metabolized from whole cereal grains burns slowly and produces caloric energy lasting longer. In this respect, a low-calorie diet centered around grains and vegetables is far superior to a high-calorie diet centered around meat and sugar.

Carbohydrates

Carbohydrates are generally known as sugars, but in speaking of sugar we should specify the variety. Single sugars or *monosaccharides* are found in fruits and honey and include glucose and fructose. Double sugars or *disaccharides* are found in cane sugar and milk and include sucrose and lactose. Complex sugars or *polysaccharides* are found in grains, beans, and vegetables and include cellulose. In the normal digestive process, complex sugars are decomposed gradually and at a nearly even rate by various enzymes in the mouth, stomach, pancreas, and intestines. Complex sugars enter the bloodstream slowly after being broken down into smaller saccharide units. During the process, the pH of the blood remains slightly alkaline.

In contrast, single and double sugars (together known as simple sugars) are metabolized quickly, causing the blood to become overacidic. To compensate for this extreme yin condition, the pancreas secretes a yang hormone, insulin, which allows excess sugar in the blood to be removed and enter the cells of the body. This produces a burst of energy as the glucose (the end product of all sugar metabolism) is oxidized and carbon dioxide and water are given off as wastes. Diabetes, for example, is a disease characterized by the failure of the pancreas to produce enough insulin to neutralize excess blood sugar following years of extreme dietary consumption.

Much of the sugar that enters the bloodstream is originally stored in the liver in the form of glycogen until needed, when it is again changed into glucose. When the amount of glycogen exceeds the liver's storage capacity of about 50 grams, it is released into the bloodstream in the form of fatty acid. This fatty acid is stored first in the more inactive places of the body, such as the buttocks, thighs, and midsection. Then, if cane sugar, fruit sugar, dairy sugar, and other simple sugars continue to be eaten, fatty acid becomes attracted to more yang organs such as the heart, liver, and kidneys, which gradually become encased in a layer of fat and mucus.

This accumulation can also penetrate the inner tissues, weakening the normal functioning of the organs and causing their eventual blockage as in the case of atherosclerosis. The buildup of fat can also lead to various forms of cancer, including tumors of the breast, colon, and reproductive organs. Still another form of degeneration may occur when the body's internal supply of minerals is mobilized to offset the debilitating effects of simple sugar consumption. For example, calcium from the teeth may be depleted to balance the excessive intake of candy, soft drinks, and sugary desserts.

In order to prevent these degenerative effects, it is important to avoid or minimize the consumption of refined carbohydrates, as well as naturally occurring lactose and fructose in dairy foods and fruits, and to eat carbohydrates primarily in the form of polysaccharides found in grains, beans and bean products, vegetables, and sea vegetables.

Protein

Modern nutrition tends to greatly overemphasize the need for protein. While it is true that the human body consists in large part of protein—such as muscle, nails, and hair—the protein required by our body does not necessarily come from the

Table 8　Protein Content in Various Foods

Meat, poultry, dairy food, and seafood are noted for their protein content. Whole grains, beans, and bean products are also high in protein, and some plant foods such as soybeans contain almost 50 percent more protein than a comparable amount of animal food. Protein requirements vary. The U.S. RDA recommends 0.8 grams of protein per kilogram body weight per day, or about 52 grams for an average male and 44 grams for a female. The FAO/WHO international standards are lower, 37 and 29 grams respectively. (Figures per 100 grams, unit g. 100 g.=3.5 ounces, a typical serving.)

Whole Cereal Grains	Brown rice, various types	7.4–7.5
	Wheat, various	9.4–14.0
	Oats	13.0
	Barley, various	8.2–8.9
	Rye, various	12.1–12.7
	Millet, various	9.9–12.7
	Buckwheat, various	11.0–14.5
	Corn, various	8.2–8.9
	Sorghum	11.0–12.7
Beans and Bean Products	Azuki beans	21.5
	Broad beans, various	25.1–26.0
	Kidney beans	20.2
	Lima beans	20.4
	Mung beans	23.0–24.2
	Peas, dried, various	21.7–24.1
	Soybeans, various	34.1–34.3
	Natto	16.9
	Tempeh, various	18.3–48.7
	Tofu	7.8
Seeds and Nuts	Various	11.0–29.7
Meat and Poultry	Beef, various	13.6–21.8
	Pork, various	9.1–21.5
	Chicken, various	14.5–23.4
	Other birds and poultry	18.5–25.3
	Eggs, various	12.9–13.9
Dairy Food	Cheese, various	13.6–27.5
Fish and Seafood	Fishes, various	16.4–25.4
	Shellfish, various	10.6–24.8
	Seafood, various	15.0–20.0

Sources:　U.S. Department of Agriculture and Japan Nutritionist Association.

protein we eat. Within the body, there is a constant interchange among protein, carbohydrate, and fat, so that reserves of carbohydrate and fat are often mobilized to supply the protein needed for body functions. Moreover, daily food is used primarily for energy in carrying on regular activities and only secondarily for the formation and maintenance of bodily functions. The ratio of food used for body construction to food used for daily activity is, on average, about 1: 7, which, of course, fluctuates according to our activities and climatic conditions from about 1: 5 to 1: 10. Generally, protein is used for body maintenance and carbohydrates for daily activity, though they are somewhat interchangeable. Therefore, under normal circumstances, carbohydrates are required in much greater volume in the diet than protein.

In the Standard Macrobiotic Diet, protein is supplied from whole cereal grains, various beans and bean products, sea vegetables, seeds and nuts, and the occasional use of fish and seafood (see Table 8). As part of a balanced diet, these foods supply all the essential amino acids needed by the body. Vegetable-quality protein, moreover, is more flexible than animal-quality protein in the ability to interchange between the needs of body construction and body energy for activity. Recently, medical researchers have begun to associate overconsumption of protein, as well as protein wastes from animal sources, with increased risk of cancer, heart disease, and other degenerative conditions. For example, K. K. Carroll, an internationally renowned cancer and heart disease researcher at the University of Ontario, has stated: "Epidemiological data derived from human populations show that the positive correlation between animal protein in the diet and mortality from coronary heart disease is at least as strong as that between dietary fat and heart disease. . . . The trend toward increasing mortality from coronary heart disease in the United States during this century coincides with a doubling in the ratio of animal protein to vegetable protein in the diet." Excess protein consumption has also been associated with the current epidemic of osteoporosis (thinning of the bones) and fractures in later life. Medical studies have shown that too much protein intensifies the loss of calcium in the body and possibly other minerals.

The average American consumes about 100 grams of protein a day, primarily from animal sources. Macrobiotic persons consume about 40 to 60 grams a day, primarily from plant sources. Generally, beans and legumes have about the same amount of protein as a comparable volume of meat, poultry, and dairy food, while whole grains have about half the amount of animal foods. Soybeans and soybean products such as tofu, tempeh, and natto are particularly high in protein, containing about one and half times more protein than a similar volume of meat and three times as much as eggs. *Seitan*, made from wheat gluten, is also very high in protein and enjoyed frequently in the macrobiotic diet.

Fat

In modern societies, fat is consumed in much larger amounts than in countries where people are eating whole grains as their principal food. For example, in the United States, about 42 percent of the ordinary diet is composed of fat, while in rural Mexico among the Tarahumara, a native people renowned for their health and longevity, the amount is only 12 percent. About 15 percent of the Standard Macrobiotic Diet consists of fat.

Lipids are the family name for fats, oils, and fatlike substances including fatty acids, cholesterol, and lipoproteins. *Fats* are solid at room temperature, while *oils* are fluid. Solid lipids tend to contain more saturated fatty acids. Fatty acids are long chains of carbon and hydrogen atoms including an oxygen molecule at

one end. *Saturated fatty acids* are bonded or saturated to hydrogen atoms.
Unsaturated fatty acids lack at least one pair of hydrogen atoms. *Polyunsaturated fatty acids* are those in which more than one pair is missing.

Fatty acids are the building blocks of fats, just as simple sugars are the fundamental units of carbohydrates. In order to help digest fats, which are insoluble in water and form large globules, the liver secretes bile, a yellowish liquid stored in the gallbladder. In the intestine, bile serves to emulsify fats and enables them to be broken down into fatty acids and glycerol by digestive enzymes.

Lipids are essential to digestion but can be harmful to the body, especially saturated acids like stearic acid, found in animal tissues, which coats the red-blood cells, blocks the capillaries, and deprives the heart of oxygen. One of the main constituents of lipids is *cholesterol*, a naturally occurring substance in the body which contributes to the maintenance of cell walls, serves as a precursor of bile acids and vitamin D, and also a precursor of some hormones. Cholesterol is not found in plants foods but is contained in all animal products, especially meat, egg yolks, and dairy products. Since cholesterol is insoluble in the blood, it attaches itself to a protein that is soluble in order to be transported through the body. This combination is called a *lipoprotein*. However, excess cholesterol in the bloodstream tends to be deposited in artery walls and as plaque eventually causes constriction of the arteries, reduces the flow of blood, and can lead to a heart attack, stroke, or peripheral artery disease. Normally, fat is absorbed by the lymph and enters the bloodstream near the heart. However, if excess lipids accumulate in the body, eventually some will become deposited in the liver. Such stored fat, primarily from meat, poultry, eggs, and dairy products, is usually the chief source of liver malfunctions. Excess fat, especially saturated fat, is also stored in and around vital organs, such as the kidneys, the spleen, the pancreas, and the reproductive organs and is a leading cause of cancer in these sites.

Because of the increased public awareness of the connection among cholesterol, saturated fat, and heart disease and cancer, many people have switched to unsaturated fats and oils, including vegetable cooking oils, mayonnaise, margarine, salad dressings, and artificial creamers and spreads. Today, these make up the largest single source of fat in the American diet. However, unsaturated fats, especially those of a refined quality, serve to redistribute cholesterol from the blood to the tissues and combine with oxygen to form *free radicals*. These are unstable and highly reactive substances that can interact with proteins and cause the loss of elasticity in tissue and general weakening of cells. *Hydrogenated fats*, moreover, such as margarine, are specially treated to remain solid at room temperature, a process that converts their unsaturated fatty acids into saturated fatty acids to a significant degree.

Whole grains, beans, seeds, and nuts contain polyunsaturated fats and oils, but these are naturally balanced by the right proportion of vitamin E and selenium, which are usually lost in the refining process. Similarly, unrefined polyunsaturated cooking oils (in which the vitamin E remains) such as dark sesame oil are a balanced product and, if used moderately, will contribute to proper metabolism, including more flexible motion and thinking.

Vitamins

Vitamins exist naturally in whole foods and should be consumed in whole form as a part of the food together with other nutrients. Vitamin pills and other nutritional supplements became popular in recent decades to offset the deficiencies, and in extreme cases deficiency diseases, caused by modern food processing. In essence, the vitamins and minerals that are taken out of whole wheat, brown rice, sea salt, and other whole unrefined foods to make white flour, white rice, table salt, and other refined foods are sold back to the consumer in capsule form. When taken in this unnatural way as a supplement to our regular food, vitamin pills produce a chaotic effect on the body's metabolism.

For hundreds of thousands of years, humanity has taken vitamins in whole form. This practice is respected by the macrobiotic dietary approach and is beginning to find acceptance in some scientific quarters. For example, in its 1982 report *Diet, Nutrition, and Cancer*, the National Academy of Sciences concluded, "Adverse effects result, at least partly, from the availability (and overuse) of vitamin and mineral supplements. Certain vitamins and most of the minerals are known to be toxic above certain levels." For example, according to medical researchers, megadoses of niacin can cause a wide variety of symptoms including abnormal heart rhythms, headache, cramps, nausea and vomiting; excessive vitamin B_6 can cause severe nervous-system dysfunctions; too much vitamin C can cause mild diarrhea, abdominal cramps, and in some cases precipitate kidney stones; and large amounts of vitamin A or vitamin D can cause acute and chronic toxicity. In addition to the active ingredients, many vitamin and mineral pills, tablets, and capsules contain fillers, binders, disintegrating agents, lubricants, artificial colors and flavors, and synthetic coatings that may also cause harmful effects.

There are two general classes of vitamins: fat-soluble vitamins including A, D, E, and K, and water-soluble vitamins including thiamine (B_1), riboflavin (B_2), B_6, B_{12}, C, niacin, folic acid, biotin, and pantothenic acid. Fat-soluble vitamins are generally more yang, while water-soluble vitamins are generally more yin. (However, there are a few exceptions such as B_{12}, a water-soluble vitamin that is predominantly yang.) When our general food tends to become excessively yin in quality, with more salad, fruits, sugars, and beverages, more volume of yang vitamins with some yin vitamins such as thiamine and riboflavin are required. If our diet becomes excessively yang in quality, with the consumption of meat, eggs, more salted food, and more well-cooked food, more volume of yin vitamins is required. A theory is popular among some people eating a great deal of animal food—or vegetarians who previously ate a lot of meat—that the daily consumption of a large dose of vitamin C is healthful. For their overly yang condition, vitamin C (especially in whole foods rather than in vitamin capsules) may have a temporary beneficial effect. However, vitamin C doses are not suitable for people eating grains and vegetables, whose food is more balanced in quality, already rich in vitamin C. In capsule form, moreover, some vitamin C originates from potatoes, tomatoes, and other solanaceous (nightshade) plants high in this substance. As we shall see in the section on plants of tropical origin in the vegetable chapter, the solanaceous plants have traditionally been considered semi-poisonous and are associated with arthritis and a wide variety of other diseases.

Vitamin C is readily available in a range of whole foods, though many people today believe that citrus fruits are the most efficient source of this nutrient (see Table 9). Such a belief depends largely upon commercial promotion and insufficient understanding of food composition. Many green leafy vegetables contain much more vitamin C than citrus fruits, which are largely tropical and subtropical in origin and can lead to loss of natural immunity if consumed regularly in temperate regions. Also, vitamin C is not destroyed as easily in cooking as generally believed. Large amounts of vitamin C are lost when cooking lasts longer than 8 minutes at 100 degrees C., the boiling temperature of water. In macrobiotic cooking, leafy green vegetables high in vitamin C are usually boiled or steamed from 30 seconds to 1 minute and in some cases 3 to 5 minutes, thereby retaining much of the vitamin C and other important nutrients.

There is also widespread confusion about vitamin B_{12}, which many people believe is found only in animal foods such as liver and eggs. Contrary to such belief, vitamin B_{12} is found in many fermented food products of vegetable origin

Table 9   Vitamin C Content in Various Foods

Citrus fruits are well known as a source of vitamin C (ascorbic acid). However, many green leafy vegetables are very rich in vitamin C, and some temperate-climate and sea vegetables contain modest amounts. The U.S. RDA is 60 mg./day and the FAO/WHO recommendation is 30 mg./day. (Figures per 100 grams, unit mg.)

Leafy Green Vegetables	Broccoli	113
	Brussels sprouts	102
	Cabbage leaves	47
	Cauliflower	78
	Chives	56
	Collard greens	152
	Daikon greens	90
	Kale	186
	Mustard greens	97
	Parsley	172
	Turnip greens	139
	Swiss chard	32
	Watercress	79
Citrus Fruits	Grapefruit	38
	Lemon	77
	Orange	50
	Orange juice	56
	Tangerine	31
Temperate-Climate Fruits	Apricot	10
	Nectarine	13
	Strawberries	59

Source: U.S. Department of Agriculture and Japan Nutritionist Association.

Table 10 Natural Sources of Major Vitamins

Vitamins are found in abundance in whole natural foods consumed in the Standard Macrobiotic Diet and are best consumed in whole form as part of the food itself. Vitamins consumed in pill form may contribute to chaotic metabolism and other symptoms of imbalance. The major vitamins, their functions, and the best sources are listed below.

Vitamin A	Retinol and β-carotene, promotes health of the eyes, skin and inner linings; increases immunity to infection; reduces risk of tumor formation, especially lung cancer. Best sources: carrots, winter squash, rutabaga, and other yellow or orange vegetables; broccoli, kale, and other dark green leafy vegetables; and nori sea vegetable.
Thiamine	Vitamin B_1, essential to carbohydrate metabolism, nervous system function, lactation, fertility; protects against beriberi. Best sources: whole grains, beans, vegetables, seeds and nuts, and sea vegetables, especially nori and wakame sea vegetables.
Riboflavin	Vitamin B_2, essential to carbohydrate and protein metabolism; protects eyes, skin, and mucous membranes; facilitates antibody and red-blood cell formation. Best sources: whole grains, beans, leafy green vegetables, nori and wakame.
Vitamin B_6	Pyridoxine, assists in carbohydrate and protein metabolism. Best sources: whole grains, beans, cabbage, nuts.
Vitamin B_{12}	Cobalamin, assists in red-blood cell formation and maintenance of nerve tissues; protects against pernicious anemia. Best sources: fermented soybean products such as miso, tamari soy sauce, natto, and tempeh; sea vegetables especially nori, kombu, and hijiki; fish and seafood.
Niacin	Contributes to the health of the tongue, skin, and other organs and tissues; aids in fat synthesis, carbohydrate utilization, and tissue respiration; protects against pellagra. Best sources: whole grains; beans; vegetables, especially shiitake mushrooms and green peas; sea vegetables, especially nori and wakame; seeds and nuts.
Folacin	Aids in red-blood cell formation. Best sources: leafy green vegetables and sea vegetables, especially nori and hijiki.
Vitamin C	Ascorbic acid, assists in formation of connective tissue; contributes to healing of wounds and broken bones; aids in red-blood cell formation; protects against capillary wall ruptures, bruising easily, and eventually scurvy; linked with decreased risk of stomach cancer. Best sources: broccoli, mustard greens, kale, and other leafy green vegetables; strawberries, cantaloupe, and other fresh, seasonal, temperate-climate fruits.
Vitamin D	Calciferol, promotes calcium absorption essential in formation of bones and teeth; protects against rickets. Best sources: sunlight, fish liver oils.
Vitamin E	Tocopherol, prevents oxidation of unsaturated fatty acids, vitamins A and C, and other substances in the body; lowers serum cholesterol and facilitates blood circulation; strengthens fertility and potency; inhibits tumor formation. Best sources: green leafy vegetables, unrefined vegetable-quality oils, whole grains, beans.
Vitamin K	Contributes to normal blood clotting. Best sources: leafy green vegetables.

such as miso, tamari soy sauce, tempeh, and natto, as well as in some sea vegetables. In modern society, B-complex vitamins are commonly recommended for various conditions of health, but this practice too has resulted from eating white bread, white flour products, and other refined grains as well as observing other imbalanced dietary habits that do not supply vitamins naturally within each food.

Table 10 lists some common dietary sources of individual vitamins in the macrobiotic diet and shows how they compare with foods in the usual modern diet. A balanced whole foods diet, containing various kinds of whole cereal grains, beans and bean products, vegetables, sea vegetables, fruits, seeds and nuts, and occasional animal food if desired, and using good quality unrefined sea salt and unrefined vegetable-quality cooking oil, supplies all essential nutrients in natural form.

Minerals and Trace Elements

The human body contains various kinds of minerals such as calcium, phosphorous, potassium, sulfur, chlorine, sodium, magnesium, and iron as well as minute amounts of trace elements such as iodine, manganese, copper, nickel, arsenic, bromine, silicon, selenium, and others. Approximately 80 percent of the body consists of water, in which these minerals and trace elements are found, and our bloodstream and other bodily fluids are similar in composition to the primordial ocean in which life began.

Minerals and trace elements are essential to form bones, muscles, and other body structures. Like seawater that neutralizes various toxins streaming into the ocean from the land, the minerals in our circulatory system serve to maintain smooth metabolism by harmonizing the influx of excessive dietary factors. For example, excessive sugar intake results in the condition of acidosis in the blood, which is neutralized by using such minerals as calcium and is ultimately eliminated from the body in the form of carbon dioxide and water. Therefore, a constant supply of various minerals in the form of good quality unrefined sea salt, whole grains and vegetables, and especially mineral-rich sea vegetables is necessary and highly recommended for daily life.

Modern refined table salt is nearly pure sodium chloride, to which trace amounts of mineral compounds, dextrose (a form of refined sugar), and usually potassium iodide have been added. This product is unsuitable for meeting metabolic requirements and is a primary reason why many modern people take mineral supplements. Another reason is to supplement minerals and vitamins lost from foods grown in mineral-poor soil that has been depleted by chemical fertilizers, pesticides, and other sprays. Scientific tests show that organic fruits and vegetables contain up to three times more minerals and trace elements than inorganic produce (see Table 11). Unrefined sea salt, the traditional type of salt used in macrobiotic cooking and food preparation, retains all the natural mineral compounds and trace elements (about sixty in number) found in the sea.

Table 11 Nutrients in Organic and Inorganic Foods

Studies have shown that organic food retains more nutrients than food that is grown with chemical fertilizers and pesticides. This table summarizes the result of one such study, analyzing the mineral contents of selected organically grown produce from a natural foods store and inorganic produce from an ordinary supermarket. The study, conducted by researchers at Rutgers University, found that supermarket vegetables had as little as 25 percent as much mineral content as the organic vegetables.

	Percentage of dry weight		Mill equivalents per 100 grams dry weight				Trace elements parts per million dry matter				
	Total ash or mineral matter	Phosphorous	Calcium	Magnesium	Potassium	Sodium	Boron	Manganese	Iron	Copper	Cobalt
Snap Beans											
Organic	10.45	0.36	40.5	60.0	99.7	8.6	73	60	227	69.0	0.26
Inorganic	4.04	0.22	15.5	14.8	29.1	0.0	10	2	10	3.0	0.00
Cabbage											
Organic	10.38	0.38	60.0	43.6	148.3	20.4	42	13	94	48.0	0.15
Inorganic	6.12	0.18	17.5	13.6	33.7	0.8	7	2	20	0.4	0.00
Lettuce											
Organic	24.48	0.43	71.0	49.3	176.5	12.2	37	169	516	60.0	0.19
Inorganic	7.01	0.22	16.0	13.1	53.7	0.0	6	1	9	3.0	0.00
Tomatoes											
Organic	14.20	0.35	23.0	59.2	148.3	6.5	36	68	1,938	53.0	0.63
Inorganic	6.07	0.16	4.5	4.5	58.8	0.0	3	1	1	0.0	0.00
Spinach											
Organic	28.56	0.52	96.0	203.9	237.0	69.5	88	117	1,584	32.0	0.25
Inorganic	12.38	0.27	47.5	46.9	84.6	0.8	12	1	19	0.3	0.20

Source: "Variations in Mineral Content in Vegetables," Firman E. Baer Report, Rutgers University, 1984.

It is also commonly believed that milk and other dairy foods can supply more calcium than any other foods and that the best source of iron is liver or other animal-quality foods. Tables 12 and 13 show that many other foods contain these nutrients and often in proportionately greater amounts than meat or dairy foods.

Taken in supplemental form, megadoses of minerals—like vitamin pills—can sometimes block the absorption of other essential nutrients or at other times increase the body's normal requirements. Excessive amounts of zinc, for example, can cause anemia by inhibiting copper absorption and in some cases can interfere with proper calcium absorption. Similarly, too much iron or selenium can cause a zinc deficiency. As part of a balanced whole foods diet, these and other nutrients are naturally found in their proper proportion and measure.

Table 12 Calcium Content in Various Foods

Dairy foods are known as a source of calcium, but many other foods are also rich in this element and often contain more than dairy foods. Calcium needs vary with age and other factors. The U.S. RDA varies from 800–1,200 mg./day. (Figures per 100 grams, unit mg. 100 g.=3.5 ounces, an average serving unless otherwise noted.)

Leafy Green Vegetables	Beet greens	100
	Collard greens	203
	Daikon greens	190
	Kale	179
	Mustard greens	183
	Parsley	200
	Spinach	98
	Watercress	90
Beans and Bean Products	Broad beans	100
	Chick-peas	150
	Kidney beans	130
	Soybeans	226
	Miso	140
	Natto	103
	Tofu	128
Grains	Buckwheat	114
Sea Vegetables*	Agar-agar	400
	Arame	1,170
	Dulse	567
	Hijiki	1,400
	Kombu	800
	Nori	400
	Wakame	1,300
Seeds and Nuts*	Sesame seeds	1,160
	Sunflower seeds	140
	Sweet almonds	282
	Brazil nuts	186
	Hazelnuts	209
Fish and Seafood	Carp	50
	Haddock	23
	Salmon	79
	Shortneck clams	80
	Oyster	94
Dairy Food	Cow's milk	118
	Eggs	65
	Goat's milk	120
	Cheese, various	250–850
	Yogurt	120

* A typical serving will usually be from about one-fourth to one-half this amount.
Source: U.S. Department of Agriculture and Japan Nutritionist Association.

Table 13 Iron Content of Various Foods

Foods noted for their iron content include liver and other organ meats, spinach, and molasses. However, whole grains, beans, green leafy vegetables, and seeds generally contain comparable amounts of iron, and sea vegetables contain about two to four times the amount found in animal food. The U.S. RDA varies from 10–18 mg./day. (Figures per 100 grams, unit mg. 100 g.=3.5 ounces, a typical serving unless otherwise noted.)

Whole Grains	Buckwheat	3.1
	Millet	6.8
	Oats	4.6
	Soba	5.0
	Whole wheat, various	3.1–3.3
Beans	Azuki beans	4.8
	Chick-peas	6.9
	Lentils	6.8
	Soybeans	7.0
Green Leafy Vegetables	Beet greens	3.3
	Dandelion greens	3.1
	Mustard greens	3.0
	Parsley	6.2
	Spinach	3.1
	Swiss chard	3.2
*Seeds**	Pumpkin seeds	11.2
	Sesame seeds	10.5
	Sunflower seeds	7.1
*Sea Vegetables**	Arame	12.0
	Dulse	6.3
	Hijiki	29.0
	Kombu	15.0
	Nori	23.0
	Wakame	13.0
Fish and Seafood	Herring	1.1
	Sardines	2.9
	Abalone	2.4
	Oyster	5.5
Meat and Poultry	Beef	3.6
	Chicken	1.6
	Egg yolk	6.3
	Beef liver	6.5
	Calf liver	8.7
	Chicken liver, various	7.9
Refined Sugar	Molasses	6.0

* A typical serving will usually be from one-fourth to one-half this amount.

Source: U.S. Department of Agriculture and Japan Nutritionist Association.

Acid and Alkaline

Our blood, under normal circumstances, is slightly alkaline, having a pH between 7.3 and 7.45. Acids are constantly produced in the body during metabolic processes, yet the blood remains relatively constant by the elimination of excessive acid conditions in the form of carbon dioxide through the lungs, the elimination of urine by the kidneys, and through the action of buffers in the blood that change strong acid into weak acid.

As a result of these reactions, some people today believe that food containing more acid (pH factor less than 7.3) should be avoided in daily eating. Sometimes this belief leads them to avoid consuming whole grains because they appear to be more acid than alkaline when reduced to ash in laboratory testing. In practice, however, living metabolism is different from laboratory experiments such as those measuring acid and alkaline content. Some alkaline foods such as sugar and fruits, for example, often produce excessive acid conditions, though acid foods such as meat and eggs also produce acid conditions. Whole cereal grains, though showing an acidic pH in the laboratory on account of their phosphorous content, produce an overall mild alkalizing condition in the blood, and the compound in whole grains containing phosphorous is used as a buffer to eliminate strong acids from the body.

In general cereal grains (acid in the laboratory) produce alkaline conditions in the body. Most vegetables (alkaline) produce alkaline conditions. Some vegetables, especially those of tropical origin (alkaline), produce acid conditions. Sugar (alkaline) produces acid conditions. Meat and other animal food (acid) produce acid conditions. Fat and oil (acid) produce acid conditions. Minerals (alkaline and acid) produce alkaline in some cases, acid in other cases, and buffer effects in still other cases.

In practice, yin and yang are much more useful concepts than acid and alkaline in evaluating the energy and nutrients of food, as well as their effect on living organisms. In general, we may say that excessively yin and excessively yang foods such as meat and sugar, dairy products and chemicalized foods, and tropical fruits and vegetables, produce acidic conditions in the body, including weak unhealthy blood. Meanwhile, balanced foods such as whole grains, beans and bean products, vegetables, and sea vegetables produce alkaline conditions in the body, including strong and healthy blood.

Nutritional Studies

When macrobiotics first became popular in the United States, Canada, and Europe in the 1960s, concern was expressed about the nutritional adequacy of the diet. Some doctors and nutritionists of that period questioned the value of any vegetarian or semivegetarian diet that did not include meat and dairy products.

In addition, macrobiotics incorporated many foods of Far Eastern origin with which dietitians were unfamiliar. Complicating matters, macrobiotics was sometimes poorly taught and understood, and some early practitioners mistook a temporary healing diet consisting of 100 percent whole cereal grains for the ideal daily diet. As a result, some individual cases of undernourishment and vitamin deficiencies resulted.

In the several decades since then, however, the adverse effects of high meat and dairy food consumption, sugar intake, and chemical additives have been widely recognized. The wisdom of eating whole grains and vegetables high in complex carbohydrates, fiber, and including vitamins and minerals in whole form have become national and international dietary policy. Brown rice, whole grain bread, tofu, tamari soy sauce, and many other macrobiotic foods are now carried in many supermarkets. The physical and psychological benefits of breastfeeding have been rediscovered, and more and more mothers are bringing up their babies in a more natural environment, including natural way of eating.

Recent studies by scientists, medical doctors, and public health officials have found that the Standard Macrobiotic Diet is completely sound and meets all the nutritional standards of the Recommended Dietary Allowances (RDA), published by the National Academy of Sciences, and the international guidelines put forth by the Food and Agricultural Organization and the World Health Organization (FAO/WHO). For example, a study published in the *Journal of the American Dietetic Association* in 1980 found that macrobiotic subjects received acceptable amounts of iron, vitamin C, vitamin A, thiamine, riboflavin, vitamin B_{12}, and folate. The study also noted that macrobiotic people tended to weigh less than other people. While tables of recommended weights have consistently fallen in recent years, macrobiotic people still weigh about 10 to 20 pounds less than the recommended amounts. Though lean to modern observers, these weights are perfectly normal for people in traditional societies.

In 1984, the Congressional Subcommittee on Health and Long-Term Care investigated the dietary practices of several groups and concluded, "The current macrobiotic diet is essentially an almost pure vegetarian diet as compared to the predominantly lacto-ovo-vegetarian diet primarily practiced by Seventh Day Adventists. This macrobiotic diet appears to be nutritionally adequate if the mix of foods proposed in the dietary recommendations are followed carefully. There is no apparent evidence of any nutritional deficiencies among current macrobiotic practices. . . . The diet would also be consistent with the recently released dietary guidelines of the National Academy of Sciences and the American Cancer Society in regard to possible reduction of cancer risks."

During the last fifteen years, modern society has substantially improved its way of eating. Heart disease is down by about 20 percent in the United States, primarily as the result of a drop in meat and dairy food consumption and an increase in the consumption of whole grains and fresh vegetables. National and international food and nutritional organizations have issued dietary guidelines that are moving in the macrobiotic direction (see Table 14). In 1977, the Senate Select Committee on Nutrition and Human Needs issued a historic report, *Dietary*

Table 14   Dietary Comparisons

This table compares the composition of the Standard American Diet, the Dietary Goals recommended by the Senate Select Committee on Nutrition and Human Needs in 1977, and the Standard Macrobiotic Diet. The percentages of each menu represent the proportion of calories from each food group.

STANDARD AMERICAN DIET

Fats	Saturated	16%	Much of it is from meat and dairy products, including highly saturated sources such as butter, steak, and hard cheeses; some highly saturated oils (coconut, palm kernel).
	Monounsaturated	19%	
	Polyunsaturated	7%	
Proteins	Animal sources	8%	Mostly from animal sources such as meat, eggs, and dairy products.
	Other sources	4%	
Carbohydrates	Refined flour	28%	White bread, processed cereals, pastries, sugared beverages, ice cream, French fries, donuts, potato chips, some canned and frozen fruits and vegetables, alcohol.
	Refined and processed sugars	18%	

DIETARY GOALS

Fats	Saturated	10%	Animal sources with less saturated fat, i.e., margarine instead of butter; lean meat; low-fat dairy.
	Monounsaturated	10%	
	Polyunsaturated	10%	
Proteins	Poultry and fish	8%	Poultry, fish, lean meat, low-fat dairy products, beans, nuts.
	Lean meat and other	4%	
Carbohydrates	Fresh vegetables, fruits, and whole grains	48%	Refined cereal products; whole grains and whole grain flours; honey, cane and beet sugar, molasses.
	Refined and processed sugars	10%	

MACROBIOTIC DIET

Fats	Saturated	2%	Primary sources of fat are from whole grains and beans, vegetable oils such as sesame used in cooking, seeds and nuts.
	Monounsaturated	8%	
	Polyunsaturated	5%	
Protein	Plant sources	8%	Mostly from whole grains, beans, bean products such as tofu and tempeh, and some fish, seeds, and nuts.
	Fish and other	4%	
Carbohydrates	Whole grains, fresh vegetables, sea vegetables, fruits, some naturally occurring sugars	73%	Primarily from whole grains such as brown rice, barley, rye, millet, buckwheat, corn, whole wheat, fresh vegetables, sea vegetables, and some fruit.

Goals for the United States, linking the modern diet with six of the leading causes of death in modern society. Along with other groups and individuals, macrobiotic educators, counselors, and journalists met with members of this panel and discussed national food and health care policy. In an endorsement of our book *The Cancer-Prevention Diet*, George McGovern, chairman of the committee and author of the report, characterized the macrobiotic approach "as a prudent diet in the prevention of cancer."

In its study of *Diet, Nutrition, and Cancer*, the National Academy of Sciences went even further than the Senate Committee, linking the modern food system with nearly all common forms of cancer. In its final 472-page report, the researchers concluded that Americans suffered from overnutrition for which modern nutritional science, as well as the modern food processing system, was responsible: "Just as it was once difficult for investigators to recognize that a symptom complex could be caused by the lack of a nutrient, so until recently has it been difficult for scientists to recognize that certain pathological conditions might result from an abundant and apparently normal diet." The scientists noted that about 55 percent of the food consumed in the United States today has been processed to some degree before distribution to the consumer. Looking to the future and reversing the trend toward biological degeneration, the report stated, "The dietary changes now under way appear to be reducing our dependence on foods from animal sources. It is likely that there will be continued reduction in fats from animal sources and an increasing dependence on vegetable and other plant products for protein supplies. Hence, diets may contain increasing amounts of vegetable products, some of which may be protective against cancer."

Part 2

The Contents of
the Macrobiotic Diet

Whole Cereal Grains

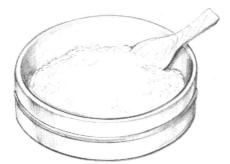

Daily Use

Within the Standard Macrobiotic Diet, whole cereal grains and grain products, including bread, pasta, and noodles, are an essential part of the daily diet. They usually comprise about 40 to 60 percent by cooked volume of the daily food intake, with the average about 50 percent.

This proportion may vary depending upon individual physical and psychological conditions; climatic and other environmental factors; the way of cooking; and kinds, volume, and preparation of supplemental food. For example, in the case of digestive disorders, the consumption of whole grains may need to be increased to 70 to 80 percent for several days. In the case of intensive mental activity, it may need to be adjusted to 60 to 70 percent for a short period. On social occasions, it may be reduced to less than 50 percent with more variety of side dishes. During intensive spiritual exercise, 60 to 80 percent may be needed for short duration, while for intensive physical activities the volume may need to be about 50 percent.

For regular consumption, whole grains and grain products should be unrefined and organic or natural in quality, avoiding as much as possible the use of petroleum, chemicals, or other artificial ingredients in fertilizers, pesticides, insecticides, preservatives, and sprays.

History

Whole cereal grains, wild or domesticated, have constituted the principal food of humanity for tens of thousands of years. Every civilization prior to our own recognized whole grain as the Staff of Life, and the different types of grain, farming methods, cooking, and other ways of preparation gave rise to the wonderful diversity and richness of the Earth's cultures and societies. Cooked whole grains and their products, in particular, have constituted humanity's staple food for millennia and, until modern times, were eaten as the main food throughout the world. For example, rice and millet were principal foods in the Far East; wheat, oats, and rye in Europe; buckwheat in Russia and central Asia; sorghum in Africa; barley in the Middle East; and corn in the Americas. Traditionally, the consumption of whole grains in bread form was more prevalent in the West than in the East where noodles were often used as a substitute for the main whole grain. Also, though corn and buckwheat are members of a different botanical family than other grains, they are traditionally included in this general category as sub-cereal plants.

Quality

Whole grains such as brown rice, millet, barley, oats, and corn are traditionally prepared in whole form, and this way of eating imparts the most healthful, balanced, and peaceful energy. The superiority of grain in whole form to cracked grain or flour products is apparent in respect to storage, preservation, and con-venience of transportation. Ideally, whole grains should remain unhulled until shortly before cooking in order to preserve their energetic and nutritional values. The hard outer hull or husk, though inedible, is rich in cellulose and fiber, and after harvesting helps protect the inner layers of the grain. Such unhulled grains can be preserved almost indefinitely without loss of vitality. Archaeologists have discovered that well-preserved whole cereal grains and other seeds will sprout after centuries under natural soil and atmospheric conditions.

Whole grains are generally sold in the natural foods store hulled (that is, with-out their hulls). Hulled whole grains will keep their vitality as long as the thin cellulose film covering the outer layer remains perfectly preserved without any physical damage. However, hulled grains are easily damaged or scratched by physical force in handling, although the surface transparent skin of the grain is very resistant to chemical invasion. During the processes of hulling, sacking, carrying, and transporting to the food store, some percentage of whole grains is damaged by physical force, resulting in a change in quality and loss of energy. Chipped grains, for example, may no longer be cultivated since their life energy has been dispersed. The lesser the degree of such damage, the higher the quality of hulled whole grains. Ideally, whole grains are hulled just before using. Small, motorized hulling machines are now available for community and household use, and some of the producers of organic brown rice in this country have recently agreed to make available sacks of unhulled grain to natural foods stores for this purpose.

Meanwhile, historically, the flouring or crushing process has been applied to some grains whose outer coats are relatively hard and require proportionately more chewing to digest. These include whole wheat berries, whole rye, and often buckwheat groats. Not only harder-hulled grains but also other softer grains such as brown rice, millet, and oats have been used occasionally crushed or in the form of flours. These flour products or crushed grains also come within the overall category of principal food, and the more common forms include pasta and noodles; breads, pancakes, and chapatis; various forms of meals; various flakes; and various half-cut, crushed grains including bulgur and rolled oats.

While these flour products and other grain products may be used from time to time for variety and enjoyment, their energy is not as complete as grain prepared in whole form. Moreover, they are nutritionally inferior to grains consumed in whole form because of oxidation and other rapid changes in the quality of their carbohydrates, proteins, fat, vitamins, and other components. To maximize the healthful quality of flour and grain products, the macrobiotic cook may observe the following guidelines:

1. Flour should be ground as freshly as possible in order to avoid the substantial change in quality of ingredients that occurs when the whole grain is processed. Similarly, when crushing grains into smaller pieces for making cracked grains, meal, or flakes, crushing should be done as close to the time of cooking as possible. A small handmill for stone-grinding grains at home is very useful for this purpose.
2. Products such as bread, pancakes, chapatis, and flakes are not to be prepared with commercial yeast, baking soda, or other additives, including chemical preservatives and flavors. They should be processed only with natural quality substances and seasonings such as unrefined sea salt, naturally fermented tamari soy sauce, and other soybean or grain products. In the case of bread and other baked products, there are wild yeasts in the air that will naturally ferment, causing the dough to rise and yielding a moderately light, tasty loaf or other naturally leavened product.

Table 15 Nutrients Lost in Refining Wheat Flour

When whole wheat flour is milled into white flour, much of the germ (embryo), bran, and surface endosperm are removed. As a result, the flour loses most of its energy and vitality as well as its natural oils and nutrients. Though a few of the vitamins and minerals are returned in enriching, the resulting quality is not the same. This table shows the typical loss of nutrients in producing white flour.

Nutrient	Loss (%)	Nutrient	Loss (%)
Thiamine (B$_1$)	77.1	Sodium	78.3
Riboflavin (B$_2$)	80.0	Chromium	40.0
Niacin	80.8	Manganese	85.8
Vitamin B$_6$	71.8	Iron	75.6
Pantothenic acid	50.0	Cobalt	88.5
Vitamin E	86.3	Copper	67.9
Calcium	60.0	Zinc	77.7
Phosphorous	70.9	Selenium	15.9
Magnesium	84.7	Molybdenum	48.0
Potassium	77.0		

Source: Henry A. Schroeder, "Losses of Vitamins and Trace Minerals Resulting from Processing and Preservation of Foods," *American Journal of Clinical Nutrition*, 1971.

3. When preparing flour or other grain products, natural methods of mixing, stirring, pressing, heating, diluting, and other forms of processing should be observed. Electricity, microwave radiation, and other modern technical methods that tend to destroy the organic structure of food molecules should be avoided. Flour is traditionally made by grinding whole wheat berries with millstones at a very slow speed and a cool temperature. This process, known as stone grinding, preserves the precious wheat germ, allowing the grain to ferment naturally, and retains the normal acidity and oxidation levels of the whole grain.
4. White flour should be avoided (see Table 15).

Varieties

Rice

Brown rice, now grown virtually around the world, is divided into three types. *Short-grain rice* is the smallest and hardiest of the three, as well as contains the most minerals and a high amount of gluten (the protein factor in grain). It is naturally sweet to the taste and the most suitable for daily consumption. *Medium-grain rice* is slightly larger and cooks up slightly softer and more moist. It too is excellent for daily consumption. *Long-grain rice*, a longer variety, is light and fluffy when cooked. It is prepared more in tropical and subtropical areas or during the hotter time of the year in temperate climates.

There is another type of rice called *sweet rice*. It is more glutinous than regular brown rice and slightly sweeter to the taste. It is primarily used in making *mochi*, amazaké, cookies, crackers, and other special preparations. Brown rice products include puffed brown rice, used as an occasional breakfast cereal or in rice cakes; brown rice flour or sweet brown rice flour used in baking; and brown rice flakes. *Wild rice*, an uncultivated cereal grass used by traditional North American peoples, is not a member of the same species as regular rice but shares similar qualities. Because of its scarcity and price, it is used sparingly, usually in holiday or festive cooking.

Barley

Barley is the traditional staple of ancient Egypt, Greece, Rome, and the Middle East. In the Far East there is a special type of whole barley called *pearl barley* that is smaller, whiter, and more compact than ordinary barley. Especially delicious and soothing, pearl barley is traditionally used for medicinal and cosmetic purposes. Like wild rice, its price is high and can thus be used only occasionally. There is another type of barley called *pearled barley*, which is to be carefully distinguished from pearl barley. Pearled barley is a milled form of the grain from which some vitamins and minerals have been removed. For ordinary, everyday

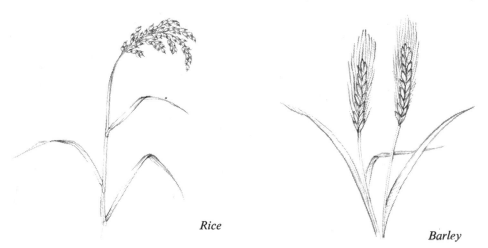

Rice   *Barley*

use unhulled or hulled organic whole barley is recommended. Barley flour, puffed barley, and other barley products may be used occasionally.

Millet

Whole millet is the traditional staple of northern Asia and some parts of Europe and Africa. There are many varieties. Those grown in the United States and Canada are primarily yellow in color, while those in the Far East are often red. Because of its small, compact form, millet is rarely crushed or split. However, it may be ground into flour and used in baking or puffed up. Much of the millet available in natural foods stores is organic in quality.

Oats

In antiquity, oats spread across Northern Europe and became the principal food in Scotland, Ireland, and parts of England. Oats are now grown in many other parts of the world. Three forms are commonly available. *Whole oats*, from which only

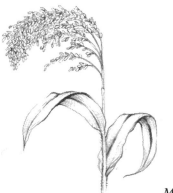

Millet

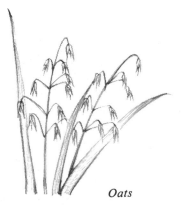

Oats

the outer husks have been removed, provide the most energy and vitality. They are preferred for everyday use, even though they take longer to prepare than the other two types. *Scotch oats* have been steamed and steel-cut into small pieces. They make for a very chewy dish. *Rolled oats* have been steamed and passed through rollers. Although the most common form of oatmeal eaten today, rolled oats retain less energy and nutrients than whole oats. Still, they may be prepared from time to time and are often the best quality grain available while traveling or eating out. Oats are also processed into flakes, puffed oats, and into flour for baking.

Wheat

Wheat is native to ancient Europe and Asia. Today it is cultivated worldwide and has become the Earth's chief cereal crop. In whole form, *whole wheat berries* are rather hard to digest and require thorough chewing. As a result, wheat is traditionally consumed in flour form as bread, pasta, or noodles or processed into forms that are more digestible and easier to prepare. These include *bulgur*, wheat that has been partially boiled, dried, and ground; *cracked wheat*, wheat berries that have been steel-cut; and *couscous*, wheat that has been partially refined and cracked but not bleached.

Wheat is divided into several classifications. *Hard wheat* contains more gluten than soft wheats and is used mainly for flour. *Soft wheat* contains proportionately more carbohydrate and is used for mixing with harder flours or making pastries. *Durum wheat* is used in making pasta and noodles. *Spring wheat* refers to wheat planted in the spring and harvested in autumn. *Winter wheat* is sown in the fall, sprouts beneath the snow, and is reaped in spring. *Pastry wheat*, a type of spring wheat, is low in gluten and used as flour for making pastry and crackers. Wheat is also classified by color such as red, white, golden, or silver. These categories are not mutually exclusive; for example, a popular grain for baking bread is called hard red winter wheat.

In the Far East, whole wheat was traditionally used to make noodles. Noodles made completely with wheat are known in Japanese as *udon* or in Chinese as *mïen*. A lighter wheat noodle called *somen* is also available and more suitable for use in a hot climate. Noodles that are made primarily with buckwheat and only partially with wheat are called *soba*. In addition, whole wheat was traditionally used to make seitan or wheat gluten, a product derived from flour that is cooked in a broth of kombu sea vegetable, tamari soy sauce, and water. Seitan has a rich, dynamic taste and lends itself to a variety of dishes ranging from stews and cutlets, to soups, salads, and casseroles. A staple of Zen cookery, it has now come to the West and become popular in grain burgers and croquettes as a substitute for hamburgers and other animal food entrees. At home, it can be made by separating the starch and bran from the gluten in whole wheat flour. Both spring and winter wheat may be used to make seitan, though spring wheat is softer and often preferred.

Fu, another whole wheat product similar to seitan, is made from wheat gluten

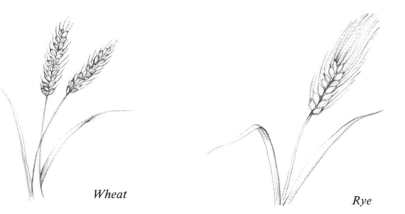

Wheat

Rye

that has been toasted, steamed, and dried. Light in consistency, *fu* absorbs liquid and expands several times in volume when cooked. Fu may be enjoyed plain, added to soups, stews, or casseroles, or cooked together with other foods. It can be made at home or bought dried and packaged in many natural foods stores.

Rye

Rye is the traditional staple in Scandinavia and other northern areas of Europe and Asia. Like wheat berries, whole rye is on the hard side and requires thorough chewing to digest. It is used principally as flour to make rye bread, crackers, or other baked products. It is also processed into flakes and used in producing some strong alcoholic beverages.

Buckwheat

The traditional staple of Russia, Eastern Europe, and parts of central and northern Asia, buckwheat is the hardiest of the cereal plants because of the cold weather it endures. Its kernels are called groats, and it is usually roasted and eaten in whole form or in coarse or fine granules. All these forms of buckwheat are known as *kasha*. Whenever available, the whole groats should be used, as they retain more energy and nutrients than the granules.

In the Far East, buckwheat has also been eaten for centuries in the form of noodles, especially in Japan, called soba. Soba comes in several varieties and is classified according to its percentage of buckwheat flour. For example, forty percent soba includes 40 percent buckwheat and 60 percent whole wheat flour. Fifty percent soba is made up of equal amounts of buckwheat and wheat. For regular use, either one of these types is fine. The traditional soba prepared on New Year's Eve in Japan was usually about 70 to 80 percent buckwheat. Modern technology has made it possible to produce a 100 percent buckwheat soba. This type is very strengthening and more expensive than the other varieties. Soba is also available mixed with other ingredients. A very strong variety is *jinenjo-soba*, combining buckwheat with flour from the long Japanese mountain potato. *Cha-soba*

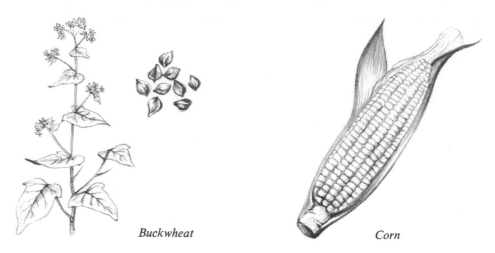

Buckwheat   *Corn*

mixes buckwheat with powdered green tea, and *mugwort soba* includes powdered mugwort leaves. In addition to these and other mixed varieties, *ito-soba*, a thin and light regular variety, is popular in summer served with a cold broth. In the West, the deep, rich taste of buckwheat flour has been enjoyed in pancakes, waffles, and dumplings.

Corn

Native Indian corn or *maize* has been grown for millennia in South, Central, and North America. The original varieties of corn were smaller, more compact, and hardier than the large hybrid varieties that have replaced them. In recent years, there has been a movement to preserve traditional strains of corn, and seeds from these original strains are available in small volume to home gardeners from selected organic seed companies. Native corn is called *open-pollinated* or *standard* to distinguish it from hybrid corn. While organically grown hybrid corn is much to be preferred over that grown with chemical methods, corn will not generally be capable of serving as a main North American grain until open-pollinated or standard varieties with full biological strength again become widely available.

Corn itself is divided into five basic types: 1) *sweet corn*, the variety most commonly eaten today; 2) *dent corn*, a whole dried yellow corn with indented crowns available in most natural foods stores and the corn from which most cornmeal is made; 3) *flour corn*, a starchy variety favored in Latin American cuisine; 4) *flint corn*, another field corn high in starch used in Latin cooking; and 5) *popcorn*, the most ancient and earliest domesticated variety of corn, whose modern descendent has become the Staff of Life in motion picture theaters.

Native American and Latin American corn cuisine were based primarily on the use of *masa* or whole corn dough. Masa is made from corn kernels taken from the cob, dried, cooked with wood ashes and water, and used as the basis for making tacos, tostadas, arepas, empanadas, and other traditional corn dishes. These whole grain preparations retain the basic energy and vitality of the whole corn. However, many of the dishes in modern Mexican restaurants or available in the supermarket today are made with refined cornmeal and other artificial ingredients rather than whole corn dough and other natural foods.

Most modern corn dishes are prepared with *cornmeal*, the flour made from whole corn. Though retaining lesser energy and nutrients than corn dough, good quality organic unrefined cornmeal that does not have any chemicals, sugar, or other refined or artificial ingredients may be used from time to time to make corn bread, corn muffins, or other dishes. A coarsely ground form of cornmeal is *corn grits*, a popular warm breakfast food in the southern United States. A crispy, flaky form of cornmeal, popular as a cold breakfast food in the northern United States, is *corn flakes*. Instead of *cornstarch*, a highly refined corn-based thickener, macrobiotic cooking uses kuzu root powder or arrowroot flour in preparing sauces, gravies, and other dishes requiring thickening.

Other Grains

In addition to the grains noted above, there are a variety of other wild and domesticated cereal grains and grasses that are eaten as staple food around the world. These include *amaranth*, the traditional grain of the Aztec civilization; *quinoa*, the staple of the ancient Incan Empire; and *sorghum*, a milletlike grain that is the staple in many parts of sub-Saharan Africa.

Cooking Methods

In China, Mesoamerica, and other parts of the ancient world, whole grains were traditionally cooked under pressure in heavy pots or caldrons. Stones set on top of thick lids often provided additional weight. When the boiling water started to produce high pressure from steam within the heavily covered pots, the fire was slowed down. This way of cooking preserved the energy and nutrients in the grain and made for easier digestion. In modern times, grains have been increasingly refined of their harder, outer layers, requiring lesser time for boiling, steaming, and other cooking. Moreover, modern forms of cooking often allow food substances to stream out of the pot, further reducing the final quality of the grain.

Pressure-cooking is the most thorough and efficient modern way to prepare whole cereal grains, especially brown rice. The natural sweetness of the grain is fully brought out under this method, and rice prepared in this way is uniformly well-cooked, easily digested and assimilated by the body, and calm and peaceful to the mind. The entire process of pressure-cooking brown rice can be accomplished within about an hour, depending upon the volume of grain cooked. Soaking the rice for several hours prior to cooking, or overnight if time permits, further softens the hard outer layers of the grain, making each grain softer and slightly reducing the actual time needed for cooking. It is also traditional to add a pinch of sea salt to the pot for each cup of uncooked rice at the beginning of cooking. This further strengthens the quality of the rice, contributing to a slightly alkalizing effect in the blood.

Besides rice, barley, whole oats, whole wheat berries, rye, millet, and whole dried corn may also be pressure-cooked using the same method, though cooking time will differ depending on the amount and type of grain. Whole grains may also be combined with one another. In the case of brown rice, 10 to 30 percent of any of the other grains may be added for a tasty and nutritious main dish several times a week. Rice and other whole grains may also be pressure-cooked with a similar proportion of other foods including beans, chestnuts, lotus seeds, other seeds and nuts, acorn, butternut, or similar kinds of winter squash, and assorted vegetables finely chopped. When mixing rice or other grain with other ingredients, slightly more sea salt is commonly added to balance the nutrients in the added food. In addition to unrefined sea salt, grains may be seasoned from time to time with a touch of tamari soy sauce, miso, or other natural seasoning. A small square of kombu, a mineral-rich sea vegetable, is often traditionally added to the bottom of a pot of rice to provide more energy, enhance taste and flavor, and improve digestion.

When a pressure cooker is not available, rice and other whole grains may be boiled. A pot with a heavy lid should be used in order to retain as much energy and nutrients as possible. Millet and buckwheat cook up much faster than the other grains and do not need to be pressure-cooked. However, to strengthen their quality, they are traditionally dry-roasted for a few minutes in an unoiled skillet prior to boiling.

Other whole grains may also be dry-roasted to improve their digestibility. Further cooking methods that may be used from time to time to prepare grains and grain products include steaming, baking, and frying.

Special Dishes

Rice

Pressure-cooked, organically grown short-grain or medium-grain brown rice is the principal staple in modern macrobiotic cooking and is generally served one or more times a day in many households. For variety, boiled rice may be prepared from time to time, and the long-grain varieties occasionally may be substituted for short-grain. As we saw in the last section, rice may also be combined with other grains, beans, seeds and nuts, and a wide variety of vegetables. Other traditional ways of preparing rice include the following:

1. **Cooked Juice.** The heavy juicy liquid that floats to the top when brown rice is cooked for a long time with several times more water than usual is referred to as cooked rice juice or *omoyu* in Japanese. This liquid may be used as a milk substitute for babies and infants or as a food substitute for sick people who cannot eat ordinary solid food.

2. Soft Rice. This form of rice, or *kayu*, is also soft in consistency but contains less liquid than cooked juice. It is traditionally eaten for breakfast in China, Japan, and other parts of Asia and is very delicious. The usual proportion is 5 or more cups of water per cup of uncooked rice, pressure-cooked with a pinch of sea salt per cup of grain. A small amount of raisins, currants, or other dried fruit occasionally may be added for variety and additional sweetness. In the case of sick persons or those needing faster energy, soft rice can be prepared with different condiments to ease digestion and promote faster absorption of nutrients. Naturally made pickles are also served often with soft rice.

3. Rice Cream. Another soft form of rice is called genuine brown rice cream. This is made by pressure-cooking brown rice with several times more water than usual for a few hours over a slow flame. Often for this dish, the rice is lightly roasted before cooking. After cooking, the rice is allowed to cool and is then placed in a cheesecloth or unbleached muslin, tied, and squeezed to remove the pulp. The creamy part is reheated and served. Rice cream makes a delicious breakfast cereal or may be used for medicinal purposes. These include use by babies and infants who need a substitute for mother's milk or solid food, sick people whose digestion is weak or whose appetite is lost, and elderly people who need more balanced nourishment.

4. Rice Potage. Rice cooked together with finely chopped vegetables and seasoned with miso, or occasionally tamari soy sauce or sea salt, is called rice potage or *ojiya* in Japanese. Another softer way of preparing rice, rice potage has been used customarily to provide substantial nourishment and energize the mind and body. Enjoyed by both healthy and sick people, rice potage makes another excellent morning dish, though it may be served at any meal.

5. Rice with Vegetables. As an alternative to plain rice, brown rice may be prepared in the standard way, mixed thoroughly with several different cooked vegetables that have been finely chopped and seasoned with a small volume of tamari soy sauce or occasionally brown rice vinegar. In such a case, this dish constitutes almost a meal in itself and supplemental dishes may be correspondingly reduced. In Japan a traditional style of cooking rice with vegetables developed called *gomoku* or "five vegetable cooked rice" consisting of such root vegetables as carrots, daikon, burdock, lotus root, and onion.

6. Paella. Rice can be cooked not only with vegetables but also with seafood and a variety of seasonings. In Spain, a rice-seafood casserole called *paella* is traditionally served for social or family occasions.

7. *Azuki* Rice. In the Far East, rice cooked with azuki beans is customarily prepared as a principal dish for birthdays, weddings, and other celebrations. Usually 10 to 15 percent partially cooked azuki beans are added to the volume of rice. These small red beans give the dish a distinctive red color, giving rise to the name red rice or *seki-han*.

8. Bean Rice. Besides azuki beans, other beans and legumes such as lentils, chick-peas, yellow or black soybeans, and black beans can be cooked together with brown rice in a proportion of about 10 to 15 percent beans to 85 to 90 percent rice. Bean rice may occasionally be substituted for regular rice at the meal. The high protein and fat content of the beans, in combination with the complex carbohydrates and other nutrients in the rice, make for an especially rich dish.

In many parts of the world, beans and rice are traditionally cooked together. In tropical areas, they are seasoned with hot spices such as chili or curry in order to help balance the extreme climatic conditions. However, in temperate zones, such strong seasonings are not advisable. A little sea salt or small pieces of kombu are commonly added for seasoning in these regions.

9. Rice Ball. Cooked brown rice, formed into various shapes and wrapped with toasted nori sea vegetable, are known as rice balls or as *musubi* or *nigiri-meshi* in Japan. In addition to round shapes, rice balls are often fashioned into triangular wedges. In the very center of the rice ball, a small amount of umeboshi plum, salty vegetable pickles, or occasionally salty broiled salmon is inserted. Rice balls have been popular for centuries in the Far East and are ideal for traveling, picnics, simple party occasions, and lunch. They require no utensils to eat and keep fresh for several days without refrigeration. Instead of nori, rice balls may be wrapped with soft wakame sea vegetable, pickled shiso (beafsteak) leaves or other naturally edible leaves, or they may be coated with ground toasted sesame seeds.

10. Sushi. *Sushi* means "vinegared rice" or "sour rice" and may be prepared in several forms. The most popular, *maki-zushi*, is the familiar rolled sushi in which cooked rice is layered with vegetables, fish, or pickles, wrapped up in toasted nori, and sliced into spiral rounds. Other types include *nigiri-zushi*, cooked rice topped with vegetables or seafood and sometimes tied together with strips of nori or cooked and seasoned dried gourd; *chirashi-zushi*, cooked rice mixed with boiled vegetables, with or without cooked or uncooked fish or seafood, and rice vinegar and served salad style; and *inari-zushi*, deep-fried tofu stuffed with rice salad or rice mixed with rice vinegar. Traditionally, sushi is not served on a daily basis but prepared for special family or social occasions as gourmet fare. Today, sushi is often prepared in Japanese households or restaurants with refined rice, sugar, and chemically processed vinegar. In macrobiotic kitchens, sushi may be made in the traditional way using whole brown rice, brown rice vinegar, and a touch of unrefined sea salt.

11. Fried Rice. Cooked or leftover brown rice can be fried with a small volume of unrefined vegetable oil and seasoned with a little sea salt or tamari soy

Sushi

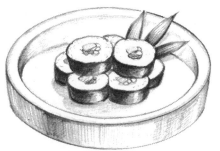

sauce to produce fried rice. A variety of vegetables, bean products, or seafood may be added during frying to create a rich, tasty dish.

12. Dried Cooked Rice. In the Far East, cooked rice was often spread on straw mats or wooden plates and placed outdoors in the shade to dry. After dehydrating, the dried cooked rice, known as *hoshi-i*, kept indefinitely without spoiling and could be eaten as is or be soaked in hot water until it expanded and softened. It was a favorite food for traveling, especially in olden times, and may be substituted for regular brown rice for some period.

13. Roasted Rice. Either dried uncooked brown rice or cooked brown rice can be roasted in a dry skillet for 10 to 15 minutes until golden brown and a fragrant aroma is released. Soaking before roasting, in both cases, makes the rice softer, and a pinch of sea salt may be added if desired. Roasting the rice with the husks still on makes for an even more energetic dish. After cooking, the roasted rice is hulled and enjoyed hot. Like dried cooked rice, roasted rice keeps indefinitely and is one of the traditional ways of carrying food for eating while traveling.

14. Pounded Rice. Cooked or steamed rice that is pounded, crushed, and prepared into small bite-size squares is called *mochi*. In addition to regular brown rice, sweet brown rice is traditionally used for this preparation because of its light, sweet taste and glutinous texture. Sweet brown rice mochi is often called "pounded rice cake." After drying, the pounded rice cakes can be preserved for long periods, prepared by baking, steaming, or boiling in soup, or soaked in hot tea. In the Far East, mochi is traditionally served on New Year's and other special occasions. During pounding, steamed beans, mugwort, and other ingredients may be added to make many unique varieties. Mochi may be enjoyed plain or served with a variety of toppings, ranging from sea salt and tamari soy sauce to brown rice syrup. Today, modern mochi is often made with white rice, white flour, sugar, and other highly refined ingredients. On the macrobiotic diet, these are carefully avoided.

Snacks may also be made from dried mochi. These are produced by drying the thin flattened slabs of pounded rice in the shade and either puffing them up or lightly roasting. Depending on the size, they are called *sembei* (for flatter and larger sizes) or *okaki* (for fatter and smaller sizes). Seasoned and flavored with a touch of sea salt, tamari soy sauce, roasted sesame seeds, and/or sea vegetable such as nori, these make chewy and healthful snacks.

15. Pounded Sweet Rice Balls. Lightly pounded sweet rice balls known as *ohagi* may also be prepared for parties and special occasions. Simpler to make than mochi, they may be coated with various ingredients including ground sesame seeds, ground roasted walnuts, azuki beans with a little rice syrup, puréed chestnuts, *kinako* soy flour, and squash purée.

16. Other Uses. Brown rice may also be baked, steamed, and prepared in a variety of other ways. Added to soups, it provides sweetness and texture. In salads, cooked brown rice may be mixed with a wide variety of fresh garden vegetables, beans, and seeds. Whole cooked rice may be mixed with a little flour and baked to form a soft rice bread known as *rice kayu bread.*

In addition to principal food, brown rice and brown rice products have traditionally been used as part of supplemental foods. Brown rice flour or sweet brown rice flour may be used in baking. Brown rice syrup is traditionally used as a sweetener for desserts, snacks, and other special dishes. Roasted brown rice, steeped in hot water, makes a soothing tea. *Amazaké* is a rice-based sweetener or beverage made from sweet brown rice and a bacterial starter that is allowed to ferment into a thick liquid. This starter, known as *koji*, is made from rice inoculated with bacteria and is also used to make other fermented foods including miso, tamari soy sauce, natto, and saké (the traditional rice wine). Koji may also be used for sushi, pickling, and for other seasoning, to add a slight alcoholic sweetness to different dishes.

Barley

Barley may be prepared in almost all of the same ways as brown rice and in macrobiotic households is especially enjoyed pressure-cooked plain, combined with brown rice (serveral parts rice to one part barley), prepared as a soft morning cereal, or used as the base for a thick, delicious barley soup or stew with various vegetables. Barley's chewy texture enhances dishes with which it is combined and produces a light, cooling effect, especially during the hotter seasons of the year. Barley may also be added to vegetable dishes, used as a stuffing for cabbages or squashes, and added in whole form to bread, muffins, and other baked goods. Toasted barley is ground into flour to make bread and pastries. Roasted barley makes a delicious tea, known in Japan as *mugi-cha*. In the West, barley hops are used in making beer, and barley malt is used as a natural sweetener in place of sugar and other more refined products in a wide assortment of desserts and baked goods.

Millet

Millet is usually dry-roasted for a few minutes and then boiled with a pinch of sea salt. It may be pressure-cooked as well but takes only about half the time of rice. Millet fluffs up when cooked, has a pleasant yellow color, and makes a light, attractive dish. Because it is rather dry by itself, millet is often topped with a miso sauce, gravy, or served mixed with lentils, azuki beans, or other beans and vegetables. Millet may also be added to soups, stews, or salads, used in croquettes and stuffings, or pounded and shaped into loaves or cakes and baked. Soft millet makes a creamy breakfast cereal. Baked with diced winter squash and cut into squares, millet makes a hearty, nourishing dish in the colder months of the year.

Oats

Oats have more fat than other grains, give a warm energy, and provide stamina and endurance. Whole oats make the best quality oatmeal and can be prepared by boiling over a low fire for several hours or ideally overnight. Oats may also be mixed in small proportions with brown rice and other grains. Rolled oats and

Scotch oats may be prepared from time to time, especially when cooking time is short or while traveling. Rolled oats or oat flour are often added to breads, cookies, and puddings to produce tasty desserts and baked goods.

Wheat

There are many ways to prepare whole wheat and whole wheat products. The main types are as follows:

1. Whole Wheat Berries.   Whole wheat berries, retaining the whole energy and nutrients of the grain, may be pressure-cooked or boiled. However, they are rather hard to eat by themselves and require especially thorough chewing. As a result, they are customarily combined with other grains, such as brown rice, in a proportion of about 10 to 30 percent wheat to 70 to 90 percent other grain. Soaking for several hours or overnight before cooking contributes to further softening of the wheat berries.

2. Processed Wheat.   Wheat berries that have been mechanically cut may be used from time to time for variety, though their energy and nutrients are reduced. Cracked wheat can be prepared into a morning cereal or small side dish. Bulgur makes a light, appetizing summer dish or salad, as does couscous which fluffs up even more. However, because of its partially refined quality, couscous should be served only very infrequently. In macrobiotic cooking it is used principally as a dessert to form a delicious couscous cake that can be prepared with a fruit topping of various kinds. Whole wheat flakes, wheat germ, and wheat bran of various kinds are available for use as cold breakfast cereals or supplemental foods. However, such products are usually so highly processed that they retain little of the wheat's original energy and nutrients and are generally avoided in macrobiotic food preparation.

3. Bread.   Bread made from whole wheat, unrefined sea salt, and water has been a staple in India, the Middle East, and Western societies for thousands of years. There are several principal varieties including: 1) flat bread such as *chapati* and *pita*; 2) round or rectangular loaves that naturally ferment and rise from wild yeast in the air and/or a sourdough starter; and 3) sprouted wheat bread. Traditional breads were not made with baker's yeast, oil, sugar, or other ingredients usually added to modern breads. Loaves of naturally fermented bread kept year

A loaf of bread

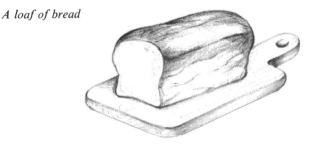

round without spoiling, their taste improved with aging, and they could be reconstituted very simply by soaking and steaming. Macrobiotic bakers have revived the traditional art of making sourdough wheat and rye, and properly made these naturally fermented breads, like miso, can have a beneficial effect on digestion and assimilation of nutrients in the body. An assortment of other good-quality breads can also be made combining wheat with softly cooked whole grains or with flour made from barley, rice, buckwheat, corn, millet, or oats. Occasionally a small amount of unrefined natural vegetable oil or a natural sweetener such as rice syrup may be added to make party breads. Good-quality bread is often prepared in macrobiotic households several times a week and is preferably served toasted by steaming or by warming in the oven rather than by electrical or microwave toasting.

4. Baked Goods.   In addition to bread, a variety of baked goods may be made using whole wheat flour and all natural ingredients. These include crackers, pizza, pancakes, muffins, rolls, biscuits, bagels, donuts, pies, cakes, and cookies. In small volume, a few times a week, foods from this category may be enjoyed by those in good health. However, as we have seen, flour products in general retain much less energy and nutrients than grain in whole form, and baked flour products in particular may be mucus-producing.

5. Pasta and Noodles.   Pasta and noodles are very delicious, come in many varieties, and are usually more digestible than flour prepared in baked form. Western pasta include whole wheat spaghetti noodles, lasagna, elbows, shells, and spirals and usually come without seasoning so the cook should add a pinch of sea salt to the water on the stove. Eastern noodles include *udon*, made from wheat; *soba*, made principally from buckwheat; *somen*, slender whole wheat noodles about half the thickness of udon; *saifun*, clear cellophane noodles made from mung bean threads; *maifun*, rice flour noodles; *ramen*, either udon or soba that has been deep-fried; and various green-colored noodles made with flour combined with mugwort, artichoke flour, or green tea. Oriental noodles customarily include sea salt and do not require further seasoning during cooking. Pasta and noodles made with eggs, white flour, or other refined ingredients and seasonings should be avoided except on rare social occasions.

Noodles

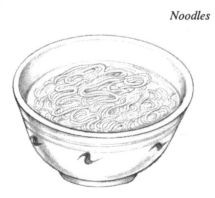

In macrobiotic households, good quality noodles or pasta are commonly enjoyed several times a week. Whole wheat spaghetti or other pasta is often made with a delicious sauce made from miso, carrots, and other vegetables. This sauce is very tasty, deep orange in color, and much more healthy than the tomato sauce commonly served. Udon or soba noodles are traditionally served in a broth made with spring water, a piece of kombu, *shiitake* mushrooms, and a small volume of tamari soy sauce. Boiled noodles may further be fried in a little dark sesame oil along with a few vegetables, such as scallions, carrots and onions, or cabbage and tofu, to make fried noodles. Somen is often prepared cold or chilled in the summer. Noodles may also be substituted for rice in making sushi.

6. Seitan and Fu. Seitan, made at home or bought ready-made at the natural foods store, may be prepared in a variety of ways. It is frequently cooked *kinpira* style with burdock, carrots, and celery; sautéed with onions; boiled with sauerkraut; deep-fried with root vegetables; made into croquettes; pan-fried into vegetable burgers; or added in small pieces to soups, stews, and salads. Similarly, fu has a wide range of uses. It is customarily served with noodles and broth; prepared as a small side dish; garnished with grated ginger and toasted black sesame seeds; added to miso or tamari broth soups; or included with stews, salads, and other vegetable dishes.

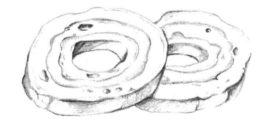

Fu

Rye

Whole rye can be prepared plain as a small side dish, either pressure-cooked or boiled as in making brown rice or barley. One of the harder grains, rye may be softened by soaking for several hours or overnight, or it may be dry-roasted prior to cooking. In macrobiotic cooking, rye is often prepared in small volume combined with brown rice, and this makes for an especially chewy dish. It is also frequently cooked together with carrots, onions, and other vegetables. Rye flour is traditionally combined with whole wheat flour to make rye bread, crackers, and other baked goods.

Buckwheat

Buckwheat or kasha has a deep, rich taste and may be prepared in many styles. The most basic method is dry-roasting for a few minutes and then boiling with a pinch of sea salt. Because of its soft, fluffy nature, it does not require soaking beforehand. For a creamy morning cereal, about twice the usual volume of water can be added. Buckwheat also goes well *gomoku* style with five or more vegetables such as celery, burdock, green peas, and onions. In the summer, it is delicious served cool in a salad, especially along with sauerkraut. Buckwheat can be milled into flour for making hearty pancakes, waffles, and muffins. Buckwheat flour is also traditionally used to make dumplings called *sobagaki* that puff up quickly.

Soba, the noodles made from buckwheat, wheat flour, and sea salt, is traditionally prepared in six ways: 1) *kama-agé*, soba served with the same water it is cooked in; 2) *zaru-soba*, soba prepared in individual bamboo baskets or strainers along with individual bowls of broth for dipping into or pouring over the noodles at the table; 3) *kake-soba*, "swimming" style soba cooked and served in a broth; 4) *yaki-soba*, fried soba cooked and served with tofu, onions, carrots, celery, or other vegetables; 5) *chirashi-zushi soba*, soba served chilled with vegetables salad style; and 6) *nori-maki soba*, noodles prepared with vegetables or seafood, wrapped in toasted nori, and served sushi style in sliced rounds.

Corn

There are hundreds of ways to prepare corn and corn products. Corn on the cob, for example, may be boiled, steamed, or baked, and each method produces a slightly different taste, texture, and energy. Whole corn kernels, freshly removed from the cob before cooking or dried and thoroughly soaked before using, may be added in small volume to a pot of brown rice and pressure-cooked for a unique blend of these two grains. Fresh or dried corn kernels may also be used in a wide variety of soups, stews, salads, vegetable dishes, puddings, and other dishes. In Italy and Southern Europe, a popular corn dish is *polenta*, made from ground fresh corn kernels baked with cooked kidney beans, carrots, onions, kombu, and a variety of seasonings. *Masa*, the traditional whole corn dough of Central and South America, is used to make *arepas*, small oval-shaped corn balls served plain or stuffed with a variety of ingredients; *bollos polones*, boiled stuffed corn balls; and *tortillas*, the thin flat corn shells that are deep-fried and filled with a variety of beans and vegetables. Cornmeal may be used occasionally along with other natural ingredients to make corn bread, corn muffins, and other baked products and desserts.

Nutritional Value

Whole cereal grains contain a balance of protein, carbohydrates, fat, and vitamins and minerals ideally suited for human consumption. In contrast, beans and legumes contain proportionally less carbohydrates and more protein than grains, while meat and other animal food lack carbohydrates and fruits and vegetables lack protein. For this reason, consumption of whole cereal grains and their products as the daily principal food in itself secures a natural balance of energy and nutrition, contributing to the maintenance of human health and social stability.

Whole grains and their products also provide more energy and calories than any other food substances. As a result, a lesser volume of food is ordinarily required on a grain-centered diet than on other diets. The complex carbohydrates—polysaccharides—in whole grains are gradually and smoothly assimilated through the digestive organs, providing a slow and steady source of energy to the cells and tissues. In the mouth, an enzyme in saliva initiates predigestive activity and is the principal reason why all foods, but especially whole grains, should be thoroughly chewed. In contrast to the gradual burning of complex carbohydrates in grains, the predominantly simple carbohydrates in fruits, milk and other dairy food, sugar, honey and other highly refined sweeteners, burn faster, contributing to rapid and uneven digestion, fluctuations in levels of physical activity, and changeable thoughts and emotions.

Whole grains are also high in niacin and other B-vitamins, vitamin E, and vitamin A. The B group, in particular, along with complex carbohydrates, contribute to mental clarity and stability. For example, the B vitamins in whole grains act as the agent for glutamic acid in the brain to produce two opposite organic chemical compounds that respectively signal "proceed" or "stop," "active" or "inactive," "advance" or "retreat." The smooth functioning of this mechanism contributes to sound mental and psychological health.

Health Benefits

Compared to whole grains such as brown rice and whole wheat berries, refined or polished grains and grain products such as white rice and white flour are inferior in their quality of energy and nutrients. The process of refining and polishing removes some degree of almost all the outer layers of the grain where various fibers, amino acids, minerals, vitamins, and enzymes are concentrated. A small percentage of these nutrients may remain, along with the complex carbohydrates, but the overall imbalance can contribute to a wide variety of disorders and degeneration.

Refinement or polishing of whole grains became popular in the late nineteenth century and spread throughout the world in the early twentieth century, especially in the areas where modern industrialization rapidly developed. In this transitory period, many deficiency diseases occurred including well-known incidences of beriberi arising from lack of B-vitamins in white rice. Besides beriberi, numerous other modern physical and psychological disorders are caused largely by the refinement and polishing of whole grains. These include hormonal imbalance, general fatigue, psychological confusion, weakened memory, loss of natural resistance, decline of natural immunity, various allergies, indigestion and resulting disorders in digestive functions.

As degenerative diseases became more widespread in the second half of the twentieth century, the protective effect of whole cereal grains became more generally recognized. Many scientific studies have shown that whole grains strengthen the heart and circulatory system, protecting against high blood pressure, heart attack, stroke, and other cardiovascular disorders that are currently the cause of about 50 percent of all deaths in modern society. Reviewing the medical evidence, epidemiologist Jeremiah Stamler, M.D., an international authority on heart disease, concluded, "People subsisting on cereal-root diets have low levels of serum cholesterol and little atherosclerotic coronary disease (clinical or morphological). This correlation has been consistently observed in every [traditional society studied] to date." In an editorial "Sensible Eating," the *British Medical Journal* commented, "Few nutritionists now dispute that Western man [and woman] eats too much meat, too much animal fat and dairy products, too much refined carbohydrate, and too little dietary fiber. Epidemiology studies of heart disease suggest that some at least of the deaths in the middle ages from myocardial infarction [heart attack] could be cut by a move toward a more prudent diet— which means more cereals and vegetables and less meat and fat."

Similarly, a wide variety of epidemiological, laboratory, and case-control studies show that as part of a balanced diet whole grains protect against many forms of cancer. The Senate Select Committee's report *Dietary Goals for the United States* (1977), the Surgeon General's document *Healthy People* (1979), the National Academy of Sciences' report *Diet, Nutrition, and Cancer* (1982), and many others all call for substantial increases in the daily consumption of whole grains such as brown rice, millet, barley, oats, and whole wheat.

A diet centered on whole cereal grains is also beneficial for the elimination of excessive fats and mucus, reducing body weight, and regaining physical and mental flexibility. These effects contribute to the prevention and relief of many other diseases and illnesses in addition to cancer and heart disease including diabetes, arthritis, asthma, Parkinson's disease, chronic skin disorders, as well as various mental and psychological disorders. It has also been found that macrobiotic people can heal themselves much faster from injury, burns, surgery, and most other forms of accidental harm or emergency medical treatment on account of their increased natural immunity and resistance to infection.

In view of longstanding dietary patterns in many traditional societies and cultures and the findings of modern nutritional studies and reports, the macrobiotic way of eating avoids as much as possible the use of refined or polished grains in the daily preparation of food. On rare social or festive occasions, these foods may be prepared for enjoyment if desired. Also, when eating out, unrefined whole grains are not always available, in which case refined grains may be taken so long as they are thoroughly chewed and mixed with saliva to help counterbalance their deficiencies with a variety of supplemental foods.

Whole grains themselves can serve to help detoxify the body from harmful effects arising from the consumption of extreme quality foods. For example, it is customary in most traditional cultures to consume cooked whole grains or their products with a small volume of salty condiments and pickles such as umeboshi pickles or daikon pickles in order to neutralize the poisonous effects from occasional overconsumption of animal food, fatty, greasy food, or extreme sweet, sour, or bitter substances. In the modern age, the harmful effects of radiation, chemicals, drugs, and consumption or exposure to other extreme substances or energies may be balanced and eliminated by the consumption of whole cereal grains and their products. The East West Foundation and other macrobiotic organizations have published case history reports of survivors of the atomic bombing in Nagasaki who healed themselves of radiation sickness on the macrobiotic diet. Similar case histories and reports have been collected from individuals who previously suffered from the adverse effects of hallucinogenic drug use, tranquilizer or amphetamine consumption, and cocaine or heroin addiction. Depending on the individual case, physical and mental damage from these substances can be overcome on the macrobiotic diet, using whole grains as the principal food, usually within a period from several months to one year.

Over time, the regular consumption of whole grains and their products as principal food will secure the following benefits to preserve physical and psychological health: 1) better digestion and elimination; 2) better blood constituents and circulatory functions; 3) better natural immunity to infection and disease; 4) better nervous system functioning including that of the brain; 5) better hormonal functions; 6) better reproductive functions; 7) improved mental clarity, psychological stability, and peacefulness in human relations; 8) strengthened physical and mental endurance; 9) heightened awareness of the environment and natural world; and 10) deeper spiritual insight and aspiration.

Soup

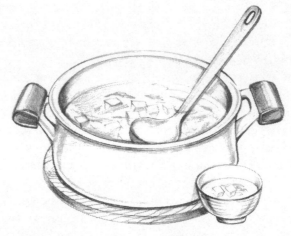

Daily Use

One or two bowls of soup seasoned with miso, tamari soy sauce, or sometimes only sea salt are recommended every day (approximately 5 to 10 percent of daily food intake). The flavor should be mild, neither too salty nor too bland. Soups may be prepared with a variety of ingredients, including seasonal vegetables, sea vegetables (especially wakame or kombu), and occasionally with grains or beans. The ingredients may be changed frequently for variety and enjoyment.

History

Soup, broth, or stock corresponds with the primordial sea in which life began. When we take soup, especially that made with a fermented base such as miso or tamari soy sauce, we are returning to our evolutionary origins, renewing our energies for the present and future. Throughout history, soup has formed an important part of all traditional cuisines. In the Far East, miso soup, kombu stock, and fish stock were customarily prepared; in India, a soup or thick broth made of lentils or chick-peas; in the Middle East and Europe, barley soup, onion soup, buckwheat soup, and others; in Africa, sorghum soup and broths made from roots and tubers; and in the Americas, squash or pumpkin soup, corn chowder, and clam chowder.

Quality

Until modern times, soups were made fresh each day with the highest natural quality ingredients, including a variety of seasonal vegetables, newly harvested grains, and the most recent catch of fish or seafood. Today, canned soup, powdered soup, and other processed types of soup have largely replaced fresh home-made soup in many households, restaurants, and dining halls. Precooked soups of this kind are deficient in both energy and nutrients and often contain refined ingredients, chemical preservatives, and other harmful substances. In the macro-biotic kitchen, only the freshest, highest natural quality ingredients should be used in preparing soup. While there now are a variety of canned and packaged soups in natural foods stores containing better quality ingredients, these items should not be used for daily meals. Occasionally, when traveling, instant miso soup or similar product may be prepared when fresh ingredients and access to a kitchen are unavailable. Also, in the case of store-bought miso, the unpasteurized varieties usually retain more energy and vitality than those that are heat-treated prior to packaging.

Varieties

There are almost an unlimited variety of soups that can be prepared in the mac-robiotic kitchen. Some are simple, mild, and quick to prepare. Others include many ingredients, are strong to the taste, and take longer to make. Each soup has its appropriate season and occasion. The basic categories of soup are as follows:

Miso Soup

The dark purée made from soybeans, unrefined sea salt and usually fermented barley or rice which have aged together is known as *miso*. After cooking, the ingredients are inoculated with koji, a special mold that stimulates fermentation, and the mixture is allowed to age in wooden kegs for usually a year or more. Miso has been a staple in Far Eastern cooking since the beginning of civilization and is now becoming popular in the West. There are now several miso-making companies in the United States making high-quality miso using local all natural ingredients and traditional methods.

Miso contains living enzymes that facilitate digestion, strengthen the quality of the blood, and provide a nutritious balance of complex carbohydrates, essential oils, protein, vitamins and minerals. According to tradition, the gods gave miso to humankind to ensure health, happiness, and peace. Sweet and delicious to the taste, subtle in flavor, and available in various hues of brown, orange, red, and yellow, miso is traditionally used as a base for a wide variety of soups. However, it is also usually very salty and should not be used in excessive volume or will create a counterbalancing desire for liquid, fruits, or sweets. In addition to soups, miso is used in pickling, preparing sauces, spreads, and dressings, and seasoning other grain, vegetable, or bean dishes as an occasional substitute for sea salt or tamari soy sauce.

There are various types of miso, and their tastes and flavors differ according to

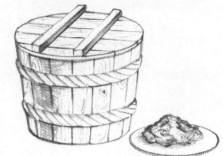

Keg of miso

the quality of their ingredients, the climate and environment in which they are prepared, the length they have aged, and the method of preparation. Traditionally, the amount of time that miso has aged is recorded in calendar years spanned rather than complete 12-month periods. Thus 3-year miso often signifies that the miso began to ferment in the autumn of the first year, aged the entire second year, and was packaged in the spring of the third year. However, today, most miso in the Far East is made quickly in an artificial temperature-controlled environment with chemically-treated ingredients. For example, red miso is commonly speeded up in modern Japanese food processing plants from one or two years with natural aging to only six weeks.

Most of the miso available in natural foods stores is good quality, traditionally prepared miso made with all natural ingredients. Long, slowly fermented miso is usually darker in color than quick, rapidly produced miso and has a rich deep aroma and taste that cannot be duplicated by modern artificial aging. Miso may also be made in the home, and many macrobiotic families prepare it with local ingredients several times a year.

The main varieties of miso are:

1. **Barley Miso.**   Miso made from fermented barley, soybeans, and sea salt is the sweetest and most suitable miso for daily cooking. It has a mild, country-style taste and mellow flavor and is enjoyed year around. Good quality barley *miso* should have aged a minimum of 18 months, preferably 24 months or longer. In Japanese, barley miso is known as *mugi miso*, and it is often marketed under this name.

2. **Soybean Miso.**   Soybean miso is made only with soybeans and sea salt and is usually sold by its Japanese name *Hatcho miso*. It is made with less water and less salt than other misos, is drier to the taste, and because of slow fermentation takes two years to mature. Heavy stones are customarily piled on top of the cedar kegs to keep moisture from sinking to the bottom. Soybean miso has a rich, hearty taste, a thick texture, and while suitable year around is traditionally enjoyed in wintertime soups. It may also be combined fifty/fifty with other misos in soup and makes good spreads and long-time miso pickles. Historically, *Hatcho* miso is said to have originated in Okazaki, a town in Aichi Prefecture, where the famous Shogun Tokugawa Ieyasu came from, and it has the reputation of being the favorite food of the *samurai*.

3. Brown Rice Miso. Brown rice miso, made from fermented brown rice, soybeans, and sea salt is usually the sweetest of the misos. The rice koji which it is made from is the same kind used to make saké, amazaké, and rice vinegar. Traditionally, rice miso or *kome* miso was made from polished rice because the hard outer bran of unpolished rice was resistant to mold. The brown rice *miso* available in natural foods stores today (often labeled as *genmai* miso) was developed in a special process by a macrobiotic food company in Osaka. It is rich-tasting, but light and enjoyed primarily for occasional soups in the warmer months or for other cooking and pickling.

4. Light Misos. In addition to the three major types of miso described above, which are ordinarily used for miso soup and regular daily cooking, there are a variety of light or sweet misos. These are usually lighter in color (yellow, white, or tan) than the other misos, and because they contain less salt they take only a few weeks to age. These sweet misos are enjoyed occasionally for light summer cooking or for festive occasions.

5. Natto Miso. *Natto miso*, made from lightly fermented soybeans and ginger, is a spicy condiment and not ordinarily used in soups.

Clear Soups and Soup Stock

Clear soup is made from kombu, vegetable, or shiitake mushroom stock and usually contains a few ingredients such as a small square of tofu, one or two slices of carrot, a radish square, and a little ginger, scallion, or parsley as a garnish. Mild in taste, soft in texture, and beautiful in appearance, clear soup creates a feeling of calm and stimulates the appetite. It is traditionally served on holidays and on special occasions as the introductory course of a large meal. Clear soup can be made with a variety of stocks including:

1. *Kombu* Stock. The most popular clear base in Japanese cooking, kombu stock is made by boiling a small piece of kombu sea vegetable in a quart of spring water. Cooking time depends on the size and thickness of the kombu, and customarily the kombu is taken out and saved for other uses prior to serving or mixing with the soup's other ingredients, though it may be retained if desired. In Japanese, this stock is known as *dashi* and is used in a wide variety of soups, noodle broths, and sauces.

2. Shiitake Mushroom Stock. Shiitake mushrooms, originally native to the Far East, are now grown in the West. They are very delicious and have been used, fresh or dried, for centuries to balance heavy animal food consumption and for other medicinal purposes. People in ordinary good health may enjoy a tiny volume of shiitake (a few slices) every day in stock, soup, stews, salads, or other dishes. However, they are not recommended or should be used very sparingly by those with weak conditions. Shiitake stock is prepared similarly to kombu stock and also may be combined with the kombu. Though traditionally used to flavor the stock, the mushrooms may be left in the soup if desired. The hardened stems are customarily removed prior to cooking.

3. Vegetable Stock. A sweet tasting, nourishing stock for soups and stews may be made using a wide variety of seasonal garden vegetables. Vegetable stock may also be made from odds and ends that would otherwise be directly composted such as vegetable cores, tough outer leaves, cabbage hearts, pea hulls, corn husks, and squash peelings. Bitter tasting remnants, such as carrot tops, spinach leaves, or Swiss chard, are usually avoided.

4. **Fish Stock.** The heads, bones, and other skeletal remains of fish or shells of seafood may be saved for stock. The fish parts may be tied in a small sack made from cheesecloth or muslin cloth prior to cooking, or they may be strained after boiling. One popular type of fish stock is made from *bonito*, a fish resembling the tuna that is traditionally smoked and flaked. Good quality bonito does not have a fishy odor and goes well with vegetables. Ideally, bonito is obtained fresh and flaked at home. Commercially prepared bonito flakes should be inspected carefully for additives or preservatives.

Tamari Broth

The delicious full taste of tamari soy sauce can be enjoyed by adding and cooking tamari soy sauce in small volume to kombu or shiitake stock. This broth may also be enjoyed by itself as one of the recommended daily bowls of soup. Cubed tofu, sliced scallions, or other small pieces of vegetables, sea vegetables, or fu may be added and changed frequently. Tamari broth is also often served with noodles.

Vegetable Soup

There are many delicious vegetable soups which can be made using only one type of vegetable or mixing different vegetables together. These include carrot soup, celery soup, squash soup, and cauliflower soup.

Bean Soup

Beans, legumes, and pulses make rich, nourishing soups. Traditional varieties include lentil soup, azuki bean soup, and chick-pea soup. Vegetables can also be cooked together with beans.

Grain Soup

Whole grains and their products can be used as the foundation for soups and stews or added in small volume to mixed soups. Popular types include barley soup, brown rice soup, fresh corn soup, and buckwheat soup. Noodles, seitan, fu, and other grain products can also be added in small volume to soups and stews. Grain soups are also often cooked with vegetables.

Medicinal Soup

Besides miso and tamari broth, there are special soups that may be prepared to help prevent or relieve sickness, overcome fatigue, and stimulate energy circulation in the body. In the Far East, for example, carp and burdock soup (known as *koi-koku*) is traditionally prepared for mothers who have just given birth or who are breastfeeding, persons low in vitality, those who have little or no appetite, or others needing a source of fresh energy. This soup is made by cooking a fresh whole carp (including the head and bones) with at least an equal volume of shaved burdock. A small bag of bancha twigs tea is nestled inside the pot for flavoring, and at the end of cooking diluted miso and grated ginger are added for seasoning. If fresh carp is unavailable, red snapper, perch, or other white-meat variety may be substituted. Carrots may be used instead of, or in addition to, burdock.

Cooking Methods

In macrobiotic cooking, soups are prepared according to principles of balance. As the usual first course, soup sets the tone for the entire meal and creates an appetite for everything that is to follow. The taste, aroma, color, and texture of the soup should complement the other courses. If the meal on the whole is light, the soup may be on the thick or hearty side, in some cases constituting almost a meal in itself. If there are many courses to the meal and much rich, nourishing fare, a simple miso soup or clear soup is usually prepared to start off with.

Similarly, the ingredients may be adjusted to take into account seasonal and climatic changes. In hot weather, more cooling soups are appealing, containing lighter ingredients such as leafy green vegetables, and requiring slightly less miso, tamari soy sauce, sea salt, or other seasoning. In cold weather, more warming soups can be prepared, including root vegetables and other heavier ingredients and slightly more seasoning.

The ingredients in the soup can complement those in the rest of the meal. If beans are not prepared as a separate side dish or part of a casserole for the meal, a bean soup might be served. If the vegetables for the meal are prepared separately, they might be complemented by a mixed vegetable soup. If they are served mixed, the soup may have a single creamy vegetable taste. If the vegetables in the meal are prepared in small cubes or diced, those in the soup may be cut in chunks or large rounds.

Soups may be made with a variety of cookware. For the ordinary household, a 4-quart saucepan made of stainless steel, ceramic, or glass is useful for making miso soup, tamari broth, or clear soups; a large 6-quart saucepan made of enamelized cast-iron is helpful for quick soups; and a heavy 8-quart kettle of cast-iron, enameled cast-iron, or stainless steel with a heavy tight-fitting lid is ideal for preparing soup stock, slow cooking soups, and large volumes of soup. Except in the cases of carp and burdock soup and some bean soups, soup is not ordinarily pressure-cooked.

Special Dishes

Miso Soup

Basic miso soup is made by heating a pot of spring water with a little dried wakame sea vegetable and some thinly sliced onions. At the end of cooking, a small volume of miso is diluted in a *suribachi*, a traditional Japanese earthenware mortar, and added to the pot to simmer for a few minutes. Just before serving, chopped scallions, parsley, or watercress or fresh grated ginger may be added as a garnish.

To this basic preparation, there are many variations, some simple and some more complex. These include miso soup with daikon and tofu, miso soup with rice and scallions, miso soup with millet and squash, celery miso soup, creamy onion miso soup, miso soup with sesame seeds and broccoli, mochi miso soup, fu miso soup, miso soup with *okara* and dried daikon, jinenjo miso soup, and many others.

Clear Soup

Clear soup is traditionally made by boiling each ingredient separately before combining in individual serving bowls and covering with stock. This preserves the bright color of the vegetables which is lost if the ingredients are cooked together. Basic clear soup is usually made with kombu or shiitake stock to which have been added a few cut up vegetable pieces such as carrots, tofu, watercress, broccoli, Chinese cabbage, or winter squash. For variety, a few clams, small shrimps, or other seafood can be added to clear soup. Toasted nori and fresh grated ginger are the customary garnish, though dried or deep-fried bread crumbs also go very well with this dish.

Vegetable Soup

Soups made from a single vegetable such as carrots, celery, or cauliflower may be prepared in several basic ways. One way is to slice up the vegetables and cook until their juice melts with the flavor of the soup. Another method is to cook the vegetables until tender and then purée them in a hand food mill (or occasionally a *suribachi*). This results in a uniformly blended soup. Kuzu or arrowroot flour may be added to make vegetable soup even more creamy.

While there are endless ways to make mixed vegetable soup, not all vegetables go well together. Those with an especially strong or bitter taste should be avoided or used in small volume to prevent them from dominating the entire dish. Similarly, when combining different foods, colors, textures, and tastes may fade and dissolve. In macrobiotic cooking, preparing mixed vegetables in soups or casseroles takes experience. Some basic combinations include onions, carrots, burdock, and celery; carrots, onions, cabbage, and broccoli; corn, onions, and carrots; corn, cabbage, and tofu; daikon, burdock, celery, Chinese cabbage, and a small taro potato.

Vegetable soups are usually seasoned with sea salt or tamari soy sauce during cooking and garnished just before serving with sliced scallions or strips of toasted nori. If desired, diluted kuzu root powder, arrowroot flour, or other natural starch (but not refined cornstarch) may be used as a thickener. In addition to the types of vegetable soup described above, vegetable soups may also be made combining land vegetables with sea vegetables, with fish or seafood, and with bread or dumplings.

Bean Soup

Lentil soup cooks up the quickest of the bean soups and is traditionally made with diced vegetables such as onions, carrots, burdock, or celery. Azuki bean soup takes a little longer and is often made with sliced carrots and onions or small pieces of winter squash. Chick-pea soup takes longer still and is usually pressure-cooked prior to final simmering with cut up vegetables. It is very delicious served cool. All other regular beans and legumes can be used to make wonderful soups. Bean soups are usually seasoned with sea salt, but depending on the type of soup tamari soy sauce may be added just before the end of cooking as well. When preparing bean soups, a small square of kombu is traditionally placed on the bottom of the pot at the start of cooking for enhanced flavor and digestibility. At the end of cooking, sliced scallions, parsley, or bread crumbs can be added for garnish.

Grain Soup

Grain soup has a rich, nourishing taste and is an excellent way to use leftover cooked whole grains. Barley soup is enjoyed almost the world over and is usually prepared with diced onions, celery, and carrots and often a small amount of lentils. Fresh corn chowder is another favorite and can be made by stripping the kernels from corn on the cob and cooking with sliced up celery, onions, or other vegetables. Brown rice or buckwheat may also be used as the foundation for a grain soup. Seasoning and garnish are similar as for bean soups.

Nutritional and Health Benefits

Miso soup has been valued in the Far East for thousands of years for its healthful properties. As a fermented food, it is easily digestible and its combination of soybeans and grains contains all amino acids considered essential by modern nutritionists. The microorganisms in the miso help stimulate the secretion of digestive fluids in the stomach and help digest and assimilate other foods in the intestines. Miso is also a good vegetable-quality source of vitamin B_{12}.

Miso helps strengthen the quality of the blood and lymph and has been traditionally used to detoxify the body from the harmful effects of excessive animal food, sugar, or other extreme substances. Following the atomic bombing in 1945, doctors in Nagasaki singled out miso soup as one of the primary foods responsible for preventing radiation sickness in a large group of survivors. Recent studies in Japan have shown that miso can help overcome the adverse effects of smoking. Thus there is reason to believe that miso is also helpful in neutralizing the body from modern contaminants such as nuclear radioactivity, industrial pollution, and artificial chemicals in the soil and food system.

Beginning in the 1960s, medical researchers for the Japanese government began a long-term study of miso soup consumption and its effects on the nation's health. Altogether the dietary habits, incidence of degenerative disease, and mortality rates of 265,000 men and women over forty years old were studied over a twelve-year period. In 1982 the National Cancer Center Research Institute released its final study showing that those who never ate miso soup had a 43 percent higher death rate from coronary heart disease and 33 percent higher death rate from stomach cancer than those who consumed miso soup daily. Those who did not eat miso also had 29 percent more fatal strokes, 3.5 times more deaths resulting from high blood pressure, and 19 percent more cancer at all sites in the body. The researchers concluded that "all causes of death were significantly lower in daily ingesters of soybean paste soup." Since then there have been other scientific studies that have confirmed the traditional nutritional and health value of miso.

Shiitake mushrooms, an ingredient traditionally used in soup stock, have also been found to have preventive and therapeutic effects. In 1970 Japanese cancer researchers reported that in animal experiments shiitake mushrooms markedly inhibited the growth of induced sarcomas resulting in "almost complete regression of tumors . . . with no sign of toxicity."

Depending on its ingredients and way of preparation, soup can have many other beneficial effects on the mind and body.

Vegetables

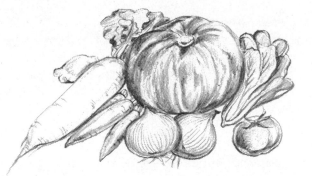

Daily Use

In the Standard Macrobiotic Diet, vegetables, served in various styles, comprise 25 to 30 percent of each meal by volume of food consumed. About two-thirds of the vegetables are generally cooked by boiling, steaming, sautéing, or other method, while one-third or less may be prepared as raw salad or as pickles. As much as possible, vegetables should be grown locally and consumed in season. Each day's menu should include a balance of root vegetables, ground and stem varieties, and leafy greens. However, the proportion and method of preparation will vary slightly with the time of year, personal needs and condition, and other factors. In autumn and winter, for example, slightly more root vegetables may be taken, and cooking and seasoning may be slightly stronger. In spring and summer more leafy green vegetables may be prepared, and more raw foods and slightly less seasoning may be used.

History

Whole grains and vegetables naturally complement each other. Traditional societies in all parts of the world cultivated many different varieties of vegetables, and they played an important role in their folklore, mythology, and healing arts as well as in daily food preparation. In the Middle East, common garden vegetables included onion, cabbage, cucumber, turnip, and lettuce. In the Far East, they included daikon, Chinese cabbage, bok choy, mustard greens, shiitake mushroom, and jinenjo mountain potato. In Africa, yams, sweet potato, and plantain were staples. In Central and South America, potato, tomato, green pepper, and avocado were produced, while North America developed acorn, butternut, and other winter squashes as well as a variety of string, wax, and snap beans.

Quality

Until modern times, vegetables were primarily consumed fresh from the garden in spring, summer, and early fall and dried, pickled, or naturally preserved in some other way for storage over the winter. Grown only with mulch, manure, or other organic materials, they retained their natural energy and nutrients. Moreover, cultivated for centuries in the same locale—often the same ancestral plot of land—common vegetables developed hardy native strains whose unique quality and biological strength differed slightly from similar vegetables grown in the same region or even the next farm or garden.

The age-old trade caravans plying the Silk Road between East and West resulted in the exchange of seeds between different cultures. While this resulted in some change in food quality, ancient and medieval societies continued to eat largely grains, vegetables, and other foods originating from the same climate zone. The Crusades resulted in the introduction of many tropical foods into Europe, though these were primarily herbs, spices, and stimulants such as tea. The discovery of the New World resulted in an influx of more exotic species into Europe, and some vegetables from the tropics, especially potato, tomato, and eggplant, took root, fundamentally changing the way of eating in harmony with the local or similar environment that had largely existed until this time.

Over the last century, the quality of vegetables and other farm and garden products has declined even further with the introduction of petroleum-based fertilizers, chemical pesticides, and other artificial sprays. Advances in refrigeration, canning, freezing, and transcontinental and intercontinental shipping have now virtually eliminated the traditional climatic and seasonal boundaries in humanity's diet, allowing families access to fruits and vegetables regardless of the environment they come from and the time of year in which they are grown.

Meanwhile, with the spread of monocropping and other modern agricultural methods, the demand accelerated for uniform crops that could be grown, harvested, packaged, and shipped quickly and inexpensively. Artificial hybridization of seeds began, so that today most traditional seed strains have disappeared and the food sold in supermarkets is largely the same in shape, size, color, and taste. Soil erosion, the evolution of insects resistant to pesticides, and other results of chemical farming have intensified the biochemical quest for the perfect species of hybrid plants. Modern vegetables and other fruits of the earth are a pale reflection of their forebears.

In the macrobiotic diet, vegetables should be organic or natural in quality as much as possible, locally grown, and consumed in the season in which they grow. Canned vegetables, frozen vegetables, and (in temperate zones) vegetables of tropical origin are strictly avoided.

Ideally, vegetables are grown at home in a small garden or even window box. However, this is not always practical in an urban environment, so for many families their chief source of vegetables will be the natural foods store, coop, or farmers' market. In many outlets, organic produce is clearly marked and certified by an organic growers' association or state agency which periodically tests soil conditions and monitors cultivation standards.

There are also several ways to evaluate produce for quality and strength. Compared to food grown with chemicals, organic food is usually smaller in size, less shiny in appearance, often harder in texture, and more symmetrical in shape and size. For example, in organically grown root vegetables, the core is generally located directly at the center. In chemically grown root vegetables, the core is usually off center and when cut will be observed to swerve to one side. Organic leafy green vegetables will often have leaves that are the same length and shape. Greens grown with chemical methods will usually have leaves that are lopsided or irregular in appearance.

In selecting organic produce, it is advisable to pick out items that are fresh, beautiful, and well proportioned, though the size may be smaller than inorganic varieties. Vegetables that are soft, limp, wilted, faded, or dull in color often lack vitality, are low in taste, and will spoil rapidly. Some of these signs show that the vegetables were harvested too late, aged too long, or have been stored at too high a temperature. Much organic produce will fall in-between, containing slight blemishes from handling, spots from aging, or evidence of tiny insects. Such produce is still usually good quality. At home, after the bad parts have been cut out before storing to prevent further spoilage, the vegetables are perfectly fine for ordinary usage.

There are many traditional ways to store and preserve organic produce to retard further natural decay such as keeping them slightly apart from each other on shelves or in containers and, in some cases, storing them under grain hulls, in sand, or in dry cool places. Greens and some vegetables may be kept fresh by spraying with water or otherwise kept cool such as by storing in the refrigerator. However, others, such as some root vegetables, absorb moisture and spoil more quickly and are better left unrefrigerated. Similarly, modern wrapping materials such as plastic bags tend to accumulate moisture and accelerate spoilage, while more natural materials, such as bamboo mats or even brown paper bags, permit the vegetables to breathe and keep their freshness.

Cutting and cooking methods also influence the quality of vegetables. Separating leaves into smaller pieces by hand or cutting stems, roots, and stalks with a knife are much superior to mechanical or electrical methods of cutting or processing whose intense energy and chaotic vibration may be absorbed by the food and transmitted to those who eat it. Similarly, electrical heat or microwave radiation should be strictly avoided in favor of wood, gas, or other more natural fuel that preserves the original energy and nutrients of the ingredients to be cooked.

Varieties

In the Standard Macrobiotic Diet, garden vegetables are usually classified into three types: root vegetables, ground vegetables, and leafy green vegetables. In addition to the typical varieties listed below, all other traditionally used vegetables may be consumed so long as they are native to the climate in which they grow. In macrobiotic cooking, wild vegetables are also used on occasion and, unless native to the local environment, tropical and subtropical varieties are avoided in a four-season temperate climate region.

Root Vegetables

Root vegetables grow below the ground and generally give stronger energy than other types of vegetables. They also take slightly longer to cook, may be prepared in a large variety of styles, combine well with other foods, and keep for a long time without spoiling. Typical members of this family suitable for daily use include carrots, parsnips, burdock, daikon, red radish, turnips, rutabaga, jinenjo, lotus root, and gingerroot. Beets, taro potato, and other root varieties may be used occasionally.

Ground Vegetables

Ground vegetables include round, stem, and climbing varieties that grow near or slightly above the surface of the ground. Vegetables in this category have properties that are usually moderate or midway between those of root and leafy green varieties. Their energy is usually intermediate in strength, cooking time is about average, and they will keep for a while but not indefinitely. Ground vegetables recommended for daily use include onions, cabbage, cauliflower, broccoli, Brussels sprouts, string beans, and fall and winter squashes and pumpkins. Those suitable for occasional use include cucumbers, summer squash, fresh beans, zucchini, green peas, snow peas, kohlrabi, and fennel. Though not strictly vegetables, mushrooms and other edible fungi may be included in this category for preparation from time to time.

Green Leafy Vegetables

Green leafy vegetables grow above the ground and consist primarily of soft green or white leaves and harder stalks. Leafy greens give an upward, rising energy, cook up very quickly, do not combine with as many other foods, and tend to spoil more rapidly than vegetables in the other categories. Vegetables in this group suitable for daily use include kale, collard greens, bok choy, Chinese cabbage, escarole, mustard greens, daikon greens, turnip greens, watercress, carrot tops, parsley, scallions, chives, leeks, celery, and endive. Greens for occasional use include all varieties of lettuce, celery, chives, endive, escarole, sprouts, Jerusalem artichoke, salsify, and Swiss chard.

Wild Vegetables

From antiquity, human beings have foraged for wild plants, including edible roots, stems, leaves, flowers, and fruits. Wild foods are much hardier than domesticated varieties and usually give strong upward energy. Because of modern people's inexperience and unfamiliarity with these powerful foods, they should ordinarily be consumed only occasionally and in very small amounts. In macrobiotic cooking, the wild vegetables most commonly cooked include dandelion roots and greens, milkweed, lamb's-quarters, wild burdock, fiddlehead ferns, wild chives, and mugwort. Because of its strong contractive effect on the mind and body, ginseng root is not recommended for use as a food or condiment. Its principal use is in a medicinal preparation known as Mu tea.

Tropical Vegetables

Tropical and semitropical vegetables may be enjoyed in their native setting but are generally too extreme in their energy and effects on the mind and body for even occasional use in temperate, four-season climates. This includes some species that originally came from southern latitudes but are now grown in northern climate zones. In most cases, they have been cultivated in the new environment for only a few centuries, which in evolutionary terms is very brief. Perhaps in several thousand years after they have more fully adapted themselves to the new type of soil, weather, and growing conditions, they will be more suitable for human consumption.

Among tropical vegetables, the solanaceous plants are especially unsuitable. These include white potato, tomato, eggplant, green pepper, red pepper, chili pepper, cayenne pepper, and paprika, as well as tobacco, belladonna, henbane, and other members of the deadly nightshade family.

In the cold mountainous region of the Andes, where the potato originated, it was used primarily as a cover crop to break up the soil for growing corn. In times of famine, when grain was unavailable, the potato's bitter taste and semi-toxic properties were neutralized to some extent by soaking in a cold mountain stream, pounding, drying and using as a meal or roasting and boiling. Only the tubers were eaten, as the leaves, flowers, stems, berries, and other parts growing above ground contain the poison solanin.

The tomato, native to the tropical lowlands of South and Central America and having some of the same toxic properties as the potato, was brought to North Africa by the Conquistadores. Along with the potato, it entered Southern Europe by the sixteenth century. The eggplant, native to India, reached Europe in the Middle Ages. However, for several hundred years all three plants were regarded as poisonous and grown only for their ornamental value.

Since antiquity nightshades had been used medicinally to stimulate and depress the nervous system, increase heart rate, reduce digestive function, and raise blood pressure. When potatoes arrived in Europe and began being eaten as food, doctors and herbalists noted an increased incidence of leprosy. While the varieties of potatoes and tomatoes consumed today are larger, weaker, and less bitter than those formerly available, regular consumption of these foods in the modern diet is a contributing factor to loss of natural immunity and may lead to a wide range of extremely expansive conditions ranging from colds and flu to skin rashes and itches, loss of sexual vitality, polio, and others. This is beginning to be confirmed by modern science. For example, Dr. Norman Childers, a professor of horticulture at Cook College in New Jersey who has worked with solanaceous plants all his life, has found that regular consumption of tomatoes, potatoes, and eggplants is a primary cause of arthritis. In his book *The Nightshades and Health*, he reports that in many arthritic patients symptoms of this potentially crippling disease go away usually in a period of several weeks to several months when they stop eating these foods.

Historically, Europeans, Americans, and other modern people have been attracted to excessively yin foods like potatoes, tomatoes, eggplants, peppers, and spices in an effort to offset their high consumption of meat, poultry, eggs, dairy food, and other overly yang items. However, such an extreme balance is unnatural and inevitably leads to illness and unhappiness. As foodstuffs, the solanaceous plants are best avoided altogether. However, their medicinal properties are still useful. In macrobiotic home care, for example, potatoes are often used externally as a compress to help draw out accumulated toxins from the body, and eggplants are baked and ground into fine powder for use as a toothpaste called *dentie*.

Another type of plant usually reduced or avoided in the macrobiotic diet is the goosefoot family and its members. These vegetables of generally semitropical origin include spinach, Swiss chard, beets, lamb's-quarters, and rhubarb. They are usually astringent to the taste, cook up dark, and do not combine well with other foods. In addition, they contain oxalic acid which prevents the body from properly absorbing calcium into the cells and tissues. In extreme cases, oxalates can lead to the formation of calcium deposits or stones in the kidneys.

Other tropical or semitropical species that are preferably avoided in temperate climates are artichoke, asparagus, avocado, breadfruit, cassava, okra, plantain, sweet potato, and yam. In their own environment, these foods are perfectly fine and form an important part of the traditional diet there.

On rare occasion, when eating out or preparing exotic vegetables in the home, the adverse effects of tropical and semitropical vegetables can be somewhat reduced by counterbalancing their extreme yin energies with more yang methods of food preparation. These include salting raw foods or marinating them with tamari soy sauce or brown rice vinegar; whenever possible cooking tropical foods rather than preparing them raw and using more long-time methods such as strong boiling, stewing, or baking; and seasoning dishes with slightly more sea salt, tamari soy sauce, or miso than usual.

Preparation Methods

Depending upon the method of preparation, different tastes, textures, and energies can be created with the same vegetable. The main methods of preparing vegetables include:

Boiling

The most basic method of cooking vegetables, boiling may be used at least once daily. Depending on the technique, boiling can take a long time or a few minutes and give either slow, steady energy or quick, fast energy. Several traditional ways of boiling are:

1. *Ohitashi* Style—Vegetables are dipped in a pot containing about 1 inch of hot boiling water and taken out quickly. In the case of leafy greens, no more than 30 seconds are usually needed, while thinly sliced root vegetables might take a minute or more. A pinch of sea salt may be added to the boiling ingredients, except in the case of bitter-tasting vegetables, in order to bring out their sweetness. *Ohitashi* style boiling, similar to blanching, produces crispy tasting vegetables with strong, deep colors.

2. *Nishime* Style— (Waterless Cooking) Vegetables are cut in large sizes and boiled slowly in their own liquid or a small volume of water for a long time. When cooked, the vegetables are very juicy and are often served together with their remaining liquid. Depending upon the ingredients, seasoning may be added at the beginning or the end of cooking. Vegetables cooked *nishime* style create strong, peaceful energy and vitality. A traditional country-style dish prepared in this way combining several vegetables in the same pot is known as *oden*.

3. *Nitsuke* Style Vegetables boiled in this way take an intermediate amount of water and time between *ohitashi* and *nishime* styles. Soft vegetables may be cooked in their own juice without water. At the end of cooking, the remaining liquid may be cooked down or served with the vegetable.

4. *Kinpira* Style—This style combines sautéing and boiling and is used chiefly with root vegetables. Thinly sliced carrots, burdock, or other ingredients are sautéed in a frying pan for a few minutes. Water is then added to lightly cover the bottom of the frying pan or half cover the ingredients. When about 80 percent done, the vegetables are seasoned to taste with tamari soy sauce, simmered a few more minutes, and any remaining liquid is boiled away.

5. *Nabe* and *Sukiyaki* Styles—*Nabe* dishes are prepared at the table on little charcoal or gas burners. They usually contain many ingredients along with a light tamari soy sauce, miso, or kuzu broth. One well-known example of *nabe* cooking is *sukiyaki*. This dish is traditionally prepared in a cast-iron skillet, then boiled in a broth at the table, and served with a special dipping sauce. In modern Japan, sukiyaki is often made with beef. However, in macrobiotic cooking sukiyaki is still made in the customary way with vegetables, noodles, tofu, and sometimes fish or seafood.

Steaming

Steaming creates vegetables with a light taste, crispy texture, and bright natural colors. It usually takes only a few minutes and vegetables prepared in this way retain less water than most other cooking methods. Actual cooking time will depend on the size and thickness of the ingredients. Steaming is an excellent way to cook some vegetables, such as carrots, cabbage, Chinese cabbage, daikon roots, onions, broccoli, cauliflower, and others, whole or in large pieces, though vegetables cut in thin rounds or other small sizes do just as well.

Vegetables may be steamed by inserting a small metal vegetable steamer inside the pot, adding about a half-inch of cold water, placing the vegetables in the steamer along with a pinch of sea salt to bring out their natural sweetness, covering, and cooking until tender. An Oriental wooden steamer that fits on top of the pot may also be used. If a steamer is not available, vegetables can be steamed in the bottom of a pot containing about ¼ inch of water. A fourth method is to insert a small ceramic dish containing the vegetables into a pot containing a small volume of water, cover, and steam. This method is similar to double-boiling and is a good way to rewarm leftover rice and other grains.

Sautéing

Vegetables sautéed or fried in a small volume of unrefined vegetable oil are delicious and crispy. The best quality of oil for sautéing is dark sesame oil, though light sesame oil, corn oil, and mustard seed oil may also be used regularly and other unrefined, traditionally used vegetable oils may be used on occasion. Nearly all varieties of vegetables, including soft vegetables, leafy greens, and thinly sliced root vegetables, may be sautéed. In macrobiotic cooking, sautéed vegetables are usually served several times a week. The main styles of sautéing are:

1. **Basic Sautéing**—Vegetables are cut into thin slices, shavings, or matchsticks and added to a hot skillet brushed with oil. A pinch of sea salt is added to the vegetables to bring out their natural sweetness. The ingredients are stirred gently to prevent burning. However, there is no need to stir or mix them vigorously. Just before the end of cooking, tamari soy sauce or sea salt is added as seasoning.

2. *Kinpira* **Style**—This technique, described above under boiling, combines sautéing and boiling and is often used to prepare root vegetables, as in the usual case of carrots and burdock roots, both thinly sliced.

3. **Stir-Frying**—Vegetables fried in a small volume of hot oil in a Chinese-style wok are especially delicious and crispy. During frying, they are stirred with a long pair of cooking chopsticks. Stir-fried vegetables may also be prepared in a regular skillet, though the effects will be somewhat different than the wok.

4. **Pan-Frying**—Vegetables sautéed in a small volume of oil for a long time over a low flame give strong, steady energy. The vegetables are generally cut in large or long slices and turned over halfway through cooking.

5. **Waterless Sautéing**—For those who need to avoid or reduce oil, vege-

tables may be sautéed in a skillet by using a little water instead of oil. Only a few tablespoons of water are usually needed.

Broiling

Broiled vegetables have a unique charcoal, slightly burnt, or bitter flavor. This method of cooking especially permits soft vegetables to keep their shape without becoming mushy. Vegetable shish kebab is one traditional method of broiling and is an appetizing and colorful way to serve vegetables at picnics or in the summertime. It is prepared by arranging and skewering large chunks or slices of onions, summer squash, carrots, tempeh, seitan, and other ingredients and broiling them in the oven or over a charcoal grill.

Baking

Baking produces vegetables with strong energy and flavor. It is the method used most frequently to cook fall and winter squashes and pumpkins. However, it can also be used for individual garden vegetables and vegetable casseroles. Whole baked carrots are particularly nourishing and tasty prepared by this method.

Pressure-Cooking

Pressure-cooking makes for strong vegetables in a very short time. However, since whole grains and to some extent beans are regularly pressure-cooked on the macrobiotic diet, daily vegetables are usually prepared in other styles. However, when time is a factor or when vegetables are mixed together in small volume with either grains or beans, this method may be used. Care needs to be taken to prevent overcooking and a bitter taste often resulting from too much pressure.

Tempula Style

Sliced vegetables dipped in batter and deep-fried in oil at high temperatures are called vegetable tempura. Tempura style cooking creates very delicious, light, crispy food, produces unique, beautiful shapes, and gives strong energy. A great many root, ground, and green leafy vegetables may be prepared in this manner including carrots, parsnips, lotus root, burdock, onions, mushrooms, winter squash, cauliflower, broccoli, cabbages, string beans, snow peas, zucchini, dandelion, celery, carrot tops, parsley, and watercress. Soft watery varieties such as daikon, turnip, rutabaga, Chinese cabbage, bok choy, and lettuce are usually not tempuraed because they turn soggy. Besides vegetables, pieces of seitan and some sea vegetables, beans, and grains, as well as fish and seafood, may also be prepared in this way.

Tempura batter is made with whole wheat pastry flour, a little kuzu powder or arrowroot powder, spring water, and a pinch of sea salt. Dark sesame oil is traditionally used for cooking, though large quantities of tempura may be made with less expensive safflower oil. At the table, tempura is served with a tamari-ginger dipping sauce. A little grated daikon is also customarily served on the side to help digest the oil. Because of the large volume of oil consumed, tempura is usually reserved only for preparation on holidays or other special occasions.

Deep-Frying

Vegetables may also be deep-fried without batter. This method is called *kara-agé* in Japan and results in sliced vegetables cooked in oil similar in appearance and taste to Western-style potato chips. Carrots, lotus root, parsnip, winter squash, carrot tops, dandelion greens, and many others can be prepared in this way. Well heated oil produces a higher temperature for cooking than boiling water.

Salads

Salads give quick, light energy to the meal and balance more strongly prepared foods such as whole grains, beans, long-cooked vegetables, and fish and seafood. Salads are easy to prepare and may be made with almost all vegetables as well as be mixed with cooked grains, beans, sea vegetables, and seafood. Different dressings and sauces give the same ingredients an entirely fresh taste, and changing them is one of the simplest ways to balance and vary the daily menu. On the macrobiotic diet, salads are enjoyed frequently in a variety of styles.

1.   **Fresh Salad**—Fresh garden salads are an excellent way to prepare lettuce, sprouts, and other soft vegetables. Typical combinations include fresh greens with grated carrots; fresh greens with sprouts; celery stalks served with a dip; sliced endive; shredded red cabbage mixed with a little sea salt; watercress served with other vegetables, deep-fried tofu, tempeh, or seitan; finely sliced parsley; and sliced jinenjo served with a little tamari soy sauce, rice vinegar, and roasted sesame seeds. Cucumber slices, red radish slices, and fresh corn kernels removed from the cob also go well in fresh salads.

2.   **Marinated Salad**—Raw vegetables may also be prepared by marinating them for a short time in sea salt or tamari soy sauce. This method draws water from the vegetables, producing a sweeter and crispier result. A little brown rice vinegar or *mirin* may be added to the marinade for a sour or sweet taste respectively. Actual marinating time will vary with the type and thickness of the ingredients, usually from 5 to 10 minutes to a half hour or more. Good combinations are sliced cucumber marinated with sea salt; shredded carrots marinated with sea salt; sliced lotus root marinated with tamari soy sauce and brown rice vinegar; rutabaga marinated with tamari soy sauce; red radish marinated with umeboshi vinegar; and cooked mushrooms marinated with tamari soy sauce and served with sesame seeds and a touch of brown rice vinegar.

3.   **Pressed Salad**—Pressing is a stronger form of marinating and may be done by putting sliced vegetables in a small pickle press and layering them with sea salt. Pressing time usually takes from 30 to 60 minutes. If a press is unavailable,

the ingredients may be layered in the bottom of a bowl, sprinkled with sea salt between layers, covered with a small dish that fits inside the bowl, and topped with another small bowl containing water on top of the dish to provide pressure. Traditional pressed salads include cabbage leaves; mustard greens or daikon greens chopped small; and carrots, grated, shredded, or cut in matchsticks.

4. Boiled Salad—Boiled salad is served frequently in macrobiotic households and is an excellent way to remove the raw, bitter taste of some garden vegetables and make the salad more digestible. Stronger flavored vegetables such as daikon, turnips, parsley, and watercress are much more enjoyable prepared in this way. The method of preparation is similar to *ohitashi*-style boiling except quicker. The vegetables are usually dipped in the hot boiling water for only a few seconds, in the case of leafy greens, to a minute or more for root vegetables. Vegetables are dipped separately in order to preserve their distinctive tastes, starting with mildest and ending with the more flavorful. Rinsing the vegetables after cooking in cold water stops their cooking and allows them to retain their bright colors. Steamed salad produces vegetables with slightly less moisture than boiled salad and also may be prepared frequently. One popular combination is boiled onion, celery, and dandelion greens with a tamari-ginger sauce.

5. Grain, Bean, and Noodle Salad—Cooked whole grains, beans, and noodles may be served in salads along with fresh greens, scallions, celery, carrots, and other sliced vegetables. Prepared cold, transparent mung bean noodles, somen, soba, or whole wheat pasta make nice summertime fare. Leftover brown rice, millet, barley, kasha, bulgur, or couscous are also very enjoyable. Kidney beans, azuki beans, chick-peas, lentils, and other cooked beans give a strong, rich taste to salads, as do small squares of cooked tempeh, seitan, or tofu.

6. Sea Vegetable Salad—Sea vegetables may be combined with vegetables and other ingredients to make nutritious salads. Favorite combinations include wakame and cucumbers with a tamari-vinegar-ginger sauce; hijiki with carrots, celery, and a tofu-umeboshi sauce; and arame with onions, carrots, tempeh, and a tamari soy sauce.

7. Fruit Salad—Seasonal, locally grown fruit may be served on a bed of lettuce on a hot summer day. Fresh strawberries, apples, grapes, and all types of melons are especially delicious. A pinch of sea salt sprinkled on top of the fruit will bring out its full natural sweetness.

8. Other Salad—Other traditionally used and commonly consumed salads may also be prepared as part of the diet.

Pickling

Pickles stimulate the appetite, strengthen the intestines, and aid digestion. Throughout history, people in all parts of the world have made pickled food from a variety of root, ground, and green leafy vegetables as well as from selected sea vegetables, fruits, fish and seafood. Pickles particularly help in the assimilation of whole cereal grains and are usually eaten together.

Pickles come in many shapes, sizes, flavors, and strengths. Some quick varieties take only a few hours to make. Others take a few days to several weeks. Together, these types are called light pickles and are usually taken in the warmer seasons of the year or recommended for people who need to restrict their intake of salt. Heavy pickles take from several weeks to several months, and, in some cases, years to make, and are strong in flavor and taste. They are traditionally consumed in the cooler parts of the year and recommended for people who lack energy or are weak. Short-time pickles will usually keep about a month in a covered container in the refrigerator, while long-time pickles will ordinarily keep much longer. In macrobiotic food preparation, a variety of pickles are made at home regularly. These include:

1.   **Salt Pickles**—One of the simplest and quickest ways to make pickles is to mix sliced vegetables with sea salt and allow them to ferment under pressure. A small pickle press is useful for this purpose, consisting of an enclosed glass or plastic container in which the sliced up ingredients are placed, layered with salt, and compressed with a pressure-plate that screws down. However, a bowl, plate, and stone or other weight can be used instead.

Quick salt pickles can be made in the morning and consumed in the evening or be left to age for 2 to 3 days. Chinese cabbage is particularly crunchy and appetizing prepared in this way. Other soft vegetables such as daikon, cucumber, red cabbage, and onion also make good quick pickles, as do mustard greens, daikon greens, and turnip greens.

Salt pickles can also be made in a wooden keg or ceramic crock over a slightly longer period, 3 to 4 days to a few weeks. Dill pickles can be made combining a few sprigs of dry dill with sea salt, spring water, and cucumbers or cauliflower, broccoli, carrots, or watermelon rinds in a slightly different way. Another traditional pickled product made with sea salt is sauerkraut. This can be made at home with shredded cabbage and sea salt mixed together in a keg or crock. The cabbage is covered with a plate or disc on which a heavy stone or weight is set. After initial adjustments for pressure, the mixture is allowed to sit in a cool dark place for $1\frac{1}{2}$ to 2 weeks.

2.   **Tamari Soy Sauce Pickles**—Tamari soy sauce pickles are also on the light, quick side. Soft vegetables such as mustard greens, celery, and watercress do especially well, but practically all others can also be used. After slicing thinly, the ingredients are immersed in a jar or bottle containing a mixture of 50 percent tamari soy sauce and 50 percent spring water. The container is covered and allowed to sit from several hours to several days. Often vegetables are dipped in boiling water prior to pickling in order to take out their raw taste and give them a fresh, crispy texture. Before eating, the pickles can be inserted briefly in cold water to rinse off excess tamari soy sauce or the salty taste. Besides the ones mentioned above, popular tamari pickles include rutabaga; turnip; broccoli and cauliflower pickled together; and onions.

3.   **Miso Pickles**—Miso pickles give a nice sweet taste and are generally a little stronger than salt or tamari pickles. They are made by simply inserting the vegetable in a jar or crock containing miso. The miso should completely surround and cover the ingredients. No additional weight or pressure is needed. The thickness

of the ingredients determines the amount of aging necessary. Thinly sliced vegetables will take from 3 days to a week. Whole vegetables pickled in miso with slits cut in their skin will take 1 to 2 weeks. Vegetables sliced into thick rounds will often take 3 to 4 months, while whole unslit vegetables may take a year or more. Root vegetables make good miso pickles, especially burdock, carrots, daikon, turnip, lotus root, parsnips, and gingerroot. Often they are dried outside for a day, pressed with a little salt, or dipped into boiling water for a few minutes prior to inserting in the miso. Green leafy vegetables are usually not pickled in miso because of their high water content. Ground vegetables such as cucumber or summer squash may be prepared in this way if pressed first in salt. Others such as broccoli must first be dipped in boiling water. Scallion miso pickles can be made in 1 to 2 days by inserting a bunch of uncut scallions directly in the miso. When done, the excess miso is rinsed off and they are sliced. Minced lemon rinds, cooked in hot water, sautéed with miso and grated ginger, and stored in a jar for 1 week also make excellent miso pickles.

4. Umeboshi or Shiso Pickles—Vegetables pickled for a few days with umeboshi plums have a unique sour taste. They also give ingredients an attractive pink coloring. Red radishes turn out exceptionally well with this method. Vegetables may also be made with shiso (beefsteak) leaves, the distinctive triangular leaves that umeboshi plums are themselves pickled in. A traditional spicy and delicious pickle is made with gingerroot and shiso leaves.

5. Bran Pickles—Bran pickles are usually aged for a lengthy time and provide strong energy. In contrast to most pickles, bran pickles may be cooked as well as eaten raw. They are made with *nuka*, the bran from polished rice or wheat. However, in macrobiotic food preparation, brown rice flour is usually preferred to bran. One long-time bran pickle made with dried daikon is called *takuan*. Strong and salty, this pickle is named after the Buddhist monk who, according to legend, trained Miyamoto Musashi, Japan's most famous *samurai*. They are usually aged from 1 to 3 years and give tremendous energy.

Short-time bran or brown rice flour pickles can also be made, and many macrobiotic families keep a large crock continuously filled with bran or flour, a variety of vegetables, sea salt, miso, and kombu. Root, ground, and green leafy vegetables are pickled together cut in various ways, and as ingredients are taken out fresh vegetables are added every few days to replace them. In this way, the pickling mixture can be kept going for several years.

6. Saké Lees Pickles—The remnants from brewing saké, the traditional rice wine of Japan, are known as saké lees (*saké-kasu*). They have a sweet, somewhat sharp taste and may be used in pickling as well as be added to other types of dishes. Usually vegetables pickled with saké lees are initially pressed with a little sea salt first. After inserting in the saké lees, as in making miso pickles, the ingredients are left to ferment for a couple of weeks before using.

7. Other Pickles—Other traditional and commonly used pickling methods using natural ingredients and seasonings may also be used.

Drying

Drying is one of the traditional ways of preserving vegetables, and there are many different methods utilizing wind and sun. Root vegetables such as carrots, daikon, and lotus root are often dried, though ground and even green leafy varieties can also be processed in this way. Before cooking, these dried vegetables can be soaked in water to soften them.

Other Methods

Other methods of cooking or preserving vegetables that are traditionally used and commonly practiced may also be used.

Cooking Styles

Vegetables can be served in an endless variety of ways. In addition to the methods noted above, they may also be cooked in soup, boiled or pressure-cooked with grains, cooked with beans, cooked with sea vegetables, served with noodle or pasta dishes, cooked with fish or seafood, or served as an ingredient in desserts and snacks. The following paragraphs describe just a few of the many ways selected vegetables are currently used in macrobiotic cooking.

Root Vegetables

1.   **Burdock**—A long thin root vegetable, burdock is dark brown in color, firm in texture, and gives very strong energy. Though consumed throughout the year, it is especially enjoyed in the cooler months. One of the most popular ways of preparing burdock is sautéing it *kinpira* style with carrots or other root vegetables. It may also be boiled, steamed, or deep-fried. Burdock also blends well with whole grains, beans, and kombu but not sea vegetables that have a dark color such as hijiki and arame. In the Orient it is traditionally made into an energizing soup along with carp, miso, and bancha tea which is known as *koi-koku*. Lightly boiled in salad, burdock is enjoyed seasoned with a little rice vinegar.

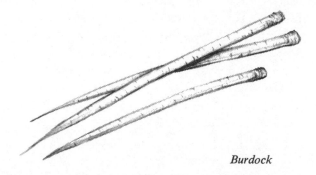

Burdock

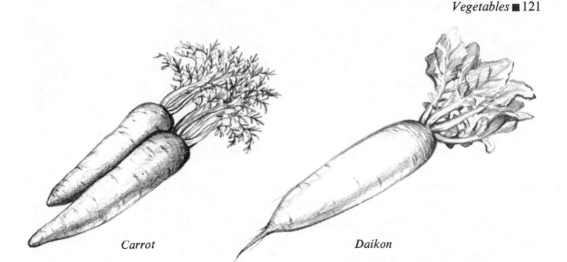

Carrot   Daikon

2. **Carrots**—Carrots have a bright orange color, crunchy texture, and sweet taste that are valued around the world. Raw, they may be enjoyed sliced or grated in salads, blended into a juice, or grated as a condiment or garnish. In soups, carrots can be enjoyed by themselves in a thick, creamy soup, or they may be added to miso soup, vegetable soups, or to *koi-koku* in place of burdock. Baked whole in a casserole dish, carrots give a unique sweet flavor and strong energy. Together with onions, carrots may be sliced thinly, boiled *ohitashi* style, and served with a kuzu sauce, or they may be cut in large pieces and boiled *nishime* style. Carrots go well sautéed with nearly all sea vegetables and other root vegetables, especially burdock and lotus root. Carrots and cabbage are another excellent combination and can be prepared in many ways. This versatile vegetable may also be steamed, broiled, deep-fried, cooked tempura style, and pickled.

3. *Daikon*—*Daikon*, or white radish, is an indispensable part of traditional Far Eastern cuisine and is now grown in the West. The smaller, thinner daikon, shaped somewhat like a carrot, grows more quickly than the larger varieties and has a strong, sharp taste. The big juicy ones grow up to several feet in length and are sweeter to the taste. This latter variety is often preferred for quick salads and goes well with a little tamari soy sauce and brown rice vinegar, lemon, or umeboshi vinegar. Grated daikon is traditionally served as an accompaniment to tempura, mochi, sashimi, and other fish or seafood to aid in digestion. When served with animal food, a little grated ginger and several drops of tamari soy sauce are customarily mixed in with the grated daikon. In soup, daikon is frequently added to miso soup along with wakame. Boiled in large slices, *daikon* may be prepared as a side dish served with a sauce, miso, or toasted black sesame seeds. It is also enjoyed cooked *nishime* style in combination with vegetables, beans, and bean products including carrots, celery, burdock, lotus root, tempeh, deep-fried tofu, turnips, rutabagas, parsnips, celery, onions, dried tofu, shiitake mushrooms, and soybeans. Dried, usually shredded daikon is also sweet to the taste and may be used regularly, boiled, steamed, or prepared in other ways.

4. Gingerroot—A light golden root with a knobby appearance, ginger has a pungent taste, firm texture, and gives warm energy. It is traditionally grated and used in small volume to garnish grain and vegetable dishes, soups, salads, sea vegetables, seitan, tempura, and oily foods including fish and seafood. Sometimes it is added raw, and other times it is added to the other ingredients at the very end of cooking and simmered for a few minutes before serving. It is especially flavorful cooked in this way with fried rice or fried noodles. In addition to grating, ginger can be prepared in juice form by squeezing the gratings in a cheese-cloth. The resulting liquid is much more concentrated than the gratings and only a few drops usually suffice. Ginger may also be cooked and used to make a spicy condiment with kombu and another with miso. It is also customarily pickled with shiso leaves and served with sushi and other rice dishes. Finally, ginger has several internal and external medicinal applications in macrobiotic health care ranging from use in medicinal teas to body compresses.

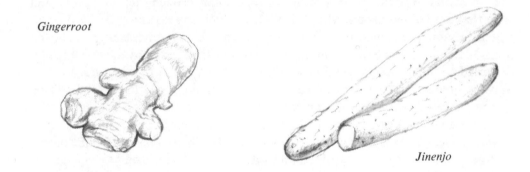

Gingerroot

Jinenjo

5. Jinenjo—This long mountain potato, native to Japan, grows up to several feet in length. It creates very strong energy and is often served in the colder months. Jinenjo is usually grated and eaten raw in small volume with a little fresh grated ginger, tamari soy sauce, and toasted nori squares. It may also be sliced and marinated with brown rice vinegar and tamari soy sauce. Jinenjo is also delicious added to miso soup or tamari broth, served on top of soba, or mixed in flour form with mochi. It is also frequently boiled in large slices *nishime* style and seasoned with tamari soy sauce or added to *oden* and *nabe* style dishes containing many ingredients. Jinenjo flour is added to a type of soba called *jinenjo soba* that is especially strengthening.

6. Lotus Root—The root of the lotus flower plant grows underwater in seg-mented lengths, is light brown in color, and contains thin hollow chambers. When sliced, these inner chambers yield many unique shapes and may be stuffed and cooked with miso, tahini, and other foods. Fresh lotus root is enjoyed in salads sliced very thinly and marinated for several hours with rice vinegar, tamari soy sauce, and/or mirin. Sautéed *kinpira* style, it may be cooked like carrots or burdock and is often cooked with other root vegetables or sea vegetables such as hijiki and arame. In large pieces, lotus root may be boiled *nishime* style along with shiitake mushrooms and daikon. It also combines well in large slices with azuki beans. Prepared tempura-style or deep-fried, lotus balls are very rich and appetizing. Lotus root is also traditionally dried for use when it is not available fresh and in powdered form is used for a soothing, medicinal tea.

7. **Parsnips**—Cultivated in East and West since antiquity, parsnips have a beautiful white color, soft texture, and strong, sweet taste. Because of their distinctive flavor and texture, they are often prepared as a side dish by themselves and may be steamed for a few minutes until crispy, prepared in a soup, or mashed, turned into a pie crust, and baked. Parsnips also combine well with carrots or onions and may be served with a sauce made from clear soup stock, kuzu powder, and grated ginger.

8. **Radish**—Red radishes have a pleasing color and shape and are enjoyable raw in salads or prepared as a garnish. Their taste is pungent like the smaller varieties of daikon, and they may be substituted in recipes calling for daikon if white radish is unavailable. Red radishes may also be cooked and go well boiled whole with umeboshi plums and served with a kuzu sauce. Along with their tops, they are also traditionally pickled with umeboshi.

9. **Rutabaga**—The rutabaga, or Swedish turnip as it is also known, is yellow-orange in color, usually large in size, and milder tasting than other members of the turnip family. Boiled or steamed by itself, it is very sweet and delicious. It may also be prepared with carrots, onions, and other root and ground vegetables. It is also tasty sliced thinly and marinated or pickled in tamari soy sauce after slicing.

10. **Taro**—Taro potato, also known as albi, is grown in the Pacific Islands, Japan, Africa, the West Indies, and South and Central America. It has a distinctive hairy skin, which is not eaten but often left on during cooking. Since taro is tropical or semitropical in origin, it is not regularly consumed in the macrobiotic diet in temperate climates. However, because of its medicinal properties, taro is used in external compresses and as food may be served very occasionally in the hot summer months. It is delicious added in small volume to soups and stews and may be cut into large slices and cooked *nishime* style with other root vegetables. Though some taros grow as big as coconuts, the smaller apple-sized ones are more suitable for use in northern regions.

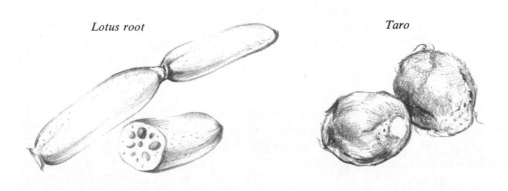

Lotus root   *Taro*

11. Turnip—Turnips come in all shapes, sizes, and colors and are one of the traditional root crops in Europe and Asia. Their sharp raw taste can be softened by pressing in salad, marinating, or pickling for a few days with tamari soy sauce. Cooked, turnips add flavor and texture to soups and stews. They also may be boiled or steamed as a small side dish or be cooked together with tofu, seitan, fish, or seafood.

12. Other Root Vegetables—Other root vegetables that are traditionally cultivated and commonly used may also be prepared as part of the macrobiotic diet.

Ground Vegetables

1. Broccoli—Broccoli has an attractive shape, bright green color, and firm crispy texture. It is enjoyed marinated for quick salads, lightly pickled, boiled, steamed, sautéed, or cooked in tempura. It is especially delicious with fried rice, fried noodles, or mixed vegetables. To prevent bruising and preserve its color, it is usually cooked separately and mixed in at the very end when combined with other ingredients. Though almost always cut into flowerets, broccoli is occasionally served whole as in some areas of Italy. Its leaves and stalk, except for the outermost fibrous layer, are also edible and may be cooked along with the flowers. At the table broccoli is often served with a creamy tofu dressing, an umeboshi sauce, roasted sesame seeds, or a dressing made from tamari soy sauce and grated ginger.

Broccoli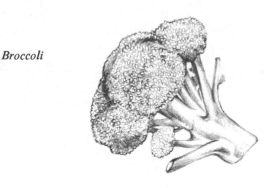

2. Brussels Sprouts—These small members of the cabbage family of vegetables are usually enjoyed cooked whole but may also be boiled or steamed sliced. Since they are slightly bitter in taste, salt is generally not used in seasoning during cooking. To bring out and preserve their bright green color, Brussels sprouts need cook only for a few minutes. Other round vegetables, such as kohlrabi and fennel, may also be used frequently.

3. Cabbage—Cabbage has been a staple food crop in Asia and Europe for thousands of years. It comes in many varieties, shapes, and colors and is valued for its mild texture and natural sweet taste. Red cabbage especially is enjoyed shredded in raw salads, while the green type goes well in boiled salads. Both

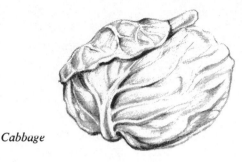

Cabbage

types may also be sautéed, steamed, or boiled as a separate side dish or combined with other ingredients. Because it blends well with many tastes, a variety of sour, sweet, or salty sauces may be prepared to accompany cabbage. With onions, celery, and carrots, cabbage is often stir-fried Chinese style. It may also be stuffed with couscous and baked as in the Middle East. Cabbage rolls filled with tempeh, tofu, seitan, arame, or hijiki, are enjoyable on holidays or special occasions. Hard cabbage is traditionally pickled with salt and allowed to ferment several weeks to produce sauerkraut. Miso or bran pickles can also be made with hard cabbages.

4.   **Cauliflower**—Cauliflower has a beautiful white color, sweet taste, and peaceful energy. To keep its crispy texture, flowery shape, and nice taste, it should not be cooked too long. The stalk and leaves may be cooked at the same time as the flowers. Raw or marinated, cauliflower makes a tasty appetizer. It may also be pickled with tamari soy sauce and rice vinegar for about two weeks. Boiled cauliflower is often enjoyed with a tamari-lemon-ginger sauce or with an umeboshi vinegar sauce and roasted sesame seeds. Thickened with kuzu root powder, cauliflower makes a creamy and delicious soup.

5.   **Cucumber**—This common garden vegetable is very cooling and usually enjoyed raw in the summertime. Its taste is enhanced by sprinkling with a little sea salt. Umeboshi or sliced shiso leaves also bring out cucumber's delicious taste and may be added to salads. Cucumber may also be marinated with a tamari soy sauce and vinegar. Pickled cucumbers are found worldwide and can be made by slicing and pressing in salt for a few hours, soaking in water with dill for a few days, immersing in miso, or covering with saké lees.

6.   **Fresh Beans**—Fresh beans of many sizes, shapes, and colors are cultivated around the world. Thought to have originated in the Americas, they are known variously as string beans, snap beans, wax beans, yellow beans, and long beans. In the summertime, they are enjoyed lightly boiled, steamed, or cooked *nishime* style and served with a mild tamari soy sauce taste, a tofu-umeboshi sauce, or ground roasted sesame seeds. Fresh beans may also be cooked with slivered almonds or other nuts.

7.   **Green Peas**—*Green peas* have a beautiful green color, round shape, and soft texture. After shelling, they are customarily boiled in a small volume of water for a few minutes with a touch of sea salt. They go well mixed together in salads with brown rice, barley, couscous, or other grain. *Chirashi-zushi* is a traditional dish made with green peas in Japan. Peas also make lovely garnishes for

clear soups, vegetable soups, and stews. *Snow peas*, whose pods are edible, are also very sweet and may be prepared occasionally. They are frequently enjoyed sautéed Chinese style with cabbages, onions, and sprouts.

8.   **Mushrooms**—Edible mushrooms are a delicacy and may be enjoyed occasionally in very small amounts. There are many varieties, both wild and cultivated. *Shiitake*, the large mushroom native to the Far East and now grown in the West, is probably used most frequently in macrobiotic cooking. It is commonly available both fresh and dried. It is delicious boiled *nishime* style as a small side dish or as a stock for kombu broth or clear soup. A few slices may be added now and then to miso soup and various grain, bean, sea vegetable, and vegetable dishes. Sautéed in sesame oil, shiitake is very crunchy. Ordinarily the tough stems are cut off before cooking, and the dried variety needs to be soaked. Recent medical studies have shown that shiitake mushrooms quickly lower serum cholesterol, which has been linked to coronary heart disease and other circulatory disorders. *Cultivated brown* and *white mushrooms* also make a nice small side dish or delicious soup. They may also be prepared with other vegetables and go especially well sautéed with seitan, added to barley soup or stew, or cooked with soybeans and grains. In salads, mushrooms are preferably marinated for a short time with tamari soy sauce and rice vinegar or pickled rather than eaten raw. For enjoyment, they may also be cooked tempura style or broiled barbecue fashion.

Shiitake mushrooms   *Cultivated mushrooms*

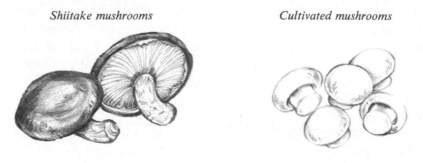

9.   **Onions**—Onions are one of humanity's oldest cultivated vegetables and have been a staple since the earliest Chinese and Egyptian dynasties. They have a strong, pungent taste when consumed raw, but cooked onions become very sweet and delicious and impart a calm, peaceful energy. In salads, red onions are milder and sweeter than other varieties. Yellow onions go well cooked with

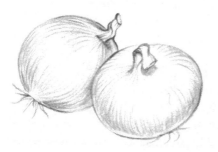

Onion

wakame in lightly boiled salad with lemon dressing. Marinated with tamari soy sauce, lightly pickled onions can be ready within an hour. In soups, onions are traditionally added to miso soup along with wakame. The small white onions may be used whole in grain, vegetable, and bean soups. French onion soup is also very enjoyable. As a side dish, onions may be prepared boiled, steamed, baked, or broiled. Cooked with other vegetables, onions provide an attractive white color, soft texture, and fresh, sweet, and mildly pungent taste. Good combinations are onions and carrots; onions, peas, carrots, and cabbage; and onions and other greens. Cooked whole and topped with miso, onions make a particularly nourishing dish. In tempura, onion rings are a favorite ingredient. *Garlic* and *shallots*, stronger members of the onion family, are occasionally pickled or used to create a hot taste, but because of their sharp, spicy taste and strong energy are not used very much in daily macrobiotic cooking. Other plants related to the onion, including scallions and leeks, are discussed in the green leafy vegetable section below.

10.   **Summer Squash**—There are many varieties of summer squash that derive from marrows and gourds first cultivated in Central America about ten thousand years ago. Because of their tropical origin, they are not used so much in macrobiotic cooking in temperate latitudes. However, in hot weather they may be enjoyed occasionally. *Yellow squash*, also known as crookneck, may be boiled, steamed, sautéed, baked, or barbecued. *Zucchini*, sliced or whole, is very delicious served with a miso sauce. *Pattypan* or *star squash* is nice boiled or steamed with a pinch of sea salt to bring out its juice and served with a creamy sauce made from kuzu root powder, tamari soy sauce, and grated ginger.

11.   **Winter Squash**—Hard round fall and winter squashes are usually deep golden in color, sweet and delicious to the taste, and contribute substantially to making a full, satisfying meal. Originally cultivated by the native peoples of North America, they have become a staple of modern macrobiotic cooking and can be prepared and seasoned in a variety of ways. In baking, a little oil may be applied on the inside or outside of the squash. However, in boiling, steaming, or pressure-cooking, oil interferes with squash's natural taste and is not ordinarily used. A plain salt taste suffices when squash is sliced into small pieces and cooked with other ingredients, though tamari soy sauce or miso be used as seasoning if desired. The skin of winter squashes (but not pumpkin) is edible and should be left on when cooking. Squash seeds may be saved for roasting. In addition to regular baked squash, squash may be cooked with onions, puréed into a creamy, delicious soup, added to miso or soup, or pressure-cooked with millet or brown rice. Squash pies, puddings, and other desserts are savory, and on Thanksgiving Day or other traditional harvest festival many macrobiotic families prepare a large squash stuffed with whole wheat bread crumbs, deep-fried onions, celery, and parsley instead of turkey.

Squashes and pumpkins come in many types. Those most commonly used include *acorn squash*, a small, round variety that is dark green or black in color. It is very sweet and usually cooked as a side dish. *Butternut squash* has a light pale skin, is oblong in shape, and its orange flesh gives a smooth sweet flavor. It is cooked as a side dish, used in soups, or made into pies. *Buttercup squash* is blocky

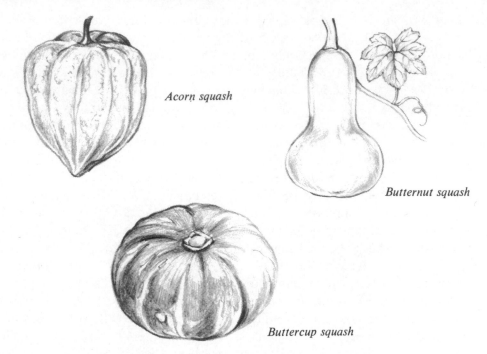

Acorn squash

Butternut squash

Buttercup squash

in appearance, dark green to black in color, it has a deep orange flesh with a strong, full flavor that makes it a favorite for soups, stews, morning cooking with soft rice, and in desserts. *Delicata squash* is usually a pale yellow or orange, zucchini-like in shape, with dark-green longitudinal ribbing. It has a sweet orange flesh. *Spaghetti squash* has a pale yellow to buff skin and a sweet, yellow spaghetti-like flesh. *Hokkaido pumpkin* actually originated in New England but owes its name to the northernmost region of Japan where it is extremely popular. Large and orange- or red-skinned, it is very delicious. *Hubbard squash*, a large bumpy hard-shell variety, comes in red, blue, and green shades and usually has a dry, solid yellow flesh. It is the squash usually stuffed for Thanksgiving Day or holiday meals. *Pumpkin*, the familiar Halloween jack-o'-lantern, makes good pies and puddings and may be cooked with other foods. It is ordinarily not as sweet as other squashes.

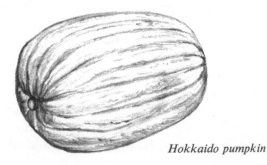

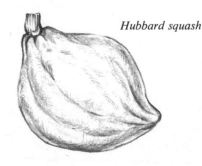

Hubbard squash

Hokkaido pumpkin

12.   Other Ground Vegetables—Other ground vegetables that are traditionally cultivated and commonly used may also be included in the macrobiotic diet.

Green Leafy Vegetables

1.   Bok Choy—A traditional ingredient of Chinese cooking, bok choy has a long white stalk and leaves that are mild tasting and blend well with strong-tasting foods such as fried tofu, fish, or seafood. It is usually sautéed and may be served with a kuzu sauce.

2.   Carrot Greens—The tops of carrots have a strong, parsley-like taste. Because they are often hard, they may need to cook longer than other greens and may lose some of their bright green color in the process. When cooking, no salt is added to prevent a bitter taste. However, they may be prepared into a very sweet condiment by sautéing in sesame oil and mixing with a little miso or a few drops of tamari soy sauce at the end.

3.   Celery—Celery's unique shape, crispy texture, and mild sweet taste makes it a popular vegetable in salads, soups, and casseroles. In buckwheat salad, for example, diced celery balances the raw taste of onions. It may also be cooked briefly, and a pinch of sea salt will bring out celery's natural sweetness. With carrots and onions, it is often prepared *nishime* style. Celery leaves are also edible and may be served raw with a dip, used as garnish for other dishes, or be dipped whole in tempura batter and deep-fried.

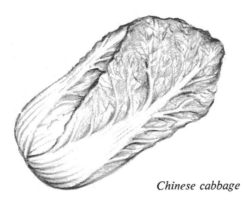

Chinese cabbage

4.   Chinese Cabbage—This white leafy vegetable is a staple in the Far East and has become increasingly popular in the West. Its soft, compact shape, mild flavor, and ability to combine well with many other foods lends itself to many cooking styles and dishes. In fresh salad, its white leaves make an attractive companion to lettuce or other greens. It may also be sprinkled with salt for pressed salad, in which case sliced kombu is often added in-between layers to absorb its drawn-out juices. Cut in halves or quarters, Chinese cabbage is also traditionally pickled for 1 to 2 weeks or longer with sea salt or salt with rice bran. Korea is famous for a spicy pickle made with Chinese cabbage called *kimchi*. Chinese cabbage's light sweet taste and natural juiciness are brought out by boiling. Leaf by leaf, it may be dipped into hot boiling water and sliced after cooking. It is also often added to miso soup or soup stock, boiled salads, or mixed vegetables. Wrapped around sliced carrots and boiled, it makes tasty Chinese cabbage rolls. This versatile vegetable may also be tied with *kampyo* strips, or dried gourd, and be added to *yu-dofu*. Chinese cabbage is often enjoyed served with a tamari-lemon sauce, a tamari-ginger sauce, or garnished with sliced scallion.

5. Chives—Chives are members of the onion family and have a stronger flavor and taste than scallions. Mixed with miso, they make a savory condiment. They may also be dipped in and out of boiling water, sliced, and served with a tofu dip.

6. Collard Greens—Collards are traditional to Native American and Black American cooking. They are soft and tender, very sweet, and give a calm, peaceful energy. They may be lightly boiled or steamed and go well with a tamari-rice vinegar sauce.

7. Daikon Greens—The large leaves of the daikon radish are very chewy and strengthening and have a slightly pungent taste. They are prepared as a small side dish often in macrobiotic cooking. To soften them, daikon tops may be cooked with diluted miso in small volume. They may also be cooked together with fried tofu and kombu in a dish combining sautéing, boiling, and steaming. Short-time daikon green pickles may be made by pressing with salt for 1 to 2 days. In this case, the greens are usually cut into small pieces. Long-time pickles, made with both root and greens, give very strong energy and may take two or more years to age. Red radish leaves are also very energizing and may be prepared in a similar way.

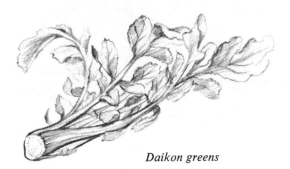

Daikon greens

8. Dandelion Greens—Wild dandelion greens have traditionally been eaten in Southern Europe and other temperate areas of the world. They may be prepared as a lightly boiled salad and are usually cooked together with their roots. They may also be sautéed in oil or a little water. Dandelion greens give strength and vitality, are a good source of fiber, and contribute to smooth digestion.

9. Endive—Endive is native to Europe, and one of the most common varieties is called the Belgium endive. The curly-leaved types may be eaten raw in salads, while the broad-leaved varieties are cooked. In macrobiotic cooking, endive is occasionally enjoyed whole sautéed in a little sesame oil and topped with miso at the end of cooking. Adding the miso sweetens and softens the endive's somewhat bitter taste. It may also be sliced and cooked in other ways. Endive goes well with a kuzu sauce or a tamari-ginger sauce.

10.   Escarole—Escarole is a soft vegetable with curly leaves, a stem that is not so tough as most other greens, and a slightly bitter taste. On account of its taste, it is usually not prepared with salt. Escarole may be served fresh or be dipped in boiling water or steamed for a short time.

11.   Kale—Kale is a hard, fibrous green and served regularly as a side dish in many macrobiotic households. It has a full sweet taste, cooks up very tender, and gives strong energy. The winter variety is very hardy, surviving from fall to spring under the snow and ice. Kale may be boiled, steamed, or sautéed. Its stems and leaves are usually cooked together. A pinch of sea salt is traditionally sprinkled on kale when boiling. Steamed, it goes well mixed with carrots. Kale is often served with a umeboshi vinegar sauce, a tofu dressing, a lemon sauce, a miso sauce, or a rice vinegar sauce.

12.   Leeks—Though bigger than scallions or chives, leeks are not so pungent. They become sweet and creamy when cooked and are traditionally enjoyed in leek soup. They may also be added in small amounts to miso or other vegetable soups. By themselves, leeks may be boiled in large or small slices, sautéed, or deep-fried. Cooking them with miso makes for an even sweeter dish. In preparing leeks, it is important to clean them thoroughly, since soil tends to accumulate in the vegetable's inside layers. This may be eliminated by cutting them in half lengthwise and rinsing well under cold water.

13.   Lettuce—The many types of lettuce include romaine, iceberg, and Boston. Soft, mild tasting, and beautiful to look at, lettuce is used primarily in fresh salads. By itself, lettuce may occasionally be eaten raw with a little tamari soy sauce, umeboshi, or roasted sesame seeds. Combined with other ingredients, it goes well with a wide variety of dressings and sauces. Lettuce may also be lightly cooked but its leaves turn dark when boiled.

14.   Mustard Greens—Mustard greens have fine, delicate leaves, a sweet taste, and give strong, hearty energy. The plant from which they come grows through the winter and blooms in the spring. Mustard seed oil, processed from the mustard

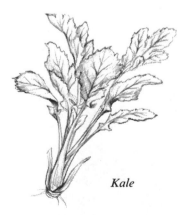

Kale

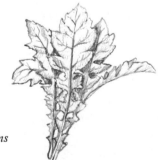

Mustard greens

plant, yields a high-quality cooking oil that may be used daily. The greens are frequently boiled *ohitashi* style for a few minutes and served as a small side dish with a light rice vinegar or tamari-ginger sauce. Salt is usually not added during cooking to prevent a slightly bitter taste from coming out.

15. **Parsley**—Parsley is known chiefly as a colorful garnish, but it may also be prepared as a small side dish or be added to soups, salads, and grain and vegetable dishes. It combines especially well with yellow or orange foods such as corn, millet, and squash. Dipped in boiling water for only a few seconds, parsley's bright green color turns even deeper. The plant's stems are a little tough and may be boiled or sautéed a little longer than the leaves.

16. **Scallions**—Scallions stimulate the appetite and senses. They yield pleasing shapes when cut, have a nice pungent taste, and give warm energy. As a garnish, they go well with whole grains, noodles, soups, stews, beans, and vegetables. They may also be boiled or sautéed for a few seconds, and they are traditionally prepared into a sweet condiment with miso. The small white roots of the scallion are very high in energy and nutrients and should always be preserved. They may be chopped and eaten with the sliced white and green parts of the plant or saved and added to other dishes.

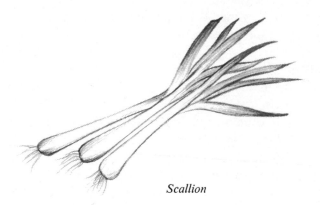

Scallion

17. **Sprouts**—Vegetable, bean, and grain sprouts can be grown at home or are widely available at most food outlets. The soft ones like alfalfa may be enjoyed raw from time to time with a little brown rice vinegar or tamari soy sauce. The harder ones like bean sprouts can be sautéed Chinese style with other vegetables.

18. **Turnip Greens**—Turnip greens are soft, beautiful in color, and milder in taste than radish tops. As a small side dish, they go well served with a sesame-tamari sauce. Turnip greens may also be pickled, along with the whole turnips, by pressing in salt.

19. **Watercress**—Watercress is native to Europe, Asia, and North America. Its pungent, slightly bitter taste is enjoyed in fresh salads. It may also be cooked for salads by dipping in hot boiling water for a few seconds. Cooking softens its strong flavor, brightens its deep green color, and creates a fresh taste and energy. Watercress salads are often enjoyed with a creamy sesame or tofu dressing. With

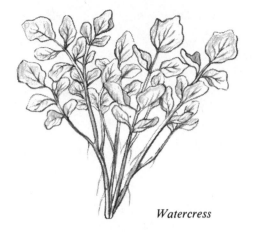

Watercress

corn and tofu, prepared scrambled egg style, it goes well added at the end of sautéing. Watercress may also be added raw or cooked to soups, stews, or sushi. It is also sometimes prepared into rolls by boiling for about half a minute, wrapping with toasted nori, and serving with a dip made of tamari soy sauce, water, and fresh grated ginger.

20. Other Leafy Green Vegetables—Other traditionally cultivated and commonly used leafy green vegetables may also be prepared.

Nutritional Value

Fresh vegetables are high in complex carbohydrates, fiber, vitamins, and minerals. As part of a balanced whole foods diet, they help provide all of the essential nutrients necessary for optimal health and vitality.

Beets, broad beans, burdock, dandelion greens, gingerroot, green peas, lotus root, shiitake mushrooms, onions, parsley, parsnips, and winter squash are especially high in complex carbohydrates.

Broad beans, broccoli, Brussels sprouts, burdock, carrots, cauliflower, collard greens, daikon leaves, dandelion greens, gingerroot, green peas, kale, lotus root, mustard greens, parsley, parsnips, pumpkin, scallions, and winter squash are high in fiber.

Broccoli, carrots, daikon, dandelion greens, kale, mustard greens, and winter squash are high in vitamin A (see Table 16).

Broccoli, Brussels sprout, cabbage leaves, cauliflower, chives, collard leaves, watercress, kale, mustard greens, turnip greens and Swiss chard are good daily sources of vitamin C.

Broccoli, collard greens, daikon leaves, dried daikon, dandelion greens, kale, mustard greens, parsley, Swiss chard, turnip greens, and watercress contain substantial amounts of calcium.

Table 16   Vitamin A Content in Various Foods

In addition to carrots, a variety of land and sea vegetables are a rich source of vitamin A or β-carotene which is converted into vitamin A in the body. The U.S. RDA is 5,000 I.U./day*. (Figures per 100 grams, unit I.U.)

	Beet greens	6,100
	Brussels sprouts	2,500
	Carrots	11,000
	Collard greens	6,500
Vegetables	Dandelion greens	14,000
	Kale	8,900
	Mustard greens	7,000
	Parsley	8,500
	Spinach	8,100
	Swiss chard	6,500
	Winter squash	3,700
Animals Products	Fortified milk	1,130
	Liver	10–100,000

* Vitamin A is increasingly measured in Retinol Equivalents. One I.U. from animal sources equals 1 retinol equivalent, while 6 I.U. from plant sources equals 1 retinol equivalent. About 800 to 1,000 retinol equivalents are recommended daily.

Source: U.S. Department of Agriculture and Japan Nutritionist Association.

Broad beans, dandelion greens, gingerroot, green peas, kale, mustard greens, parsley, and Swiss chard are very high in iron.

Health Benefits

Vegetables are an essential part of a healthy diet and as a complement to whole cereal grains contribute to smooth digestive, circulatory, and nervous system functioning.

In general, root vegetables give very stabilizing energy, contribute to physical vitality and endurance, focus the thinking, and strengthen the will. They are especially beneficial to the intestines, heart and circulatory system, and lungs. Green leafy vegetables give an upward, rising energy, calm the mind, stimulate mental and psychological processes, and lead to peace and tranquility. They are especially strengthening to the liver, gallbladder, and in some cases kidneys and urinary system. Ground vegetables give energy and affect metabolism at an intermediate level between root vegetables and green leafy vegetables. They are especially beneficial to the stomach, spleen, and pancreas.

The specific qualities of different vegetables and their effects on mind and body have long been studied by traditional Far Eastern medicine, traditional Western medicine, folk medicine, and many families and individuals. For example, carrots are traditionally good for alleviating eye and liver conditions. Burdock provides strength and vitality and has often been taken to improve sexual functioning. Daikon facilitates the digestion of whole grains and vegetables. It also helps eliminate excess water and animal fats from the body. Jinenjo gives strength and vitality. Lotus root is very beneficial to the lungs and large intestine, helps relieve coughing and internal bleeding, and assists in loosening and discharging accumulated mucus in the sinuses. Fresh ginger stimulates circulation of blood and other body fluids.

Among ground vegetables, onions give balanced, peaceful energy when cooked and, prepared with squash and carrots, are highly recommended for diabetic persons who must watch their intake of simple sugars. Cabbage is good for the stomach and spleen. Broccoli and cauliflower are very strengthening for the lungs. Winter squashes and pumpkins are excellent for the pancreas.

Leafy green vegetables are high in fiber and very important for digestion. In most cases they are strengthening to the liver, sometimes to the lungs, and occasionally to the kidneys and sexual organs.

The way vegetables are prepared greatly affects their energy and nutrients. Cooking usually brings out their natural flavor and taste, aids digestion, and improves the proportion of nutrients effectively utilized by the body. Each style of cooking has a different effect on the energy and composition of the food. One of the most important food processing methods is pickling. Pickles stimulate the appetite, aid digestion, and strengthen the intestines and blood quality. During the fermentation process, enzymes and bacteria change the sugar in pickled foods into lactic acid. Lactic acid strengthens the villi in the intestines that assimilate metabolized foodstuffs into the bloodstream.

The importance of fresh vegetables has been recognized by almost all modern scientific and medical bodies. Their importance in preventing and relieving degenerative diseases is now just beginning to command official attention. In its report *Diet, Nutrition, and Cancer,* the National Academy of Sciences recommended daily consumption of yellow and orange vegetables such as carrots and winter squashes high in β-carotene (a precursor to vitamin A) and green leafy vegetables, especially cabbage, broccoli, cauliflower, and Brussels sprouts, as part of a prudent diet to help prevent against cancer. The American Heart Association, the American Diabetes Association, and many other organizations have issued guidelines on vegetable consumption that are similar in direction to the macrobiotic diet.

One of the few studies that examined overall effects of vegetable-quality foods on health involved the Tarahumara Indians of Mexico. The Tarahumara consume primarily whole corn, beans, squash, and other local vegetables and fruit. They eat almost no animal foods. In the *American Journal of Clinical Nutrition,* medical researchers who studied the Tarahumara reported that they displayed no signs of high blood pressure, obesity, coronary heart disease, stroke, or other circulatory disorders. The Indians' high intake of vegetable protein, unsaturated fat, and fiber from cereal and vegetable sources was further associated with substantially lower concentrations of cholesterol in their blood. "The customary diet of the Tarahumara is adequate in all nutrients," the scientists concluded.

Beans and Bean Products

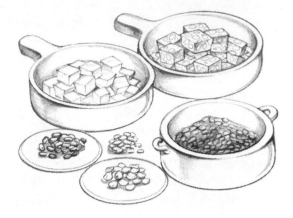

Daily Use

In the Standard Macrobiotic Diet, whole dried beans and bean products are usually eaten daily or otherwise several times per week and comprise about 5 to 10 percent of the volume of total food consumed. Beans that are more northerly in origin, smaller in size, and contain less fat and oil than other varieties, such as azuki beans, lentils, and chick-peas, are eaten most frequently. Medium-sized beans such as pintos, kidneys, and whole soybeans are used occasionally. Large beans such as limas that are more southerly in origin and higher in fat are prepared less frequently. In addition to, or as a substitute for, beans in whole form, soybean products such as tofu, tempeh, and natto may be used almost daily or several times a week.

History

Beans have been cultivated around the world since ancient times. Along with vegetables, they are a traditional complement to whole cereal grains. In South and Central America, for example, beans wrapped in tortillas made from whole corn have been the staple for thousands of years. Popular varieties include black beans, kidney beans, and pinto beans. In India, rice or chapatis are traditionally eaten with *dhal*, a thick sauce made from dried and split lentils or the yellow pigeon pea. In Asia, azuki beans, soybeans, and mung beans were staples; in Africa, chick-peas, black-eyed peas, and locust beans; in Europe, broad beans, lentils, and dried peas. In addition to being dried, some beans are also eaten green and prepared as vegetables. In some cases, sprouts, pods, leaves, and flowers are consumed as well as the seeds. Besides serving as a cooked side dish or main ingredient in soups or salads, some beans are parched and ground into a flour for baking, roasted as a beverage, processed into a cooking oil, or fermented and made into a variety of condiments, pastes, and seasonings.

Quality

Since beans are often rotated with other crops, it is important to determine the quality of the soil in which they are grown. True organically grown beans are grown in soil that has not been subjected to chemical fertilizers or pesticides for at least a minimum of several years. This consideration arises because most commercially grown beans are not directly sprayed but alternated with crops that have been sprayed and thus cultivated in chemically-depleted soil. Nonorganically grown beans are thus slightly better quality than nonorganically grown grains or vegetables but still inferior to organically grown beans.

After harvest, beans are cleaned and bagged. About 10 to 15 percent are lost in the process to damaging or cracking. At the natural foods store or market, beans should be well-formed, uniform in size, smooth skinned, and generally full and shiny in color. Spots, streaks, flecks, wrinkles and pits show that the beans have lost their vitality. Beans that are open at the seams are called fish-eyes. These show oxidation from drying too quickly. Good quality beans should have only 1 to 2 percent broken skins and surface chips. However, batches of organic beans will sometimes include proportionately more odd, misshapen, and discolored beans than nonorganic batches. This is because most commercially sold beans are run through an expensive electronic sorting process that removes irregular appearing beans for cosmetic purposes. Another consideration is proper dryness. Good quality beans will crackle and shatter when bitten into with the teeth. Dried beans that produce only a dent when bit have not dried adequately.

At home, beans keep extremely well because they are less susceptible to insects and rodents than other dry goods. They should be stored in closed, airtight containers and be kept in a cool, dark place. Preserved in this way, beans will retain their energy and nutrients for many years. Different types of beans should be stored in separate containers from one another, and different batches of the same bean should not be mixed or cooked together because they will have dried for slightly different periods and may cook up unevenly if mixed together.

Varieties

Azuki Beans

Azuki beans are small and compact in size, oblong in shape, and red or brown in color. They contain less fat and oil than other beans, and in the Far East where

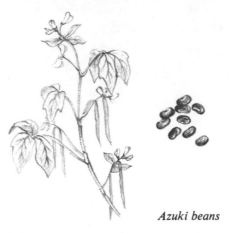

Azuki beans

they originated are considered an honorary grain. They are enjoyed as a small side dish, in soup, cooked in small volume with grains, and sweetened or slightly salted as a dessert. Now grown in North America, encouraged by macrobiotic education, azuki beans have become a staple of the macrobiotic and natural foods movements.

Black-Eyed Peas

Black-eyed peas are medium in size, oblong in shape, and have a distinctive black spot on their light surface. Since their pods often grow up to three feet or more in length, they are sometimes known as yard-long beans. Native to Africa, black-eyed peas were brought to Europe, South America, and North America, where they became part of the traditional Black diet.

Black Turtle Beans

Black turtle beans, often called Mexican beans, are small to medium in size, round in shape, and black in color. A member of the kidney bean family, they are traditionally cultivated in the Americas and can be boiled or baked.

Broad Beans

Broad beans are wide, flat, and usually white in color. Prior to the discovery of America, they were the major legume cultivated in Europe, where they are also known as fava, Windsor, and straight beans. The young and tender broad beans may be cooked in their pods. Older ones are shelled first. In South America, where they are now also popular, dried broad beans are boiled, refried, and eaten with various corn dishes, as well as roasted and ground into a flour for baking.

Chick-Peas

Chick-peas are small, hard, and compact. Their unique nutlike seeds have a small point at each end. In North America, the peas are usually light yellow or brown in color, but in the Middle East and Mediterranean areas where they have been cultivated for thousands of years the seeds can also be white, red, and black. Chick-peas can be prepared in many ways, as a small side dish, cooked in small volume with grains, and in salads and soups. Ground into a paste and mixed with lemon, oil, and tahini, chick-peas are made into a delicious spread called *hummus*. In Spanish, chick-peas are known as *garbanzo*s.

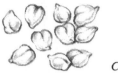

Chick-peas

Great Northern Beans

Large in size, flat and circular in shape, and white in color, great northern beans are members of the kidney family of beans. They may be prepared in the usual ways.

Kidney Beans

Kidney beans have been cultivated in Central America, South America, and Mexico for thousands of years. The most familiar modern variety is kidney-shaped, medium in size, and red in color. However, kidney beans come in a multitude of shades, shapes, and sizes, and their family includes great northern beans, Mexican black beans, and navy beans. String beans, French beans, snap beans, and other bush or climbing varieties that are prepared fresh as a garden vegetable are also members of the kidney clan.

Lima Beans

Lima beans are native to Peru and go back to pre-Inca times. The seeds are large, flat, and kidney-shaped and vary in color from white to red, brown, and mottled. This variety is also known as butter beans or pole beans and is now grown in the Philippines, Africa, and other parts of the world. There is another, small variety called sieva beans that is also popular in tropical climates. Many modern people prefer the tender, young green beans ("baby limas") that are harvested early, frozen, and shipped to supermarkets. However, their energy and nutrients are less than the mature, dried variety.

Lentils

Lentils are mentioned frequently in the Bible as a principal food and entered the cooking of Southern Europe in ancient times. Lentils were also staples in India and parts of South and Southeast Asia, where they are prepared into *dhal* and eaten on top of rice or with flat, whole wheat bread. At the turn of the twentieth century, lentils came to the western hemisphere and are now grown worldwide. There are two main varieties. The Middle Eastern is green to brown in color and the Indian is orange to red. Both types are soft and cook up very quickly. However, the orange variety tends to lose its shape and dissolve into the broth or other ingredients with which it is cooked, while the green type keeps its shape.

Lentils

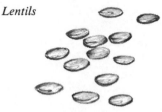

Mung Beans

Though better known as fresh sprouts in Chinese style cooking, mung beans are also traditionally dried and used in various dishes. In the Far East they are mixed with a little sweet rice and made into a porridge, and in India the dried seeds are roasted and prepared into a flour. Mung bean seeds are small, hard, and convex and range in color from yellow and gold to green and black.

Navy Beans

Navy beans, a member of the kidney family, are usually medium in size, round, and white. They may be boiled, baked, or pressure-cooked and are especially delicious in a soup with a little scallions or onion.

Peas

Peas are one of humanity's oldest cultivated foods, dating back to ancient Sumerian and Egyptian times. They were also used in Greece and Rome and by the Middle Ages had become the most common legume in Europe. The garden pea, which is eaten fresh and served as a vegetable, has yellow or green seeds, while the field pea, which is dried and prepared whole or split, is grey or spotted. The dried variety is traditionally made into a thick nourishing soup containing small amounts of sliced carrots, onions, celery, burdock, or other vegetables.

Pinto Beans

Another member of the kidney family, pinto beans are medium in size, oval in shape, and usually brown in color. They are often served as refried beans in Mexican cookery and put inside tacos or on top of tostadas.

Soybeans

Soybeans and their products have been used in the Far East and Southeast Asia since the beginning of civilization. In modern times, samples were brought to the West from Japan by scientists and travelers, including Commodore Perry. Today, most of the world's supply is grown in the United States. The two main types are the *vegetable soybean* used for regular cooking and making miso, tofu, tamari soy sauce and other products and the *field soybean* used for processing into soybean oil, flour, and meal. In appearance, soybeans are round, medium in size, and range in color from white to yellow, brown, grey, and black. Because they contain more protein and fat than other beans, soybeans are usually easier to digest in naturally processed form such as miso, tofu, or tempeh rather than in whole form. However, if properly prepared, they are very sweet cooked whole and should give no problem with gas. The main products made from soybeans include:

    1. Miso—Miso is a paste made from fermented soybeans, usually barley or brown rice, sea salt, and an enzyme starter called *koji* containing *Aspergillus oryzae*. In macrobiotic cooking, miso is used as a base for daily soups, in sauces, dressings, and spreads, and as an occasional seasoning for grain, bean, and vegetable dishes. (The types of miso are discussed in the soup chapter and its use in sauces and seasoning is discussed in those respective sections.)

    2. Natto—Natto is a fermented soybean product that resembles baked beans connected by long sticky strands. Its strong odor takes some adjusting to but once appreciated is enjoyed regularly as a small side dish or condiment. It is very beneficial to digestion and may be enjoyed regularly on the macrobiotic diet. It can be made at home or be obtained ready-made in selected natural foods stores.

    3. Okara—The pulp leftover from making tofu is known as *okara*. It is beige in color, fine grained in texture, and high in fiber. In Far Eastern cooking, it is traditionally used to flavor and give body to grain and vegetable dishes, casseroles, and soups.

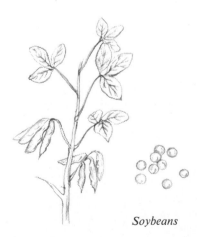

Soybeans

4. Soy Flour—Soy flour is commercially available in several forms: fat free, low fat containing about 5 to 8 percent fat, and full fat containing about 20 percent fat. It is used in small volume for adding to breads and baked goods, soups, and casseroles. Because of its highly processed quality, soy flour is used very infrequently in macrobiotic cooking. A traditionally made soy flour called *kinako* is available in some natural foods stores and may be used occasionally to coat rice balls, flavor noodles, or serve as a condiment for other dishes.

5. Soy Grits—Soy grits or granules are made from fresh soybeans that have been cut mechanically into smaller pieces. Because they cook up quickly, they are preferred by some people in place of soybeans or are used for making soybean patties and loaves. However, soy grits are lower in energy and nutrients than soybeans consumed in whole form or soybeans processed by natural methods, and as a consequence they are rarely used in macrobiotic cooking. Similarly, textured vegetable protein (TVP), a soy protein or soya concentrate processed to simulate beef, chicken, and other animal products, is avoided.

6. Soy Milk—Soy milk is traditionally used in the Far East as a beverage or base for soups, puddings, and other dishes. It is now available ready-made in some natural foods stores. The unsweetened variety made with a little pearl barley, kombu, a bit of sea salt, and sometimes barley malt is more suitable than the types sweetened with honey or other strong sweeteners.

7. Soy Oil—Soybean oil is used commercially in a wide range of modern food preparations. However, its strong taste and flavor do not blend well with many foods. For occasional home use, only the unrefined quality should be selected.

8. Tamari Soy Sauce—High quality tamari soy sauce is an essential ingredient of the macrobiotic kitchen. (It is discussed in the seasoning chapter.)

9. Tempeh—Tempeh, a whole fermented soy food developed originally in Indonesia, is chewy, delectable, and satisfying. It produces strong, dynamic energy and can be used in a wide variety of dishes. Now made in the United States, Canada, Latin America, Europe, and Japan, tempeh is especially appealing to those in transition from animal foods because its taste and texture somewhat resemble pork and chicken, though it has a unique flavor all its own. It is also enjoyed by long-time vegetarians and macrobiotic people and can be used daily or several times a week. Tempeh can be made at home or bought ready-made in many natural foods stores. (The starter containing the enzyme *Rhizopus oryzae* for making tempeh at home is available from the Farm, 156 Drakes Lane, Summertown, Tenn. 38483.)

10. Tofu—Tofu's discovery is attributed to a Taoist alchemist in ancient China. It was brought to Japan by Zen monks and quickly became popular among all types of people. About a century ago, tofu came to the West with Chinese and Japanese immigrants and has been popularized in this century by Seventh Day Adventists and by the macrobiotic and natural foods movements.

Though somewhat bland by itself, tofu combines well with other foods, absorbing their flavors and aromas. Tofu can be prepared in endless recipes and styles. It can be added to miso and other soups, cooked with grains, noodles, and vegetables, marinated in salads, pickled, or used in sauces, dressings, and spreads. At home, tofu can be made quickly and easily in a couple hours, or purchased ready to eat at the natural foods store or supermarket it can be prepared in a few minutes.

Tofu is usually prepared in square or rectangular white cakes, weighing between $\frac{1}{2}$ and $1\frac{1}{2}$ pounds. Just before using, these cakes may be cut in a variety of ways and boiled, steamed, sautéed, broiled, baked, deep-fried, or occasionally prepared raw.

In making or purchasing tofu, several considerations of quality need to be kept in mind. Traditionally, tofu is solidified from soy milk with a mineral-rich substance called *nigari* in a way that is somewhat similar to the curdling of dairy cheese with rennet. *Nigari* is the concentrated residue, rich in magnesium and other mineral compounds, remaining from sea salt that has been extracted from seawater. Another good quality natural solidifier is unrefined calcium sulfate, which is obtained in the mountains from gypsum. Today most of the tofu available in the Far East and Oriental food stores is made with vinegar, alum, refined calcium sulfate, or other low-quality ingredients. Good-quality tofu should be made with organic soybeans and real nigari or natural calcium sulfate. If these are unavailable, lemon juice is the best substitute.

Fresh tofu is usually prepared in two consistencies: soft and firm. The soft variety is used mainly for miso soup, salad dressings, and short-time cooking. Firm tofu is used more for deep-fried tofu, *nishime* style tofu, scrambled tofu, pickled tofu, fermented tofu, and other long-time preparations. Immersed in cold water and stored in the refrigerator or cool, dark place, tofu will keep about a week. In cool weather, the water should be changed every few days; in warm weather, daily. Tofu that has turned slightly filmy, sour, or moldy can still be used if the bad parts are cut off, though if spoilage is extensive it should be disregarded.

In addition to being made fresh, tofu can also be prepared frozen and dried. At home, *frozen tofu* can be made by pressing the water out of fresh cakes of tofu, slicing into about $\frac{1}{2}$-inch thick slices, and placing individual slices without touching on a plate in the freezer. After freezing for up to 24 hours, the frozen slices are transferred to a cellophane bag and kept in the freezer. When needed, they can be reconstituted by placing in hot or cold water for a few minutes, rinsing, and squeezing. *Dried tofu* has a unique texture and flavor and combines well with thinly sliced root vegetables and other dishes. Traditionally, tofu is dried outdoors for several weeks in temperatures that fluctuate between freezing at night and thawing by day. Modern dried tofu is made in a process involving ammonia gas and results in light beige cakes that are similar in appearance to dehydrated camping food. The ammonia can be washed out by soaking in hot water for several minutes, rinsing in cool water, and pressing with the hands to squeeze out excess liquid. Frozen or dried tofu can be substituted for fresh tofu in any recipe.

11. Viilia A soy yogurt has been developed from viilia, a cultured dairy product traditionally prepared in Finland. Instead of cow's milk, soy milk is added to the starter. The consistency of soy viilia is custardlike and its flavor is pleasant and lightly sweet. A little barley malt or rice syrup may be added for additional sweet-ening if desired. (The starter is available from GEM Cultures, 30301 Sherwood Rd., Ft. Bragg, CA 95437.)

12. *Yuba*—Yuba is the skin that forms on the surface of soy milk during the tofu making process. It is traditionally prepared in large flat sheets up to 15 inches square and enjoyed by itself with a little tamari soy sauce or cut and folded into rolls, dumplings, and cutlets and stuffed with cooked vegetables, miso, or sea vegetables.

13. **Other Soy Products**—Other soybean products that are traditionally made and commonly used may also be prepared frequently.

Other Beans

Other beans and bean products that are traditionally prepared and commonly used may also be incorporated into the macrobiotic diet.

Cooking Methods

To improve their digestibility and reduce their hardness, most beans require soak-ing in cold water prior to cooking. Soaking time will vary with the kind and qual-ity of beans, climate, soil conditions, season of the year, altitude, and other factors. In general, chick-peas, black soybeans, and other hard beans require from 6 to 8 hours soaking, or preferably overnight, if boiled and a minimum of 2 hours if pressure-cooked. Azuki beans, pintos, kidney beans, navies, whites, yellow soy-beans, black turtle, and other medium-sized beans need at least 2 to 4 hours if boiled and 1 hour if pressure-cooked. Lentils, split peas, and other light beans require no soaking in either case. Some beans may also be soaked in hot water just below the boiling point, and this method generally takes slightly less time than soaking in cold water. A pinch of sea salt is sometimes added to the hot water, especially toward the end of cooking, but not to the cold.

In order to allow the inside and outside of the beans to cook evenly, beans are usually seasoned toward the end of cooking. Seasonings used for beans include sea salt, miso, and tamari soy sauce and occasionally mirin, barley malt, rice malt, or vegetable oil. In the Far East, a small strip of kombu is traditionally added to the bottom of a pot of beans. The mineral-rich sea vegetable adds flavor to the beans, which are rich in protein and fat, and improves their digestibility. Beans may also be cooked with diced vegetables such as carrots, onions, or acorn or buttercup squash, with chestnuts, with root vegetables in casseroles, or with dried fruit and served as a dessert.

Garnishes generally used with beans and which are all helpful for better diges-tion include grated fresh gingerroot, grated fresh daikon, grated fresh radish, grated fresh horseradish, chopped fresh scallions, chopped fresh onions, and other traditionally used and commonly consumed garnishes.

After sorting out for pebbles and debris, washing, and soaking, the beans are ready to be cooked. The main ways to prepare beans include:

1. Shocking—Shocking is a traditional method of preparing beans in the Far East. The soaked beans are placed in a cast-iron pot containing $2\frac{1}{2}$ cups of spring water per cup of beans. The beans are allowed to cook slowly in the uncovered pot over a low flame until the water boils. After the water has lightly bubbled for a few minutes, a small drop top is set inside the beans. This may be a wooden or metal lid that fits loosely inside the pot, keeps the beans from hopping, and lowers their cooking time. During cooking, the beans will expand causing the lid to jiggle. When the water returns to a strong boil, the lid is removed and cold water is added down the side of the pot to bring down the boiling. The lid is reinserted. This process of "shocking" the beans with cold water is continued each time the water boils, until the beans are about 80 percent cooked. At this point, seasoning is added, the cover is taken off, and the beans are cooked until done, with more cold water added when necessary. At the end of cooking, the flame may be turned up to boil off excess liquid. The natural taste of the beans will be fully brought out by this method, and the result will be perfect beans, soft, smooth, delicious, and easy to digest.

2. Boiling—Beans may be boiled after soaking using about $3\frac{1}{2}$ to 4 cups of cold spring water or soaking liquid per cup of beans. After bringing to a boil, the beans are covered, the flame is lowered, and the pot is allowed to simmer until beans are 80 percent done. After seasoning at this time, beans are recovered and cooked until done.

3. Pressure-Cooking—Pressure-cooking is the fastest method of preparing beans, gives very strong energy, and may be used when time is limited. However, in macrobiotic cooking, beans prepared by themselves are not usually pressure-cooked. The reason for this is because whole grains are usually pressure-cooked for the main course of the meal, and the other dishes are ideally prepared in a variety of complementary ways such as boiling, steaming, and sautéing. When beans are cooked together with vegetables or added in small volume to rice or other grain and cooked together, they may regularly be pressure-cooked. When pressure-cooking beans, 2 cups of spring water or soaking liquid are used per cup of beans.

4. Baking—Baking in a ceramic pot or crock makes beans that are very delicious and energizing. Navy beans and pinto beans are traditionally prepared in this way. Usually the beans are initially boiled on top of the stove for 15 to 20 minutes to loosen their skins prior to being put in the baking dish or crock and baked in the oven. Total cooking time is 3 to 4 hours and seasoning is added when beans are about 80 percent done. About half way through cooking, diced carrots, onions, and other vegetables, or raisins, dried apples, or other fruit, may be added if desired.

5. Roasting—Some beans may be roasted in an oilless frying pan prior to cooking by other methods or prior to being ground into a flour for baking or use as a beverage.

6. Other Methods—Tofu, tempeh, and other bean products may be sautéed, steamed, deep-fried, and broiled as well as boiled, pressure-cooked, and baked. Other traditional methods of preparing beans and bean products may also be used.

Special Dishes

A few of the dishes that are frequently prepared with beans and bean products in contemporary macrobiotic cooking are listed below.

Azuki Beans

Azuki beans are most frequently enjoyed as a small side dish cooked with the shocking technique. They also make a delicious soup. In the Far East azuki beans are traditionally cooked with brown rice on holidays and special celebrations. The color of the beans gives the rice a beautiful red hue, giving rise to the name Red Rice for this dish. In the autumn, azuki beans cooked with cubed buttercup squash or other winter squash makes for an especially smooth, sweet dish. Azukis are also frequently prepared with lotus seeds and lotus root, quartered and cut in large chunks. This dish is said to give longevity and vitality. Azuki beans cooked with chestnuts provide warming energy, especially in the autumn and winter. *Omedeto* (meaning "congratulations"), a porridge made from azuki beans and roasted brown rice, is very sweet tasting and makes a delicious morning cereal. The sweetness of these beans makes them suitable for use in desserts, sometimes enhanced with a little barley malt or rice syrup. During cooking, azuki beans are usually seasoned with sea salt.

Chick-Peas

Chick-peas make a tasty and satisfying side dish, or they may be prepared with a wide range of vegetables. They go especially well in salads with celery, carrots, and corn. They may be cooked together in small volume with brown rice or other whole grain. They are also enjoyed in mixed vegetable casseroles, in soup, with salty seitan, and mashed and mixed with scallions, parsley, and celery and pan-fried into patties. Chick-peas are traditionally ground into a paste with lemon juice, oil, and tahini to make a thick spread known as *hummus* that can be used in salads, sandwiches, and dips. During cooking, chick-peas may be seasoned with sea salt or a touch of tamari soy sauce.

Lentils

Lentils make a soothing soup or side dish. They may be cooked with cut up carrots, onions, celery, winter squash, and other ingredients. Burdock gives lentils an especially strong taste and energy. Lentils are usually seasoned during cooking with sea salt or a little tamari soy sauce.

Soybeans

Yellow soybeans are hard and require thorough cooking. They should be soaked overnight with a strip of kombu and then pressure-cooked for a short time prior to boiling. Properly cooked, yellow soybeans are very soft and delicious and give no problems with gas. A delicious dish called Colorful Soybean Casserole is made from yellow soybeans, kombu, shiitake mushroom, lotus root, dried tofu, daikon, carrot, burdock, and celery. The yellow variety also goes very well served with hijiki sea vegetables. Black soybeans, also known as Japanese black beans, have a strong, delicious taste. They may be prepared plain or cooked with rice. To sweeten black soybeans, a little barley malt, rice syrup, or mirin is often added. Black soybeans are usually cleaned by rubbing with a damp towel to prevent their skins from falling off under water. During cooking, some of the skins from these beans may float to the surface and should be skimmed off. Foam also arises and needs to be discarded. Yellow soybeans are nice seasoned during cooking with a little tamari soy sauce or miso. Black soybeans are usually seasoned with tamari soy sauce.

Tofu

In macrobiotic cooking, fresh tofu is usually cooked rather than eaten raw. Tofu has a natural cooling energy and cooking improves its digestibility. Even the tofu used in salad dressings is usually dipped in boiling water for a few minutes prior to puréeing. Similarly, because tofu is high in protein and oil, it naturally balances with a salty taste such as miso or tamari soy sauce rather than a sweet taste, which intensifies its normal cooling energy. For this reason, macrobiotic cooking does not recommend combining tofu with natural sweeteners to make desserts, although tofu ice cream, tofu cheese cake, and similar products have become popular and are suitable for those people in transition from dairy food.

In miso or clear soup, soft tofu is usually cut into small cubes and added at the very end of cooking. They will sink to the bottom and then rise to the top. At this point, seasoning should be added and the ingredients allowed to simmer a few more minutes before serving. The tofu will become hard and rubbery if boiled too long. As a small side dish, boiled tofu may be served with a parsley-ginger sauce.

Short-time methods of cooking also include preparing tofu scrambled egg style.

Tofu

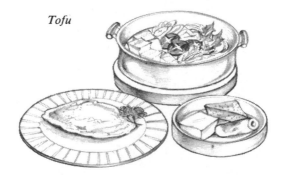

The tofu is crushed by hand, sautéed for a few minutes in a little dark sesame oil, mixed with fresh corn or chopped greens, and seasoned with tamari soy sauce. Tofu may also be added to fried noodles or fried rice in this way. Tofu is also frequently sautéed with carrots, celery, scallions, and scallion roots.

Long-time methods include cutting firm tofu into big slices and cooking over a low flame with vegetables in *nishime* or *sukiyaki* styles. Pan-frying the tofu first for a few minutes allows moisture to escape and improves its taste. A traditional stew known as *oden*, consisting of tofu, daikon, and a wide variety of other ingredients prepared in a broth, is very popular during the colder months. *Yu-dofu*, or simmering tofu, is also very strengthening. It consists of sliced tofu simmered in a kombu-shiitake-ginger sauce and served with Chinese cabbage, scallions, watercress, or other suitable leafy vegetable, a little hot tamari-ginger sauce, and chopped scallions as a garnish.

Deep-fried tofu is called *aburage* and goes well with *kinpira* style vegetables such as carrots, burdock, and lotus root and may be served with a kuzu sauce. Deep-fried tofu also combines well with hijiki, arame, and kombu cooked *nishime* style. One of the traditional forms of sushi is *inari-zushi* or fox-style sushi made from deep-fried tofu stuffed with vegetables. Tofu may also be baked in large slices with a delicious lemon-miso sauce. Tofu is also very enjoyable baked or pan-fried in sandwich form with a miso and tahini filling and a wrapping of toasted nori. A wonderful tofu cheese can be made by pickling raw tofu in miso for about 24 hours.

Frozen or dried tofu may be substituted for fresh tofu in any recipe. Their unique textures and tastes make for many further variations.

Tempeh

Tempeh is delicious, crispy, and energizing and may be enjoyed frequently sliced in small squares or rounds and prepared with grains, vegetables, or sea vegetables. Depending on the recipe, it may be cooked for as little as a few minutes or up to about an hour but should never be eaten raw. Popular styles include steaming, pan-frying, boiling, broiling, and deep-frying. It is usually seasoned with a little tamari soy sauce or miso dressing.

In miso soup tempeh goes well with daikon and wakame. In clear soup, it is enjoyed with carrots, onions, and burdock. With vegetables, it may be cut into small cubes, pan-fried in dark sesame oil, and served with a tamari-kuzu sauce.

Tempeh

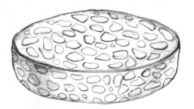

Celery, watercress, or tofu are very tasty prepared with tempeh in this way. On top of layered vegetables such as cabbage, carrots, daikon, onions, celery, kale, or collards, tempeh may be boiled *nishime* style in a large pot. Tempeh is also enjoyed fried with rice or noodles; rolled in cabbage leaves, tied with strips of *kampyo*, or dried gourd, and boiled; added to barley stew; sautéed *kinpira* style with burdock; and prepared with arame or hijiki. For summer picnics, boiled or broiled tempeh makes wonderful vegetable shish kebab along with skewered carrots, burdock, red radishes, broccoli, and cauliflower.

Natto

Natto, a fermented preparation made from cooked whole soybeans and koji, is usually served as a small side dish without further cooking. It is customarily eaten with a little tamari soy sauce, grated ginger, grated daikon, horseradish, mustard, sliced scallions, jinenjo mountain potato, or raw egg yolk. It is also nice mixed with brown rice, served on top of soba, or spread on mochi. Natto may also be cooked by lightly sautéing or deep-frying and be added to other dishes.

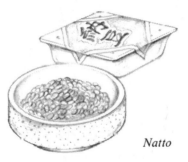

Natto

Nutritional Value

Beans and bean products are proportionately higher in protein and fat than whole grains and lower in complex carbohydrates. With grains, they make a complete protein and provide all of the amino acids needed by the body.

Legumes are also very high in calcium, phosphorous, iron, thiamine, niacin, and vitamin E. Although they contain only modest amounts of vitamin A, beans contain phosphatides that increase the absorption of carotene, the precursor to vitamin A found in carrots and other yellow and orange vegetables. Fermented soy foods, especially tempeh and miso, also contain vitamin B_{12}, an important nutrient otherwise found primarily in animal foods, and eating these foods regularly ensures an adequate supply.

Health Benefits

Beans have formed a central part in the cuisine of all traditional cultures, and their nutritional superiority to animal foods is beginning to be recognized by modern scientists. Beans and bean products contain about twice as much protein as a comparable amount of meat or dairy food, their fat is unsaturated in quality, and they are entirely free of cholesterol. Beans and bean products are also very high in calcium. Tofu, for example, contains more calcium by weight than dairy milk.

Among beans, soybeans are the highest in protein and have been studied more by researchers than other beans. Beginning in the 1940s, medical researchers first reported that animals fed a diet high in soy protein remained free of arteriosclerotic lesions, while those on a diet high in protein from dairy sources contracted hardening of the arteries. Recent studies on humans directly have shown similar benefits. In 1980 European doctors reported that a diet high in soy protein significantly reduced the risk of heart disease with patients with dangerously elevated cholesterol levels. In 1982 Canadian researchers found that both cholesterol and triglyceride values dropped substantially in human volunteers when they drank soy milk but not when they drank dairy milk. Tempeh has been found to contain a microorganism, *Bacillus subtilis*, that has strong natural antibiotic effects. Finally, cancer studies have identified a substance in soybeans and some other legumes, seeds, and nuts called a protease inhibitor which protects against the development of tumors.

Beans and foods derived from beans provide a slow, steady source of energy midway between the quick, rapid energy created by most vegetables and the calm, peaceful strength produced by whole grains. Fermented bean products, such as natto, miso, tamari soy sauce, and tempeh, are especially beneficial to digestion and strengthen the quality of the blood, the lymph, and other body fluids. As part of a balanced whole foods diet, beans and bean products contribute to smooth functioning of the digestive, circulatory, and nervous systems, leading to physical, mental, and psychological health and vitality.

Sea Vegetables

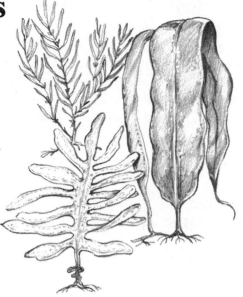

Daily Use

Sea vegetables, or edible seaweeds and mosses, are served in small quantities
and comprise about 5 percent or less of daily intake in the Standard Macrobiotic
Diet. They are prepared in a variety of ways including small side dishes, in soups
and stocks, in salads, or cooked with grains, beans, or vegetables. They are also
used in condiments, pickles, and garnishes.

History

Sea vegetables have played an important part in the cuisine of all traditional societies. For thousands of years, green, brown, red, and blue-green algae have been
harvested from oceans, lakes, and rivers for daily consumption. In the Far East,
kombu, wakame, hijiki, arame, nori, and several dozen other marine and fresh
water species have been gathered and are still popular today. In the British Isles,
especially among the Celtic and Gaelic population but also among the English,
tangle, Irish moss, sea-whistle, dulse, driftweed, purple laver, sea cabbage, and
many other varieties formed part of the regular diet until very recently. In Scandinavia, Russia and Siberia, the Mediterranean region, the Iberian Peninsula, the
African coastline, Southeast Asia, Australia, the Pacific Islands, and along the
Pacific and Atlantic coastlines of North and South America, sea vegetables have
also been regularly consumed by coastal, island, and seafaring peoples and transported inland in exchange for grains, vegetables, and other land crops. Rich in
fiber, minerals, and vitamins, sea vegetables have long been valued for their health-
giving qualities and when properly cooked are delicious and satisfying.

In addition to food, sea vegetables have been used since ancient times as fertilizer, insulation material, as a source for salt, and for ash used in the manufacture of glass. In modern times, ingredients derived from sea vegetables have been used for industrial purposes, as fillers, stabilizers, and emulsifiers for processed foods, and in cosmetics and medications. Although their use as a whole food has practically disappeared in modern times, the macrobiotic food movement has reawakened interest in these versatile plants. In North America, for example, they are now being harvested again off the coasts of Maine, California, and Nova Scotia.

Quality

Sea vegetables are generally among the least processed natural foods and the most safe. Unlike mushrooms and other wild plants, there are no toxic varieties of sea vegetables. Some species are noxious smelling, tough, and taste bad, but they are not harmful. For foragers today, the primary concern is chemical pollution, which can affect the quality of life growing below water as well as above. A clean shore away from industrial areas and possible toxic material that has seeped into the water is best.

Traditionally, after harvesting, sea vegetables are immediately washed in fresh water to desalinize them, dried outdoors quickly in the shade, and stored in dark, dry places. Treated in this way, they will keep indefinitely. However, if they are left untreated after harvesting, salt on their surface will absorb water and lead to discoloration. Similarly, direct sunlight can alter their pigmentation and cause sea vegetables to fade and deteriorate faster than plants that grow on land. To improve their digestibility and prevent deterioration, some sea vegetables are soaked in an ash solution prior to drying in a way that the Indians traditionally soaked whole corn in ashes prior to using. In the modern period, an alkaline chemical solution has sometimes been substituted for ashes in processing wakame, and chlorine compounds and other artificial bleaching agents are occasionally used to whiten agar-agar and other sea vegetables that are used in making gelatins. These type of products, of course, should be avoided, as should monosodium glutamate, a modern chemical seasoning designed to synthesize the taste of kombu.

While most sea vegetables are harvested wild, a few of the more popular varieties have long been cultivated in order to supplement the available supply. In Japan, for example, nori is farmed at the end of the summer by stretching bamboo poles and nets underwater at the mouths of rivers leading into the sea. Spores from nori settle on the poles, producing young fronds in several weeks. Altogether up to a dozen harvests can be obtained at these inlets during the year. Kombu is also now cultivated. As technology advanced, plastic poles and synthetic nets have replaced natural materials, and after harvesting, most sea vegetables, cultivated and uncultivated, are now subjected to a variety of mechanical drying, pressing, and shredding methods that also affect their energy, nutrients, and taste.

In addition to these considerations, the quality of sea vegetables depends on a variety of environmental factors. Water temperature, ocean currents, the cycle of the tides, intensity of the sunlight striking the water, and the relative roughness or calmness of the seas will also affect the natural properties of the plants as well as their taste, flavor, and texture when cooked. Growing season is also very important. Sea vegetables that have aged too long are tough, lose color, and have less taste. Traditionally, the time and season of harvesting were carefully observed in order to obtain the freshest and most delicious young fronds. In Tokyo Bay, for example, in the preindustrial era, nori picked just before sunrise in the spring was prized above all others for its tenderness and delectability. In present-day Japan, the highest grades of nori and other sea vegetables still command premium prices and are used only on special occasions.

Finally, as with other natural foods, sea vegetables are ideally consumed in whole form as much as possible rather than processed. Dulse, kelp, and nori are often manufactured into flakes, powders, and in some cases capsules and pills. Some of these products are naturally processed and may be used occasionally. However, they should not be the primary regular form in which sea vegetables are consumed. Moreover, like making flour from wheat berries at home, making sea vegetable condiments from whole sea vegetable by grinding in a *suribachi* or bowl and roasting gives a fresher quality and retains more of the energy and nutrients of the original than store-bought products.

Dried sea vegetables are often kept in glass containers. Though they do not need to be covered tightly, they should be kept in a cool, dark place. In the refrigerator, cooked sea vegetable kept in closed containers will keep about a week. Powdered sea vegetable condiments should be tightly sealed in a jar or bottle to maintain their freshness.

Varieties

Sea vegetables are classified by color into four families: green algae, brown algae, red algae, and blue and green algae. Pigmentation depends on the intensity of light from the sun reaching the plants and their depth under water. Generally, red algae grow at the greatest depths, blue and green at the shallowest depths, and brown algae in-between. Among the nearly one hundred varieties used for food worldwide, the following are commonly available in macrobiotic natural foods stores.

Arame

Arame is a brown algae native to the Pacific coast and grows on the coasts of Japan and South America. Its scientific name is *Eisenia bicyclis*. Arame's fronds are big and tough like oak leaves, and in the West the plant was traditionally known as sea oak. After drying and shredding, arame condenses to a mass of wiry black threads. It turns dark brown when cooked and has a sweet, delicate taste. Arame is frequently sautéed with root vegetables, tofu, or soybeans and served as a small side dish. It may also be added to soups and salads.

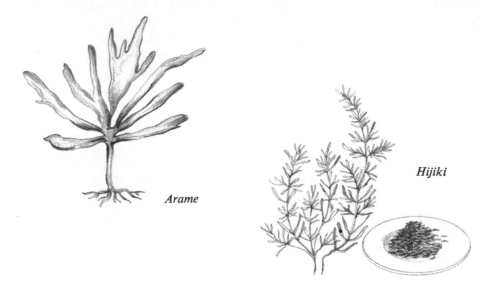

Arame

Hijiki

Hijiki

Hijiki, a member of the family of brown algae, is black in color and shaped like a pine-needle. It grows in Far East Asian seas off the coasts of China and Japan. Harvested in the spring, dried hijiki has a strong flavor of the sea when cooked and is popular for its nutty aroma. Its long stringlike strands are crisp and tender and give a beautiful black contrast to the meal. Hijiki is commonly sautéed as a small side dish. It may also be baked, boiled, steamed, or deep-fried with other foods and used in soups and salads.

Kombu

Kombu, a brown algae, belongs to the *Laminaria* family of sea vegetables which includes some kelps, oarweed, tangle, and other deep-sea varieties. The color of Japanese kombu ranges from dark brown to black and the plant has wide, thick fronds. It is gathered off the southern coast of Hokkaido, Japan's northernmost island. Harvested in middle to late summer by boatmen with long poles, kombu is initially wind- and sun-dried and then stored for two to three years in a dark place before being packaged and sold in a variety of grades and sizes. Over one hundred different kinds are available in Osaka, a trade center known for its superior kombu.

Used to make *dashi*, the broth traditionally used as a stock for soup and noodle dishes, kombu is also prepared as a side dish, cooked with grains, beans, and root vegetables, and made into condiments, pickles, snacks, candy, and teas. In natural foods stores, Japanese kombu is most commonly available in long, dried flat strips, about 3 to 18 inches in length. It is also sometimes available pre-cut into strands (*natto kombu*) and in a finely shaven, paper-thin form that has been soaked and softened in brown rice vinegar (*tororo kombu*). Kelp, which is related to kombu and may be used to replace it in cooking, is found all over the world. There are several varieties of kelp from the coasts of Maine and the northwestern Pacific that are now available in natural foods stores.

Alginic acid, a polymer derived from the cell walls of kombu and other brown algae, has a wide range of industrial applications including use as a bonding agent for mortar and cement, an electrical insulator, a mixing agent for the production of rubber, a stabilizer for ice cream and confections, and a metallic salt used in printing, textile manufacture, and pharmaceuticals.

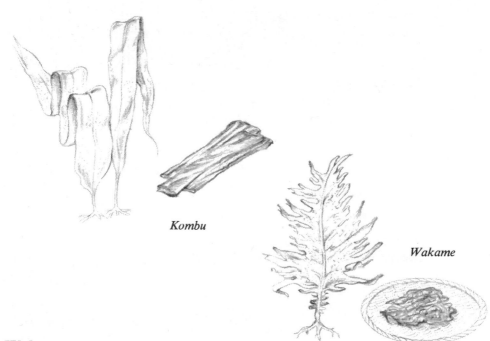

Kombu

Wakame

Wakame

Wakame is a brown algae found in temperate waters off the coasts of northern Japan, China, and Korea. Its scientific name is *Undaria pinnatifida*. Though still harvested wild, much of the wakame in the Far East is now cultivated. Originally, only the soft upper portions of the plant were consumed, but now the hard middle stipe and tougher lower parts are commonly used after softening with an ash or enzymatic solution. When cooked, wakame turns a beautiful, translucent green. It is the sea vegetable most commonly used in miso soup and cooks up more quickly than other types. It may also be enjoyed as a small side dish, added to salads, made into a condiment, and deep-fried as a snack. *Alaria*, a sea vegetable similar to wakame, is distributed worldwide and formed part of the cuisine of Ireland, Scotland, and Scandinavia. In addition to Japanese wakame, natural foods stores often stock Alaria from the North American coast, and it may be substituted in any recipe calling for wakame.

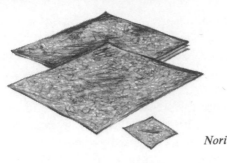

Nori

Nori

Nori, a sea vegetable with long, thin fronds, is cultivated along the temperate coasts of Japan. After gathering, the nori is washed, chopped, and dried into thin sheets which are folded in half and sold usually ten to a package. These wafer-thin sheets are used primarily to wrap sushi and rice balls. Shredded nori and powdered nori are also available for use as a condiment or garnish. A member of the *Porphyra* family of red algae, wild nori is traditionally harvested in waters around Ireland and the British Isles where it is known as *sloke* and *laver*. In European cooking, it was customarily boiled down into a gel and fried with oatmeal to make a laver bread. Other varieties grow wild along both coasts of North America, and native laver from Maine is now available in some natural foods stores as well as the imported varieties of nori from Japan.

Dulse

Dulse is found in colder waters of the Atlantic and Pacific and was a popular sea vegetable in the British Isles, Ireland, and the east coasts of the United States and Canada until the early twentieth century. Its scientific name is *Palmaria palmata*. Harvested in the summer months, dulse has a purplish-red hue and is tufted in appearance. Its flavor is mild but zesty. Dulse is most commonly dry-roasted and crushed or ground into a powder and sprinkled on salads, soups, or vegetables. It may also be baked, fried, and sautéed.

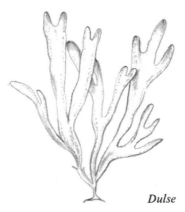

Dulse

Agar-Agar

The agar-agar stocked in macrobiotic natural foods stores is a sea vegetable product derived from *Gelidium*, a family of red algae growing in Japanese waters. After harvesting by women divers, the many species of *Gelidium* are intentionally exposed to sunlight and water in order to speed up their deodorization and discoloration. The fronds are then processed into agar-agar, which is sold in the form of light translucent bars, flakes, or powder. In the kitchen, these products may then be dissolved in hot liquid, poured over fruit, vegetables, beans, or nuts, and allowed to gel into a delicious dish called *kanten*. Various species of *Gelidium* are found on both sides of the Atlantic and along the Pacific basin from British Columbia to Baja California. Agar-agar is also used as a gelatin base for jams, marmalades, and other confections, as well as in cosmetic preparations and assorted industrial and scientific applications. There are processing plants in many nations, including Portugal and South Africa. The name agar-agar itself originally comes from Malaya.

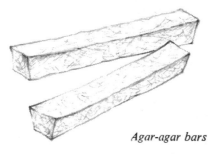

Agar-agar bars

Irish Moss

Like agar-agar, Irish moss is used primarily as a gelatin or thickening agent. A red algae, its scientific name is *Chondrus crispus*, and its flat, leaflike fronds come in many sizes, shapes, and colors. The active ingredient in this sea vegetable is called *carrageen*. The name comes from an Irish village where the sea moss was traditionally gathered and valued for use in cooking and folk medicine. Today, carrageen is processed in large amounts from several species in addition to Irish moss. Its strong viscosity is favored by the modern food processing industry as a stabilizer, emulsifier, and filler for cheese, ice cream, syrups, puddings, pies, and other products. It is also widely used in the manufacture of cosmetics, textiles, and glue.

Mekabu and *Nekombu*

Mekabu is the flowering sprout of wakame. It has a strong, sweet, and creamy taste and is traditionally brewed into a tea or cooked in small amounts with other foods. Nekombu is the root of kombu. Tougher than mekabu, it is used principally for tea.

Corsican Seaweed

Corsican seaweed has a foxtaillike shape and is harvested in warmer seas off the Atlantic and Pacific Oceans. It is traditionally brewed into a medicinal tea used to prevent or relieve intestinal parasites. In Japan it is known as *makuri*.

Other Varieties

Other sea vegetables that are traditionally harvested and commonly used may also be incorporated into the Standard Macrobiotic Diet.

Cooking Methods

When properly prepared, sea vegetables are delicious and appetizing. However, many Westerners initially find their taste, smell, and texture unfamiliar and hesitate to cook them. For those new to these foods, the milder tasting sea vegetables are recommended to begin with. Arame is sweet to the taste, soft and tender, and has almost no fishy aroma. It is usually the sea vegetable enjoyed most in the beginning. Dulse and nori, which toast up quickly and can be added as a garnish to soups, salads, and grain and vegetable dishes, are also readily enjoyed.

Gradually, the stronger and more flavorful varieties can be introduced. Wakame, kombu, and hijiki, for example, can be added in small volume to miso soups or be cooked with root vegetables or whole soybeans. In the Far East, a small piece of kombu, about 3 to 6 inches long, is customarily added to the bottom of a pot of brown rice or beans to enhance their taste, improve their digestibility, and shorten their cooking time. Another good way to make the acquaintance of this sea vegetable is to use it in the preparation of kombu stock or noodle broth. In these preparations, the kombu is often just used to flavor the liquid and removed before serving.

To prevent a gritty taste, sea vegetables should be thoroughly rinsed and, in some cases, soaked prior to cooking. (Dried nori, which comes in thin sheets, is an exception and needs no cleaning.) The method of cooking usually depends on the plant's size and thickness. Arame, wakame, and other thinner varieties need only moderate cooking, while kombu, hijiki, and thicker types require longer preparation. Nori and dulse toast up quickly and need no further cooking.

Long-time cooking also affects the taste, aroma, and texture of the thicker varieties. Their ocean flavor often disappears and over the flame they become very tender. In cooking, oil is usually not used in preparing sea vegetables that are naturally oily such as kombu and wakame. Hijiki and arame, however, go very well with oil and are frequently sautéed. Despite their origin in the sea, sea vegetables are not salty to the taste and do not have a high sodium content. Nevertheless, they are usually seasoned with tamari soy sauce in small volume at the beginning of cooking in order to bring out their naturally sweet taste. Sea salt usually makes for too sharp a taste and too salty a flavor. For tough varieties, a little brown rice vinegar or mirin may occasionally be used to help in softening.

Sea vegetables combine especially well with root vegetables such as carrots, onions, burdock, lotus root, and daikon. Sautéed together with other foods, wakame is usually prepared on the side, while other types are placed on the bottom of the frying pan and layered with the other ingredients.

In planning menus, the unique colors of cooked sea vegetables should be kept in mind to add to the aesthetic enjoyment of the meal.

Special Dishes

Arame

Arame is principally served as a small side dish. Prior to cooking, it is cleaned by removing loose dust and rinsed quickly under cold water three times. The third rinsing water is customarily saved for use in cooking. Arame comes shredded and usually requires no further cutting. When cooked, arame doubles in volume. It is sautéed *kinpira* style with sliced onions in a little dark sesame oil and seasoned with tamari soy sauce. For variety, it may be prepared with carrots cut into matchsticks, burdock, lotus root, dried tofu, dried daikon, or cubed tempeh. Roasted sesame seeds, chopped very fine, make a nice garnish. Arame is also very delightful in salads.

Hijiki

Hijiki is cleaned similarly to arame and needs no further cutting. When cooked it expands to about five times its original volume. Hijiki is enjoyed frequently as a small side dish sautéed *kinpira* style with onions and seasoned with tamari soy sauce. It may also be cooked with a variety of other ingredients including finely cut root vegetables, deep-fried or dried tofu, or tempeh. Hijiki rolls, made by rolling up cooked *hijiki*, sliced vegetables, and tofu in a whole wheat pie crust and baking, is very delicious and a popular hors d'oeuvre at parties or a good way to enjoy sea vegetables while traveling. Hijiki may also be steamed, boiled, and deep-fried. Freshly cooked or leftover hijiki is nice in salad, along with carrots, celery, onions, and parsley, with a umeboshi-tofu dressing.

Kombu

Kombu is cleaned by soaking in cold water for a few minutes or rinsing thoroughly. The tiny white flecks on its surface are mineral salts and complex sugars and should not be rubbed off. They come out when the plant loses moisture and enhance its taste and energy. Kombu should soak only long enough to soften or it becomes slippery and hard to slice. After soaking it will double or triple in volume.

Kombu may be prepared in a wide variety of ways. A small piece is traditionally used to flavor *dashi*, the stock used in making clear soup and broths for noodles. Depending on the kombu's strength and flavor, the sea vegetable is removed from the stock after simmering for several minutes and saved for use in other dishes. A small square or piece of kombu is also traditionally added to the bottom of a pot of rice or beans to improve its flavor, digestibility, and cooking time.

Kombu may be sliced into small or large pieces, square or rectangular in shape, and occasionally in long strips for tying around other ingredients. In ordinary boiling, kombu requires 30 to 40 minutes to cook because of its thickness and will become even more tender if cooked longer. It is usually seasoned during cooking with tamari soy sauce. One of the simplest ways to prepare kombu is to slice a long strip into small pieces and boil it with sliced onions and carrots; burdock and carrots; or shiitake mushrooms and dried daikon. A very strong condiment called *shio-kombu*, or salty kombu, is made by pressure-cooking it with tamari soy sauce in a small volume of water for about 10 minutes. If not made by pressure-cooking, it takes about 45 minutes to boil, depending on the texture of the kombu. Kombu may also be baked and is frequently prepared in a casserole with carrots, onions, and cabbage. Another tasty combination is kombu rolls, prepared by rolling up lengths of kombu around sliced carrots, tying them with gourd strips or other strips of kombu, boiling for up to an hour, and slicing into round sections. Kombu may also be baked in an oven until charred and ground in a *suribachi* to make roasted kombu powder for use as a condiment in soups, salads, and other dishes.

Kombu is also traditionally deep-fried and made into chips for snacks and parties. Pressed in salt with sliced turnip, it makes quick pickles. Kombu may also be used in salads either freshly cooked or in the form of leftovers, such as the pieces saved from kombu stock or saved from cooking with grains or beans. If kombu is unavailable, kelp may be substituted in recipes calling for kombu and, depending upon its thickness, usually takes slightly less cooking time.

Wakame

Wakame is rinsed under cold water to remove surface dust and then soaked for several minutes. After soaking, it turns a lovely translucent green. In this softened state, the thin outer fronds can be cut into small squares or rectangles and the thick central vein chopped very finely. Wakame cooks up more quickly than most sea vegetables but still requires about 20 to 30 minutes to tenderize the hard vein. Its most popular use is in daily miso soup with onions, daikon, or other ingredients. Wakame may also be prepared into a small side dish by boiling with onions or scallions and serving with a sour tofu dressing or a miso-brown rice vinegar sauce. It also goes well with carrots, cauliflower, parsnips, burdock, celery, daikon, and cabbage and is enjoyed in summer salads served cool with cucumbers. It is usually seasoned during cooking with tamari soy sauce.

Nori

Nori needs no cleaning prior to using. To improve its digestibility it is ordinarily toasted by holding the shiny side a few inches above a low flame and twirling the sheet for about half a minute until it turns from purple to green. Nori may also be roasted by baking in a moderate oven for a few minutes. The sheets are used whole to prepare a bed for sushi, rolled up, and sliced into spirals. The sheets are also customarily torn into quarters and used to wrap rice balls. Cut into thin strips with a scissors, nori may be used as a garnish for salads, soups, fried noodles, fried rice, or casseroles. It may also be crushed by hand and ground into a powder. In addition to sheets, nori is also available in some macrobiotic natural foods stores prepared in strip or powder form. As a condiment, nori is toasted and served with a little fresh grated gingerroot, tamari soy sauce, and mirin. It may also be cooked down into a thick paste by boiling in spring water and a little tamari soy sauce.

Fresh nori, or laver, can be gathered along coastal regions. The best time to forage is at low tide. Since the sea vegetable is very slippery, wood ashes are recommended for dipping the hands into to facilitate picking. To remove the sand and grit, the nori should be washed afterward in fresh water many times before using. At home or for a barbecue at the beach, it may be prepared by slicing into small pieces, seasoning with tamari soy sauce, and boiling until the liquid is nearly gone, about 30 to 40 minutes. It is very tasty served with roasted and chopped sesame seeds.

Dulse

Dulse has a rather salty taste and is usually rinsed and soaked for a few minutes to reduce its salty flavor. It is usually prepared by dry-roasting for about 10 minutes in a skillet, crushed or ground into a powder, and used as a zesty garnish in soups, on salads, and in vegetable and grain dishes. It may also be added to breads, fritters, and porridges or be brewed in a tea. Whole or shredded into bite-size pieces, dulse may be enjoyed boiled, sautéed, or deep-fried. It goes well with carrots and celery.

Agar-Agar

Agar-agar comes in a variety of bars, flakes, and powders. The amounts of agar and water to be used differ with each manufacturer, so directions on the package should be followed carefully. The proportion usually varies from 1 to several bars per quart of liquid or 1 teaspoon to 2 tablespoons of flakes or powder per quart. To prepare, the recommended amount of agar is added to hot water, simmered for about 10 minutes, and poured into molds or cups over several pieces of cooked fruit, nuts, or vegetables. The containers are then refrigerated for about an hour until the agar has gelled.

A delicious fruit gelatin prepared in this way is called *kanten* and may be made with strawberries, cherries, blueberries, pieces of melon, peaches, apricots, and other fruits and nuts. When made with beans or vegetables, agar gelatin is called an aspic. Azuki beans and raisins are very popular cooked with agar in this form. Other good aspics include split peas and fresh peas, lentils and celery, and carrots and onions. By itself, agar-agar is also tasty and may be served with a sweet and sour miso sauce, grated ginger and tamari soy sauce, or chopped scallions or other greens.

Irish Moss

Like agar-agar, Irish moss is also used to make gelatins. It is customarily soaked for a short or long time, depending on its toughness, and cooked with the other ingredients with which it is to be combined for about a half an hour. After cooking, the sea vegetable is removed, excess liquid is squeezed out, and the mixture is poured into molds or dishes and chilled until served. The squeezing out process may be facilitated by wrapping the Irish moss in cheesecloth after soaking and inserting it into the pot during cooking.

Other Sea Vegetables

Other sea vegetables that are traditionally harvested or cultivated and commonly used may also be prepared regularly.

Nutritional Value

Sea vegetables are among the most nutritious foods and have long been valued for their health-giving properties. Dried sea vegetables are high in complex carbohydrates, fiber, protein, vitamins, and minerals and low in fat. Polysaccharides

Table 17   Iodine Content of Various Foods

The main source of iodine in the modern diet is from the potassium iodide added to artificially refined table salt. However, iodine is naturally available in mineral-rich sea vegetables as well as fish and seafood in general. The U.S. RDA is 150 micrograms/day. (Figures per 100 grams, unit microgram.)

	Agar-agar	160
	Arame, various	98–564
Sea Vegetables	Hijiki	40
	Kombu, various	193–471
	Wakame, various	18–35
	Shellfish	0.29
Sea Animals	Crustaceans	0.15
	Fish, various	0.07

Source: Seibin and Teruko Arasaki, *Vegetables from the Sea*, Japan Publications, Inc., 1983.

account for about 50 to 60 percent of their weight, protein up to 7 percent, and minerals and vitamins up to 30 percent. The remaining 10 to 20 percent is water, and only about 1 to 2 percent is fat.

Sea vegetables contain proportionately more minerals and vitamins than any other type of food. Nori, for instance, has from 2 to 4 times more vitamin A than carrots and 10 times more than spinach. Hijiki, wakame, and arame have from 11 to 14 times more calcium than milk. Kombu, wakame, arame, hijiki, and nori have from 3 to 8 times more iron than beef.

In the Far East, sea vegetables are the main source of iodine in the diet, so that refined, chemically iodized salt is not necessary (see Table 17). Sea vegetables are also proportionately higher in vitamin A, thiamine, riboflavin, vitamin B_6, vitamin B_{12}, and niacin than most land vegetables and fruits. Nori is also high in vitamin C and protein.

Health Benefits

In order to maintain health and vitality it is necessary to balance foods that grow above the ground with those that develop beneath the sea. Human blood has a slightly salty composition similar to the deep ocean, from which primordial life originated. The complex carbohydrates and fiber in sea plants are softer than in land plants and more digestible. This is because sea plants sway with the rhythms of the tides and currents, while land species tend to grow more rigidly. Traditional civilizations have long recognized the importance of sea vegetables in the diet in contributing to the flexibility of body and mind. This understanding may have developed in ancient times by observing wild bears, deer, foxes, and other animals living on coastal regions who naturally nibble seaweed and mosses on the rocks and seashore at low tide.

In traditional medicine, sea vegetables have been especially identified with strengthening the blood, the heart, and the circulatory system. They are also excellent for the kidneys, the urinary system, and the reproductive organs. They give elasticity to arteries, veins, and organ tissues, contributing to flexibility and the smooth functioning of the body's many interrelated systems.

Each type of sea vegetable, moreover, is believed to have restorative properties as well as preventive ones. Arame, for example, is traditionally used to help relieve female disorders. Hijiki is taken to strengthen the intestines, produce beautiful, shining hair, and purify the blood. Kombu is taken to reduce high blood pressure and relieve edema. Wakame has long been used for cleaning the blood after childbirth. Nori is associated with relieving beriberi and wens. For centuries, Irish moss has been used in Europe to alleviate respiratory ailments.

Recent scientific studies have upheld many of these folk customs and confirmed that sea vegetables have strong antibacterial, antifungal, antiviral, and antitumoral effects. In laboratory experiments in Japan, common sea vegetables such as kombu, wakame, nori, and hijiki have been shown to reduce cholesterol levels in the blood, inhibiting the development of high blood pressure, protecting against the development of arteriosclerosis, and improving fat metabolism. Several varieties of sea vegetable also have been discovered to have blood anticoagulants similar to heparin, the body's natural blood thinner which is often given intravenously to heart patients to prevent clotting.

Modern researchers have also discovered that the highest incidence of longevity in Japan is found on Oki Island, an area noted for its large consumption of sea vegetables on which its local economy depends. Residents of this region also have strikingly low rates of stroke compared to other Japanese. Okinawans also have high longevity rates, and one of the main dietary variables between them and other Japanese is their higher consumption of sea vegetables.

Sea vegetables have also been reported to be effective in eliminating tumors. In 1974 scientists stated in the *Japanese Journal of Experimental Medicine* that several varieties of kombu, a common sea vegetable eaten in Asia and used as a decoction for cancer in traditional Chinese medicine, were effective in the treatment of tumors in laboratory experiments. In three of four samples tested, inhibition rates in mice with implanted sarcomas ranged from 89 to 95 percent. The researchers reported that "the tumor underwent complete regression in more than half of the mice of each treated group." Similar experiments on mice with leukemia, cancer of the blood, showed promising results when treated with sea vegetables. In 1984, medical researchers at Harvard University reported that a diet containing 5 percent kombu significantly delayed the inducement of breast cancer in experimental animals. Extrapolating these results to human subjects, the investigators concluded, "Seaweed may be an important factor in explaining the low rates of certain cancers in Japan." Japanese women, whose diet normally includes about 5 percent sea vegetables, have from three to nine times less breast cancer incidence than American women, for whom sea vegetables are not part of their usual way of eating.

Plants from the sea may also be protective against nuclear radioactivity. In addition to the testimony of medical doctors in Nagasaki who helped save their patients on a traditional diet of brown rice, miso soup, and sea vegetables after the atomic bombing in 1945, scientists at McGill University in Canada reported in the 1960s and 1970s that common edible sea vegetables contained a polysaccharide substance that selectively bound radioactive strontium and helped eliminate it naturally from the body. The substance, sodium alginate, was prepared from kombu, kelp, and other brown sea vegetables found off Atlantic and Pacific coastal waters. "The evaluation of biological activity of different marine algae is important because of their practical significance in preventing absorption of radioactive products of atomic fission as well as in their use as possible natural decontaminators," the researchers concluded in an article in the *Canadian Medical Association Journal*.

Sea vegetables are an integral part of the macrobiotic diet. By including a small volume of this ancient life form in our diets each day, we maintain our health and vitality, experience more of the energy of the earth as a whole, and develop toward universal consciousness.

Fish and Seafood

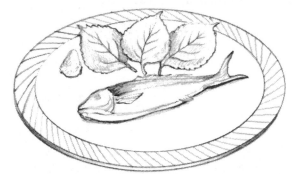

Occasional Use

For variety, enjoyment, and nourishment the Standard Macrobiotic Diet includes the occasional consumption of fish and seafood by those who are in ordinary good health. The frequency of eating fish or seafood varies according to climate, age, sex, and personal needs and can range from once in awhile to several times a week. The norm, however, is about twice a week. The kinds of fish and seafood recommended are those with less fat and cholesterol and those that are most easily digestible. As a separate side dish, fresh fish or seafood is usually prepared in a small to moderate amount as a supplement to whole grains and vegetables, which still comprise the major volume of the meal. It may also be served in soups and cooked with other foods.

In cold, northern climates, where the agricultural growing season is shorter, a slightly higher percentage of fish and seafood may be taken. Conversely, in warm, southern regions, a lesser proportion of animal food in the overall diet is generally more in harmony with the local environment. In accordance with their biological development, men and boys in most traditional societies have also consumed relatively more animal food than women and girls. Babies and infants are usually not given any fish or seafood for a few years except occasionally as necessary for special nourishment, while older persons may take correspondingly less as their level of activity diminishes.

For those engaged in high levels of physical activity and for some persons who are weak or lacking in vitality, fish and seafood may be consumed more frequently. Also, those in transition from the modern diet to one centered around whole grains and vegetables may take a larger portion of fish and seafood in place of meat and dairy products until they have more fully adjusted to the new way of eating. However, for those with some forms of illness, including many types of cancer and heart disease, no animal food of any kind is recommended during the initial period of from one month to several months until the condition stabilizes. For mental and spiritual development, little or no animal food is usually recommended.

Far inland, where freshwater or seawater fish and seafood are not available, in extreme or unusual climates or environments, or under other special circumstances, wild animals, such as birds, may be taken instead occasionally and in small volume as supplemental animal food.

History

Fish and seafood have been the primary source of supplemental animal food in most cultures and civilizations. In the Far East and Southeast Asia, tiny fish were traditionally cultivated in the rice fields. Carp and other freshwater varieties were raised in ponds, and numerous white-meat species were gathered from the oceans, as well as shrimps, crabs, eels, octopus, and other seafood. Similarly, in the ancient Near East and the Hellenistic world, fish and seafood supplemented the basic diet centered around barley, wheat, olives, lentils, and other vegetable-quality foods. In the Americas, the native peoples enjoyed trout and salmon from freshwater streams and lakes and cod, flounder, haddock, clams, oysters, and lobsters from the seas. In cold semipolar regions, herring, mackerel, sardines, and other varieties have been traditionally salted, smoked, and dried for preservation during the long winters.

Quality

In the past, fish was one of the most uncontaminated and least processed foods. However, in modern times, its quality has been greatly affected by pollution, and seafood has been subjected to many potentially harmful industrial processing techniques. Chemicals from farm and factory and improperly treated sewage have poisoned many rivers, streams, and lakes where freshwater fish breed. Pesticides, PCBs, and mercury have also contaminated coastal regions where shellfish are traditionally harvested. Sea- and airborne pesticides, oil spills, and the dumping of radioactive toxic wastes into the oceans have begun to kill off or weaken many deep-sea varieties.

In the food chain, pesticides and other toxic substances accumulate at increasingly higher levels of life. Thus humans are more affected than animals, and animals are more affected than plants. Even small doses of chemicals in the environment can have a large adverse impact. In the Great Lakes, for example, it has been discovered that fish may concentrate pesticide residues at levels several thousand times higher than those to which they are exposed in the water. Environmental pollution and chemically treated feed, in the case of rainbow trout raised in hatcheries, have been associated with recent outbreaks of liver cancer in some species that have reached epidemic levels.

Meanwhile, once caught, fish and seafood are often exposed to a further round of chemicals on the way to market or in the marketplace itself. On oceangoing fishing trawlers, "fresh fish" is often frozen for up to two weeks in ice or a dipping solution containing antibiotics or chemical preservatives. Similarly, between the docks and the supermarket, "fresh fish" may be exposed during refrigeration to sodium nitrite, hydrogen peroxide, or other chemicals to prevent spoilage.

Finding a reliable source of truly fresh and uncontaminated fish and seafood is very important for people who wish to include these foods in their diet. As a general rule, seawater varieties are less polluted than freshwater varieties. Among deep-water species, moreover, white-meat fish are less fatty and less oily than red-meat and blue-skinned varieties. Similarly, among shellfish, those that are slower-moving like clams and oysters are usually lower in fat and cholesterol and may be taken more often than faster-moving ones such as crabs, lobsters, and shrimp that are generally higher in fat and cholesterol. Furthermore, store-bought fish and seafood should be obtained fresh as much as possible rather than frozen, smoked, canned, prestuffed, prebreaded, concentrated, or otherwise commercially processed. However, fish or seafood that has been dried, pickled, or naturally processed without artificial preservatives may occasionally be used.

Quite apart from the dangers of modern chemicals and elevated fat and cholesterol, all animal food, including fish and seafood, tends to decompose quickly, producing protein wastes and other toxins that can have a harmful effect when eaten. To balance these side effects, fish and seafood are traditionally prepared with a small side dish of grated daikon or grated radish and a few drops of tamari soy sauce and a touch of grated fresh gingerroot. For stronger red-meat varieties, a little mustard, horseradish, or *wasabi* (the green Japanese horseradish), may be consumed to further aid in digestion. These strong garnishes or condiments help concentrate and naturally discharge toxins from the body. In addition, the fish's liver, gallbladder, and other excretory organs which naturally store and filter poisonous substances, may be removed prior to cooking. In fish markets, the proprietor will usually cut these out at no additional charge if requested.

When selecting fresh fish, things to look for include good color, smooth skin, clear eyes (rather than cloudy), good odor (a fishy smell shows decay), clean and intact gills, and resiliency when poked.

In the kitchen, fish and seafood should be stored, cleaned, and cut apart from vegetables, fruit, and other plant foods, even though they may later be cooked together. Using a separate knife and cutting board for this purpose prevents the heavier animal-quality vibrations from interfering with the lighter energy of vegetable-quality foods. Traditionally, a special set of cookware, plates, and utensils was used to prepare and serve animal food, and after the meal it was thoroughly washed and cleaned with wood ashes.

Finally, in planning the menu, if fish is served as a separate side dish, it should be consumed with a regular serving of whole grain and from two to three times the usual volume of hard leafy green vegetables such as kale, daikon greens, mustard greens, or collards. Apart from also helping to neutralize possible toxic side effects, these foods help to balance the strong contractive energy of fish and seafood.

By observing these common sense guidelines and procedures, the dangers of eating fish and seafood can be minimzed and their enjoyment enhanced.

Varieties

There are several thousand different kinds of fish and seafood that are commonly eaten around the world.

Among fresh white-meat varieties from the ocean, the most frequently prepared include cod, flounder, haddock, halibut, mullet, perch, red snapper, shad, smelts, and sole. In New England, fresh *scrod* is also very popular and usually of good quality. This is not a separate species but the first catch of the day of young cod. Scrod is a contraction of "sacred cod." Spelled with an *h*, as in *schrod*, it signifies young haddock.

Freshwater varieties of white-meat fish include bass, catfish, pike, trout, and whitefish.

Fish used less frequently in macrobiotic food preparation include bluefish, herring, mackerel, salmon, sardines, swordfish, tuna, and other blue-skinned or red-meat varieties.

In the Far East, small sardinelike dried fish known as *iriko* and very tiny dried fish called *chirimen-iriko* are traditionally consumed and are also frequently used in modern macrobiotic cooking.

Shellfish and seafood for occasional use include abalone, clam, crab, lobster, mussel, octopus, oyster, prawn, scallop, shrimp, squid, and various others.

Cooking Methods

Fish and seafood may be prepared in a wide variety of cooking styles. On occasion, as in Japanese sashimi and sushi, they may be prepared raw and fresh. They may be marinated with various combinations of miso, tamari soy sauce, mirin, saké, kombu or shiitake mushroom stock, and grated fresh ginger. Plain or after marinating, fish may be steamed, boiled, baked, sautéed, pan-fried, deep-fried, cooked tempura style in a batter, dried and then boiled, dried and then steamed, and dried and then baked. Fish and seafood may also be flaked, pickled, smoked, and prepared in other traditionally used and commonly practiced cooking styles.

Dark or light sesame oil, corn oil, safflower oil, mustard seed oil, olive oil, or other unrefined vegetable oil is preferred for frying. However, because fish and seafood are generally oily and fatty to begin with, methods that do not require oil such as steaming, baking, or boiling are used more frequently.

Garnishes used to balance fish and seafood dishes include grated daikon, grated radish, chopped scallions, grated gingerroot, *wasabi* paste, grated horseradish, shredded daikon, raw fresh salad, lemon, orange, fresh shiso (beefsteak) leaves, and other traditionally used and commonly consumed garnishes.

Seasonings for fish and seafood include sea salt, tamari soy sauce, miso, brown rice vinegar, unrefined vegetable oil, mirin, umeboshi vinegar, black or red pepper, tofu sauce seasoned with some of these ingredients, kuzu sauce seasoned with some of these ingredients, oil sauce seasoned with some of these ingredients, and other traditionally used and commonly consumed seasonings.

Special Dishes

Fish and seafood can be prepared in soup, as a separate side dish, in stew, with grains, with vegetables, with sea vegetables, as a raw fresh salad, as fish cakes, or used as flavoring and seasoning in soup, vegetable dishes, and other dishes. A few ways they are commonly used in macrobiotic cooking are described below.

Baked White-Meat Fish

Baked halibut, cod, red snapper, scrod, trout, and other white-meat varieties are very tender and appetizing. The fish may be seasoned just prior to baking with plain sea salt sprinkled on both sides or with a combination of tamari soy sauce, a little mirin, and a touch of grated ginger. For an even richer flavor, a marinade may be prepared consisting of barley or Hatcho miso, white miso, mirin, and saké in which the fish is allowed to soak for several hours before baking. A marinade that takes an hour or less can be made with tamari soy sauce, mirin, kombu stock, and grated ginger. Quickest of all is a sauce made of barley miso or white miso, mirin, and kombu stock or spring water that is spread on top of the fish after it is about two-thirds cooked. Baking time will depend on the type of fish, its thickness, and whether it is cooked whole or in fillets, though it usually averages about 15 to 20 minutes in a very hot oven. Marinated fish are sometimes pierced with thin wooden skewers and suspended over the bottom of the circular stand on which a wok rests (or other object with raised sides) and placed on a baking sheet in the oven to catch drippings. Whole fish are usually incised with shallow diagonal slices along the top. After cooking, the baked fish may be served with grated daikon.

Steamed Fish

Steamed fish is very delicate and tender. Sole is particularly enjoyed, though other white-meat varieties may also be steamed. One way is to place a small strip of kombu in a ceramic cooking dish, add the fish, and season with a small amount of saké. Shallow cross cuts on both sides of the gill allow the cooking wine to be absorbed. A few shiitake mushrooms are placed next to the fish. The ceramic dish is then covered and inserted, double-boiler style, in a larger pot in which water is boiling and steamed for 15 to 20 minutes. Broccoli flowerets may be added during the final several minutes of steaming, and the fish may be garnished with lemon slices and served with a tamari-ginger sauce for dipping.

Deep-Fried Fish

In Japan, whole red snapper is traditionally steamed, baked, or deep-fried on New Year's Day and other happy occasions. It is very crispy and delicious. Carp, smelts, sole, and other white-meat varieties may also be prepared in this way. In a frying pan containing several inches of dark sesame oil, the fish is deep-fried over a low frying temperature, about 300 degrees F. To soften its bones and make it more digestible, the fish is allowed to fry about a half hour. Before cooking, it may be rolled in pastry flour, and after cooking it is served with grated daikon and a sweet and sour dipping sauce made from tamari soy sauce, brown rice vinegar, mirin, kuzu, grated ginger, and kombu stock.

Broiled Fish

Broiling brings out the fish's juiciness in contrast to baking or steaming which cooks with dry or moist heat. Prior to broiling for several minutes until browned, the fish may be seasoned with a little sea salt; marinated for a short time with tamari soy sauce, spring water, and grated ginger; or sprinkled with fresh lemon juice and a touch of tamari soy sauce.

Pickled Fish

Red-meat fish such as sardines, mackerel, and herring may be pickled by sprinkling with sea salt for a half hour or more and then marinating with brown rice vinegar for another hour before serving. For example, pickled herring is very popular in Holland.

Raw Fish

Small slices of fresh raw fish are very popular in sashimi and seafood sushi. Only fish that are caught the same day are customarily used. To prepare raw fish properly requires special cutting techniques to debone the fish and often specially sharp knives. Serious digestive problems can result if the fish is not prepared correctly. For this reason, these dishes are usually better prepared by experienced chefs in a good macrobiotic or Japanese restaurant than at home.

Fish Soup

In macrobiotic cooking, fish and seafood are occasionally prepared in soup and soup stocks. *Koi-koku*, an especially strengthening soup made from carp and burdock, is traditionally prepared for weak and sick persons, new mothers, and those requiring a source of energy and vitality. Bonito fish flakes are sometimes used in soup or added to broths for noodles.

Seafood

Mollusks, shellfish, and other seafood are occasionally prepared in macrobiotic cooking. Small shellfish such as clams and mussels are good in soups. Oysters may be prepared, *gomoku*-style, together with brown rice. They may also be baked in the shell and served with a dipping sauce. Shrimp are traditionally used in seafood tempura, Spanish paella, or shrimp cocktail. Squid is also enjoyed in tempura or boiled quickly and served with wakame and cucumber in salad. After its insides are removed, whole squid may be stuffed with sweet rice or with sushi rice. In addition to cooked seafood, fresh raw shellfish such as cherrystone clams or oysters are enjoyable prepared in moderate amounts with a garnish of horse-radish, ginger, or wasabi and seasoned with tamari soy sauce.

Nutritional and Health Benefits

Fish and seafood are high in protein, contain unsaturated rather than saturated fat, and have plenty of B vitamins. In northern regions where the growing season is short and whole grains and vegetables are less plentiful, these foods are an important supplementary source of these nutrients.

Traditional societies that consumed high volumes of fish and seafood such as the Inuit (Eskimo) remained relatively healthy and active. Medical studies have shown that such cultures showed no signs of heart disease, cancer, or other degenerative disease until modern civilization brought them into contact with sugar, white flour, and other processed foods.

In the industrialized nations, nutritionists and scientists have recommended that meat and dairy foods be substantially reduced and replaced in the diet with fish and seafood that are low in fat and cholesterol. Researchers have recently iden-tified a fatty acid found in fish, in some marine oils, and possible in sea vegetables that is protective against thrombosis, the formation or presence of a blood clot inside a blood vessel or the heart itself. The substance in the fish, EPA or eicosapentanoic acid, was shown to lower serum cholesterol up to 17 percent in healthy persons and 20 percent or more in heart patients. These anticlotting factors have been confirmed by other studies.

In traditional Oriental and Western medicine, specific fish and seafood also have therapeutic uses. For example, a carp plaster is used to treat pneumonia. However, excessive consumption of fish and seafood on a daily basis can lead to imbalance, including a variety of physical, mental, and psychological disorders. For example, on a national level, Japan's aggressive militaristic behavior in the first half of this century resulted biologically in large part from overconsumption of fish and seafood, as well as polished rice, sugar, and MSG or monosodium glutamate. In contrast, the aggressiveness of the Western nations and their stub-born, short-sighted foreign policies can be viewed biologically as arising from the daily overintake of meat, poultry, and dairy foods in combination with sugar, chemically processed foods, and other extremely expansive substances.

For those in normal good health, a small to moderate amount of good quality fish or seafood may be enjoyed, if desired, as part of a balanced macrobiotic diet.

Seeds and Nuts

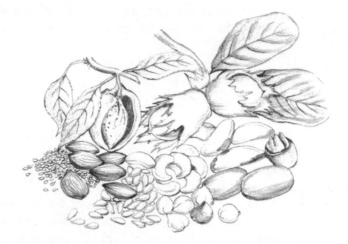

Occasional Use

The Standard Macrobiotic Diet includes lightly-roasted seeds and nuts, lightly salted with sea salt or lightly seasoned with tamari soy sauce, as occasional snacks. From time to time, seeds and nuts may also be cooked in grain and vegetable dishes, baked in breads and pastries, processed into oil, prepared in seed and nut butters, and used as condiments and garnishes. Seeds are lower in oil and fat than nuts and generally used more frequently.

History

In prehistoric times, prior to the rise of agricultural civilization, seeds and nuts constituted one of humanity's principal foods. They were easy to forage, kept well throughout the year, and could be ground into flour, pressed into oil, dissolved to form nut milk, and prepared in many other ways. In Europe, pine nuts, hazelnuts, and almonds were traditionally eaten. In the Middle East and parts of Africa, walnuts, pistachios, and sesame seeds were commonly consumed, while in Asia, chestnuts, almonds, and sesame seeds were popular. Peanuts originated in ancient Peru, and cashews and Brazil nuts played a role in the diet of the Amazon basin. In North America, native peoples found many ways to use acorns and hickory nuts, and they roasted the seeds from sunflowers, pumpkins, and squashes. The home of macadamia nuts was originally in Australia. With the development of agriculture, the use of seeds and nuts diminished and became a relatively small, supplementary part of the diet as whole cereal grain, a more evolved form of seed, became the Staff of Life.

Quality

As with other categories of foods in the macrobiotic diet, seeds and nuts that are smaller in size, contain less oil and fat, and usually originate in a temperate climate are more suitable for consumption than those that are larger, more oily and fatty, and are native to the tropics. Sesame seeds, sunflower seeds, squash and pumpkin seeds, chestnuts, almonds, peanuts, walnuts, and pecans are among those used more often. Cashews, Brazil nuts, macadamia nuts, and other larger varieties are used less frequently, unless they are growing in the environment in which they are consumed.

Spoilage is a problem with nuts and seeds because of their high fat content. After a time their oils begin to turn rancid. Unhulled seeds or whole unshelled nuts keep best, up to a year or more, if stored in a cool, dark place. Seeds whose hulls have been taken off or nuts that have been shelled will keep for several months, and they should be stored in an airtight bottle or jar and also may be refrigerated if desired. Nuts that have been chopped into pieces, slivered, or ground also spoil more quickly, as well as retain less energy and nutrients of the nuts in whole form. Seeds and nuts that have been preroasted are also apt to go bad faster than the unroasted variety. Because harvesting, processing, transportation, and warehousing can take from several weeks to even months in some cases, shelled nuts and hulled seeds have sometimes begun to turn rancid by the time they reach the store. Securing a fresh source of nuts and seeds is essential. Good quality nuts and seeds should be firm, not rubbery. If shelled, their surfaces should generally be smooth and regular with a minimum of scratches, chips, or cracks. They should not be too hard or dried out, and an off smell or color is usually an indication of rancidity.

Whenever possible, nuts and seeds that have been grown organically are to be preferred. Most of the commercially grown nuts in the United States are produced with artificial fertilizers and subjected to intensive spraying with insecticides and fungicides. Moreover, after harvest, many commercially sold nuts are treated with a further round of chemicals in order to retard spoilage and extend their shelf life. For example, walnuts to be shelled are customarily exposed to ethylene gas to loosen their shells. After shelling, they are coated with the fumigant methyl bromide to protect them from the residues of ethylene. They are then blanched in a solution of glycerine and sodium carbonate or hot dye and rinsed in citric acid to remove their inner skins, which contains a layer of nutrients. Finally, walnut pieces are usually treated with sodium carbonate and lime chloride to lighten their color for cosmetic purposes.

In the macrobiotic diet, the use of nut and seed butters is minimized because they are relatively high in oil and fat and difficult to digest. Nevertheless, there are a variety of delicious spreads such as organic, all natural peanut butter, sesame butter, and cashew butter that can be made at home or be purchased at the natural foods stores for infrequent use. The taste, texture, and overall quality of these products is vastly superior to those that are sold commercially. For example, supermarket peanut butter is usually laced with refined salt, sugar (up to 10 percent by weight), and preservatives. In addition, commercial peanut butter is hydrogenated during processing in order to keep the oils solid at room temperature. This process (also used in making margarine) saturates the fat, destroys much of the energy and nutrients, and reduces the flavor and taste.

Varieties

Sesame Seeds

Sesame seeds have been a staple in Oriental, Middle Eastern, and Mediterranean cooking for thousands of years. The tiny round seeds come in two main varieties: white (actually light brown in color) and black. They are traditionally roasted and ground with sea salt into a flavorful and highly nutritious condiment called *gomashio*. Unrefined dark sesame seed oil, pressed from these seeds, is the preferred oil in daily macrobiotic cooking and has a wonderful nutty aroma and flavorful taste.

Hulled sesame seeds are used in making *tahini*, a mild, sweet sesame paste, used in sauces, spreads, and custards, and the unhulled variety is used to make a stronger tasting sesame butter. Plain roasted sesame seeds are often used as a condiment or garnish for soups, salads, and grain and vegetable dishes. They may also be ground into a flour and used in baking or be combined with other ingredients to form dishes such as *hummus*, a thick spread made with tahini, chick-peas, and various seasonings, and *baklava*, a traditional Greek pastry.

Sunflower Seeds

Sunflower seeds are chewy and delicious. In addition to being roasted with tamari soy sauce and used as a snack, they can be sprinkled on morning cereals, grain and vegetable dishes, soups, salads, and other dishes. They may also be added to bread, cookies, and other baked flour products. Sunflower butter makes a thick, tasty spread, and unrefined sunflower oil, pressed from these seeds, may be used on occasion for cooking.

Squash and Pumpkin Seeds

Seeds from fall and winter squashes and pumpkins are flavorful and crispy when roasted and seasoned with a little sea salt or tamari soy sauce. The variety of large, flat green pumpkin seeds sold in macrobiotic natural foods stores comes from a Central American gourd specially cultivated for its seeds. They are often sold as *pepitas*.

Almonds

Almond kernels are oval in shape, smooth to the touch, and sweet to the taste. Their durable outer brown skin protects them to some extent from spoiling, and so they are commonly available in the natural foods store shelled. The skins also retain some nutrients. White almonds whose skins have been removed through blanching should be avoided. Roasted with a little tamari soy sauce, almonds make great snacks with raisins and other small seeds or dried fruits. Halved, quartered, or slivered, they may be added to grain, bean, or vegetable casseroles. Almonds are also processed into almond butter and blended into almond milk for puddings or beverages.

Cashews

These white, medium-sized, kidney-shaped nuts come from Central and South America, India, and other tropical regions. Soft and sweet to the taste, they contain almost 50 percent fat. Dry-roasting with tamari soy sauce makes them more digestible.

Chestnuts

Low in fat and high in complex carbohyrates, chestnuts are probably the most widely used nut in macrobiotic cooking. They are sweet and delicious, have a smooth, chewy texture, and combine well in cooking with grains, beans, and other ingredients. With the decline of the native American chestnut tree, most chestnuts come from European, Oriental, or hybrid varieties. Chestnuts may be purchased fresh or dried. The fresh type, encased in dark red-brown shells, is commonly roasted or baked in the shell. The dried type, which is shelled and hard and shriveled in appearance, requires soaking for several hours or overnight. It is slightly sweeter tasting than the fresh type and is used regularly in cooking with other ingredients.

Hazelnuts

Hazelnuts are light to the taste, round in appearance, and medium brown in color. Celebrated in Celtic, French, and Scandinavian mythology, they are used for both eating and baking. Hazelnuts are very similar to filberts, which grow wild throughout the United States and are also cultivated commercially.

Peanuts

A member of the legume family, peanuts are the main ingredient in peanut butter, the source of a vegetable cooking oil, and the Staff of Life for circus elephants. In addition to nut butters and snacks, they may occasionally be cooked in sauces and gravies. However, like most nuts they are very high in fat and should be used only occasionally.

Pecans

Pecans have a rich, sweet taste which lend themselves well to baking in pies, cakes, and other desserts. However, they have the highest fat content of any ordinary nut and should be used sparingly.

Pine Nuts

The seeds of the pine tree have been prized since antiquity in China and Japan where they supplemented the regular diet and were a favorite food of forest sages. Pine nuts contain the highest amount of protein of all the ordinary nuts. They may be roasted and enjoyed as snacks, cooked whole or chopped with grains and vegetables, ground into a sauce or gravy, or pressed into a milk. The two varieties usually found in the natural foods market are *piñons* from small pines in the southwestern United States and *pignolias* from Spain and Portugal.

Pistachios

Pistachios are naturally light gray or tan in color but dyed red, green, or blue by commercial processors for cosmetic purposes. Natural foods stores usually stock the undyed ones. The pistachio's small oval kernel has a hard double-skin which must be removed before eating. In addition to snacks, these sweet nuts are occasionally used in desserts. Most of the supply available comes from California and the Middle East.

Walnuts

Walnuts are believed to have originated in the Middle East, though they are commonly marketed as English walnuts and are now grown around the world. Rich and oily, walnuts may be cooked in small volume with brown rice and other grains, added to waffles and pancakes, and baked in cakes and pies. One of the most processed of the commercial nuts, walnuts should be obtained whole, in their shells, and organically grown whenever possible. The regular variety is less bitter and easier to shell than the black walnut.

Other Seeds and Nuts

Apricot seeds, plum seeds, poppy seeds, umeboshi seeds, alfalfa seeds, acorns, beechnuts, Brazil nuts, ground nuts, macadamia nuts, and other traditionally used and commonly consumed seeds and nuts may also be used from time to time.

Cooking Methods

To bring out their full flavor and increase their digestibility, seeds and nuts may be dry-roasted on top of the stove or baked in the oven for a short period of time until they turn slightly golden or brown in color and a nutty aroma is released. They should be stirred gently to prevent burning.

As snacks, seeds may be dried and served alone, roasted plain, roasted with sea salt, roasted with tamari soy sauce, baked with flour products such as cookies, crackers, breads, cakes, and other baked flour products, used as an ingredient in natural candies, and prepared in other traditionally used and commonly consumed ways.

As condiments, seeds may be dried and ground, roasted and ground, roasted and ground with sea salt, roasted and ground with umeboshi powder and sea salt, and roasted and ground with miso.

As garnishes, seeds may be sprinkled on grains, soups, vegetable dishes, beans, fish and seafood, fruit, and desserts.

Seasonings commonly used with seeds include sea salt, tamari soy sauce, miso, barley malt, rice syrup, and other traditionally used and commonly consumed seasonings.

Nuts may be prepared in a variety of ways. As snacks, they may be roasted plain, roasted without sea salt, roasted and seasoned with tamari soy sauce, roasted and sweetened with barley malt or rice syrup.

Nuts may also be used whole or be chopped, slivered, or sliced and cooked in small volume with whole grains, beans, vegetables, or other dishes; ground into nut butter; shaved and served as a topping, garnish, or ingredient in other dishes; cooked in breads, biscuits, muffins, cookies, cakes, pastries, pies, and other baked products; served with dried fruits as a snack; mixed with water and ground or puréed into a nut milk; and served in other traditionally used and commonly consumed ways.

Special Dishes

In macrobiotic cooking, sesame seeds are used regularly to prepare gomashio, a sesame salt made by dry-roasting white or black sesame seeds and grinding them with a small volume of roasted sea salt. Gomashio is used as a condiment and may be sprinkled at the table on top of brown rice, in soups, on salads, or used on other dishes. (It is explained more fully in the section on condiments.)

Chestnuts are the nut most frequently used in cooking with other ingredients. They go very well pressure-cooked in small volume with brown rice or with azuki beans. They are also enjoyed prepared together with azuki beans and winter squash and make a very sweet dish. Because of their natural sweetness and low fat content, chestnuts may also be used often in desserts.

The next most commonly used nut in cooking is the almond, which can be chopped and added to rice; boiled with string beans or other fresh garden vegetables; and be used as an ingredient in puddings, pastries, and baked goods.

Nutritional and Health Benefits

Seeds and nuts contain many essential nutrients. Compared to meat and dairy products, they are a much better source of protein, and their fat and oil are either neutral or unsaturated in quality. However, compared to whole grains, their composition is not as balanced. Seeds and nuts are much higher in fat, higher in protein, and much lower in complex carbohydrates. The principal exception is chestnuts, which are more like grains, containing up to fifty times less fat than other commonly consumed nuts, less protein, and from two to four times as much complex carbohydrates.

Seeds and nuts are also very high in fiber, iron, calcium, vitamins A, B, and E, and other minerals and vitamins. Sesame seeds and pumpkin seeds are especially rich in iron, containing about five times more than meat and more than any other plant foods except sea vegetables. Sesame seeds are also a major source of calcium, containing about ten times that of a comparable amount of dairy milk.

In medical studies, cancer researchers have recently identified an ingredient in seeds called a protease inhibitor which helps protect against tumor development.

As part of a balanced whole grain diet, seeds and nuts provide variety and enjoyment, as well as serve as a source of essential nutrients for the smooth regulation of normal bodily functions. Consumed in excess, they can lead to emotional dependency, "nuttiness," and eccentric thinking and behavior. Taken in small volume and very occasionally, they can contribute to intuition, inspiration, creativity, and the development of other physical, mental, and spiritual qualities.

Fruit

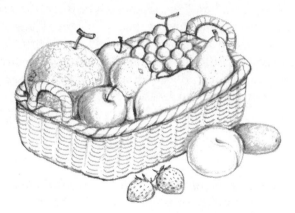

Occasional Use

Fresh fruit and dried fruit are enjoyed on occasion by those in normal good health. Frequency of consumption varies according to climate, season, age, level of activity, and personal need. The average is about two or three times a week. Ideally, fresh fruit is consumed in the season in which it is grown and is produced locally or comes from a similar environment. Cooked fruit is usually more digestible than raw fruit, and fruit juice or cider may be taken occasionally but is not recommended as a regular beverage because of its highly concentrated nature.

History

Along with nuts and seeds, fruit formed an important part of the human diet in prehistoric times. Fruit grew plentifully in the wild, kept fresh for a period of several days or longer, could be preserved in other ways for a much longer period of time, and added flavor and taste to a variety of other ingredients. With the development of agriculture, some species of fruits, seeds, and nuts began to be domesticated. However, their role in the diet diminished with the cultivation of whole cereal grains, a more evolutionary advanced plant combining the seed and the fruit together in the same kernel and providing a more complete balance of energy and nutrients.

Fruit has continued to play a supplementary role in the human diet during the last several thousand years. In some instances, species native to one area have spread around the world. For example, peaches, plums, apricots, and oranges are originally indigenous to China. Mangoes, bananas, and lemons come from India. Figs, grapes, and olives come from the Middle East. Dates, pomegranates, and watermelon come from Africa. Apples, cherries, and strawberries come from Europe. Strawberries also are native to North America, but cranberries and blueberries are unique. Papayas, pineapples, and guavas originated in South and Central America. Coconuts and breadfruit are harvested in the Pacific Isles, and kiwi fruit hails from New Zealand.

Until the middle of the nineteenth century, the only nonalcoholic fruit drink was cider made from apples, pears, or other fruits. In 1869 Thomas Welch devised a way to make grape juice that would not ferment by heating it at high temperatures to kill the microorganisms that turn the sugars in the fruit into alcohol. Apple juice was introduced about 1920, and orange juice became the most popular juice in America in the 1930s.

Quality

Fruits are an enjoyable part of a balanced whole foods diet. However, many of the fruits commonly consumed today in the modern diet are tropical or subtropical in origin and inappropriate for regular consumption in temperate latitudes. Moreover, those that are native to a four-season climate are usually grown in vast commercial orchards with chemical fertilizers, pesticides, herbicides, and growth hormones. Current law also allows spraying of antibiotics on seeds, vines, and soil prior to the appearance of the fruit. After harvesting, commercial fruit is sprayed with various dyes, gases, and insecticides and subjected to other processing and artificial preservation techniques that fundamentally alter its original energy, nutrients, texture, and taste.

In California orchards, for example, growth hormones are used to produce abnormally large grapes, strawberries, and other fruits. In some cases, hormones are also employed to delay ripening and keep crops on the bush, vine, or tree longer and grow bigger. In other cases, such as citrus fruits, crops are picked before they have fully matured in order to market them more quickly. To compensate for premature picking, citrus fruits, bananas, pears, and others are often sprayed with ethylene gas to give the appearance of freshness. Other fruits such as apples, plums, peaches, melons, and strawberries are sometimes waxed to enhance their looks. Waxing seals in chemical residues and cannot be washed off. Other fruits are given a glossy shine by dipping them in artificial color.

From plantations in California, Mexico, or Central America, fruits are shipped by air, boat, truck, or train thousands of miles to major metropolitan areas for distribution to local supermarkets and food stores. During transportation, produce is wrapped in papers or packed in boxes that are treated with a further round of fungicides, insecticides, and preservatives. For example, peaches, nectarines, and apricots are often sprayed with sulfur to prevent brown spots.

Dried fruits are also exposed to a wide variety of potentially harmful substances. Commercially dried fruits are usually exposed to sulfur dioxide and required to carry a warning label on their packages to this effect. This substance gives them a glossier, juicier look, but like other chemicals alters their nutrients and damages their taste. Some dried fruits, such as the lighter or golden varieties of raisins, are bleached to obtain their uniform color. Dates are fumigated with a toxin called methyl bromide. By law, all dried fruits imported from abroad into the United States must be fumigated chemically.

Modern freezing and canning methods are also inferior. Commercially frozen fruits are commonly cleaned in detergents and blanched by microwaving. Since their natural sweetness is destroyed, they are often mixed with sugar or other refined sweetener. Commercially canned fruits are often dipped in lye or other harmful solution prior to peeling. Canning causes them to lose about half of their nutrients, and small amounts of iron from the can are absorbed during storage.

Commercial fruit juice also goes through various processing methods that alter its quality. To prevent fermentation and extend shelf life, nearly all juices with the exception of fresh apple cider are pasteurized. Pasteurization causes chemical changes in the fruit's composition and loss of some nutrients. Commercial juices are then commonly filtered with enzymes or diatomaceous earth to produce a clear liquid. These substances can alter the aroma and taste of the juice. Synthetic ascorbic acid (vitamin C) is frequently added to the final product to break down and remove the natural pectins that collect on the bottom of the bottle and darken the final product. Sodium benzoate or other preservative is also frequently added.

Obtaining good quality fruit is essential because of the exceptionally poor quality of most commercially available supplies. Whenever possible, organically grown fruit should be obtained. Growing your own or picking your own at an organic farm or orchard is ideal. However, for many people the most practical source will be their local macrobiotic natural foods store or coop. Organic or more naturally grown fruit will generally be slightly smaller in size, duller in appearance, and contain more blemishes and evidence of nibbling by small insects than commercially grown fruit. However, it will generally have a more symmetrical shape, fresher aroma, and sweeter taste than the other kind. Because it is more perishable than nonorganic fruit, organic fruit is apt to go bad quickly and should be used as soon as possible. Aging is indicated by wateriness, puffiness, spots, and browning. A thick sweet aroma shows the start of rotting on the inside. Good fruit is delicate but firm to the touch, feels slightly heavier than it looks, and has a light, fruity bloom.

In the macrobiotic diet, fresh fruit is generally preferred over other types, and cooking makes fruit more digestible than consuming it raw. Naturally dried fruit (prepared without exposure to sulfur dioxide) is also acceptable, again preferably cooked. However, dried fruit is a concentrated product, requiring about 5 to 10 pounds of fresh fruit to produce one pound of dried fruit. Fruit juice is even more concentrated. One glass of apple juice, for example, requires about six to ten apples to make. While good quality organic, unfiltered fruit juice is available in natural foods stores, it should be used only sparingly. All commercially canned, frozen, or irradiated fruit should be strictly avoided.

Finally, fruit should be obtained and consumed as much as possible in whole form. At the store, cantaloupes or watermelons that have been halved or sliced already have lost some energy and nutrients on the shelf. Whole dried fruits are preferable to sliced dried fruits. Juice or cider that is pressed by hand or a simple mechanical method has smoother energy and retains more nutrients than that which is subjected to the high vibrations and chaotic energy of an electric blender or a juicer.

Varieties

Apples

Crab apples formed a part of humanity's early diet in Central Asia. By the Middle Ages cultivated apples were the major fruit crop in Europe. They came to America with the Pilgrims and were spread westward by Johnny Appleseed and other pioneers. There are several hundred varieties. *Cortland* are red with green streaks, have a light, tart flavor, and make excellent pies as well as fresh snacks. *Golden delicious* are bright yellow, have a sweet taste, and are also very good fresh or in baking. *Red delicous* are bright red, sweet to the taste, and primarily eaten raw. *Granny Smith* are bright green, tart in taste, and are good both fresh and baked. *McIntosh* are red and green in tone, slightly tart, and favored for pies or a fresh snack. *Newton pippin*, a yellow-green variety, are slightly tart and considered one of the best for making applesauce. *Rome beauty* are bright red with occasional yellow streaks, slightly tart, and especially popular in baking. *Jonathans* are bright red, tart, juicy, and tender and usually used for everything except baking.

Apricots

Apricots spread westward from China in ancient times and are now cultivated in warmer temperate zones around the world. Higher in vitamin A than any other fruit, they have a strong, slightly tart sweet taste that goes well as a cooked filling or topping for gelatins, puddings, cakes, croissants, and other desserts. Undyed dried apricots are sweet and chewy and make delightful snacks. Although referred to as a plum, the umeboshi is actually a type of Japanese apricot that is naturally dried, salted, and pickled for about six months to several years and used as a principal condiment, seasoning, and sauce in macrobiotic cooking.

Berries

Edible berries are enjoyed the world over for eating fresh, baking into tarts and pies, and for making jams and jellies. *Blackberries* grow wild on bramble bushes in Europe, Asia, and North America. Their deep, full flavor and taste is enjoyed fresh or valued in preserves. Members of the blackberry family include *loganberries*, a cross between a blackberry and a raspberry, *boysenberries*, and *dewberries*. *Blueberries*, native to North America, are small, round, and smooth and come in both wild and cultivated varieties. They are popular as a topping for morning cereal or pancakes, added to muffins, or baked into pies. *Huckleberries*, another American species, are mostly foraged and used in baking and preserves. *Mulberries* are dark purple, juicy, and mildly flavorful. The mulberry tree in China is traditionally valued for its leaves, which silkworms feed upon, but its fruit is also used for making a thick preserve. *Cranberries*, revered by native Americans, are rather tart but make a good sauce, ingredient for adding to muffins or bread, and juice. *Raspberries*, a sweet, delicate berry, are found on bramble bushes across temperate latitudes. They come in many colors besides red and are enjoyed fresh, baked in pastries, or in preserves. *Strawberries*, native to Europe and North America, are a member of the rose family. The small wild ones are the most delicious, and all varieties go well with shortcake, in fruit salad, in jam, or pressed into a juice and blended with apples or other fruits. Other traditionally used and commonly consumed berries may also be used.

Citrus Fruit

Citrus fruit, including *oranges*, *tangerines*, *lemons*, *limes*, and *kumquats* originated in China and Southeast Asia and spread to warmer temperate and subtropical regions. The main orange producers today are Israel, Spain, Brazil, South Africa, Florida and California. Tangerines are widely cultivated in Japan. The Mediterranean countries and the southern United States produce lemons, limes come primarily from the West Indies, and kumquats are still popular in China.

In modern society, citrus fruits are consumed today, both fresh and in juice form, primarily for their vitamin C. However, in daily macrobiotic cooking, this nutrient is primarily obtained in hard leafy green vegetables, some of which are actually twice as high in vitamin C than citrus fruits. Considering the hot, humid climate in which they grow and their exposure to chemical sprays, dyes, and waxes, citrus fruits are used very sparingly in the macrobiotic diet in most temperate regions. In very hot summer weather, an organically grown orange or tangerine is enjoyable from time to time fresh or in fruit salad. However, good quality freshly squeezed orange juice is usually too concentrated for regular use. Otherwise, citrus fruits are generally used only in tiny condiment-sized amounts as garnishes or ingredients for sauces, dressings, or dips. In addition to their pulp, citrus rinds are flavorful and are a good way to create a bittersweet or sour taste.

Cherries

Cherries are believed to have originated in Central Asia and spread to both East and West. They come in both sweet and sour varieties and are sometimes very tart. They are enjoyed fresh, prepared in preserves, and cooked in cobbler, pie, pudding, and other desserts.

Grapes

Grapes are one of humanity's oldest foods. They played a central role in the Middle Eastern diet in Bible times, and because of its abundance of wild varieties North America was originally called Vineland by the Vikings. The four most common types are the green seedless grape, the black grape, the red grape, and the white grape. Enjoyed fresh from the vine or added to fruit salad, they are also used in making grape juice and wine. In the Middle Ages, a seasoning was made from fermented sour grapes and other fruits called *verjuice* and somewhat like tamari soy sauce was used to season many dishes. *Raisins* are grapes that have dried in the sun and come in many varieties. The small seedless ones are called *sultanas* and even smaller ones *currants*. Higher in iron than any other fresh or dried fruit, they make excellent snacks and may be cooked occasionally with soft rice or other morning cereal, added to kanten, or used to sweeten other desserts.

Melons

Fresh ripe melons are cooling and delicious on a hot summer day, especially with a touch of sea salt to bring out their natural sweetness. The modern *cantaloupe* is a type of *muskmelon* that originated in Persia. It has a corrugated, usually netted skin, pale orange flesh, and small white seeds. *Casabas* are also round, with thick wrinkled skin, and golden or light green to light yellow flesh. *Crenshaws* come to a slight point at the stem and have a round base. Their skin is slightly pebbly, with green and gold tones, and their thick, juicy pulp is usually bright reddish-orange. *Honeydews* are round and have a smooth outer rind that ranges from creamy to gray. Their flesh varies from white to green and has a distinctive light, sweet aroma. *Persians* are round, with a dark green skin and ribbing. Their orange flesh is strong and thick. *Watermelons* are usually large, long, and green on the outside, though they also come in several other shapes and hues. Their bright red flesh is enjoyed as a thirst-quencher in hot summer weather. The watermelon's black seeds may also be eaten and its white inner rind pickled.

Olives

Olive trees have been cultivated by the Greeks, Italians, Spanish, and other Mediterranean peoples for thousands of years. Their fruit is eaten fresh, pickled in brine, pressed into a cooking oil, or occasionally cooked with other foods. The young green olive, ripening purple olive, and mature black olive are different stages of the same fruit. However, there are many types of olives and their flavors and oil content vary considerably. Because of their relatively high amount of fat and oil, it is preferable to consume them in moderation.

Peaches

Peaches originated in China and are revered as the fruit of immortality in the Taoist heaven. Their seeds traveled along the Silk Road to Arabia and Europe and came to the New World with Columbus. The two basic types are *clingstone* and *freestone*. The former have a firm flesh that adheres to the pit. The latter have a juicy flesh and a pit that is essentially separate. Either variety may be enjoyed plain, cut up for fruit salad, cooked for crisps and cobblers, baked for pies and pastries, used to make preserves, or pressed into a juice for sauces and dressings. Good quality dried peaches are also enjoyed in snacks and in cooking. Because peaches do not usually ripen after being picked, only mature ones should be selected. Organic quality is essential, and commercially frozen, canned, or dried varieties should be avoided.

Pears

The Greek poets extolled pears, though like peaches they actually originated in the Far East. They are now extensively produced in Europe and the United States. Pears grow in many sizes, hues, and textures. The two principal types are *European*, which are soft, sweet, and enjoyed fresh or in cooking, and the *Asian* or *Chinese*, which are hard, granular, more tart to the taste, and used primarily in preserves. Among European varieties, juicier ones such as *Bartlett* are preferred for eating raw or using in salads, while firmer ones such as *Anjou* or *Bosch* are enjoyed baked or stewed. Pear juice has a light sweet taste and fresh bouquet. In Europe wild pears have traditionally been fermented like apples to produce a pear cider called *perry*. Pears may also be dried. Organic quality pears are commonly available in macrobiotic natural foods stores.

Plums

Wild plums grow in northern latitudes around the world. The cultivated varieties are native to the Orient, though France, the United States, and Japan are among the major suppliers today. Immature plums have an unpleasant bitter taste, so they should be fully ripened when picked or bought. Plums may be eaten raw but are more flavorful cooked and make good additions to kanten, puddings, sauces, and preserves. Dried plums are known as *prunes*, which are occasionally enjoyed in stews or in the form of juice. Whole unpitted, unsulfured prunes are best.

Other Temperate Climate Fruit

Other temperate climate fruits that are traditionally cultivated and commonly consumed may also be eaten occasionally in the season during which they grow. These include fresh currants, nectarines, persimmons, pomegranates, quinces, and litchis.

Tropical Fruits

In the Standard Macrobiotic Diet, the regular use of tropical fruits is discouraged in a temperate climate. Their energy and balance of nutrients are usually too extreme for even occasional consumption. In their own environment, however, they may be consumed in small volume. Tropical fruits include bananas, breadfruit, coconuts, dates, figs, grapefruits, guavas, kiwis, mangoes, papayas, plantains, and other traditionally consumed and commonly prepared varieties.

Serving Styles

Fruit may be served in a variety of ways. These include fresh and raw; fresh, raw, and soaked in lightly salted water; grated; boiled; baked; steamed; pressed into juice for use as a beverage or flavoring; made into preserves; spread on whole grain bread or other baked flour products; as an ingredient in stuffing; as a dessert; as an ingredient and flavoring in kuzu or agar-agar gelatin; baked in bread; dried and served as a snack, dessert, or garnish; pickled; deep-fried in a batter; used as a fresh garnish; aged and fermented for use as a beverage; and other traditionally used and commonly practiced ways.

Most fruits are naturally sweet and usually require no further sweetening when cooked or baked as an ingredient in bread, pastries, or desserts. Those that require further sweetening may be combined with a small volume of good quality natural sweetener such as barley malt or rice syrup.

Special Dishes

In macrobiotic cooking, apples are generally considered the most balanced fruit because of their small size, firm texture, and mild, sweet taste. They are commonly enjoyed fresh, made into applesauce and apple butter, added to kanten to make a fruit gelatin, baked into pies and crisps, and made into apple cider.

Strawberries, blueberries, cherries, grapes, and other smaller varieties are also used frequently, either fresh or for use in kanten, as topping on shortbread or couscous cake, baked in strudels or pies, and made into spreads.

Softer, medium-sized fruits such as peaches, apricots, plums, and pears are also enjoyed fresh on occasion. They may also be served by themselves stewed or baked, cooked in cobblers and pies, sliced and added to kanten, prepared as a topping for couscous cake, and made into preserves.

Melons and other firm, large fruits are enjoyed from time to time freshly sliced or in fruit salad or punch. However, medium or large-sized fruits that are soft and delicate, have a strong aroma, or extreme taste are rarely used. These include commonly available tropical fruits and some warmer temperate varieties. Fruits that are extremely acidic and either bitter- or sour-tasting such as citrus fruits are also used sparingly. Tangerines are usually a little more balanced in energy and taste than oranges.

Among dried fruits, raisins, currants, and other small compact varieties are often preferred and are nice now and then added to cooked whole grains, breads, or puddings and desserts. In the winter and early spring, when good quality, locally grown fresh fruit is not available, dried fruit may be used instead and can be prepared cooked as well as raw. However, at these times of year, in order to harmonize with the environment, fruit is usually consumed less often and in much smaller volume than during other seasons.

Nutritional and Health Benefits

In the macrobiotic diet, fruits are regarded as supplemental foods and consumed primarily for variety and enjoyment. Compared to whole grains, beans, and vegetables from land and sea, they contain much smaller amounts of complex carbohydrates, fiber, protein, unsaturated fat, and essential vitamins and minerals. Most of their composition is water. Fructose, the primary carbohydrate in fruit is a simple sugar and enters the bloodstream more rapidly than the complex carbohydrates found in grains and vegetables. Moreover, the energy fruits give is very light and expansive and needs to be balanced by the strong centering energy of the other types of food to maintain health and vitality.

In the modern diet, fruit is consumed in large volume—often at every meal and in-between meals—as part of a physiological mechanism which helps to offset the strong contractive energy of animal products and refined salt. After eating meat, eggs, poultry, cheese, or other extremely yang food, one is naturally attracted to something expansive such as fruit, sweets, or spices. During the late Middle Ages in Europe when meat began to enter the daily diet (in contrast to the festive diet), it was customarily cooked with sliced fruit, a fermented fruit sauce, or sugar and spices in an effort to make a rough sort of natural balance. Compared to ice cream, soft drinks, and other more excessive yin food products widely consumed today, fruit is higher in quality and makes a less extreme balance for meat and cheese, and this is why it is so highly recommended by modern nutritionists. However, such an equilibrium is only temporary and sooner or later leads to the development of imbalance. Taken in excess, fruit may contribute to a wide variety of illnesses ranging from colds and flu to arthritis, rheumatism, diabetes, and heart disease.

Furthermore, as many people today make the transition away from fatty, oily, and greasy foods and away from foods that are overcooked, they often make a wide swing in the opposite direction and adopt a dietary approach that involves consuming large amounts of fruit and raw foods. In extreme cases, some people even go on an all raw fruit diet. In the beginning, such a one-sided diet may have beneficial effects in helping to rid the body of protein wastes, toxins, and the cumulative effects of past meat-eating and in increasing energy and vitality. However, in the long run, a diet centered around fruit, juice, and raw foods is very weakening and may contribute to loss of natural immunity, unfocused thinking, irritability, a tendency to talk and laugh excessively, and other symptoms of imbalance.

On the macrobiotic diet, sensitivity to the natural textures, flavors, and tastes of whole foods is gradually recovered. As the natural sweetness of whole cereal grains and vegetables is rediscovered and appreciated, the desire for fruit and sweetened foods naturally decreases or diminishes. In season, locally grown, and in small volume, good quality fruit is very delicious and cooling. Consumed properly, it can deepen our aesthetic awareness, contribute to our mental and emotional development, and further our appreciation of nature.

Snacks and Desserts

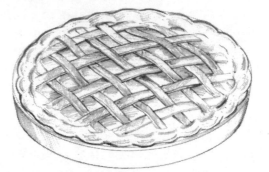

Occasional Use

For those in good health, the Standard Macrobiotic Diet includes frequent snacks and occasional desserts. Snacks are generally lighter and may be consumed in-between meals, while desserts are usually a little heavier and served at the end of a major meal. Both snacks and desserts may be grain-based, bean-based, nut-based, seed-based, sea vegetable-based, or fruit-based. If additional sweetening is needed, a high quality natural sweetener, especially one made from grain such as barley malt, rice syrup, or amazaké, may be used in small amounts. The type, frequency, and volume of snacks and desserts will vary with the climate, the season, personal condition and needs, and other factors, but on the average snacks are enjoyed in moderation daily or every other day, while desserts are commonly prepared several times a week. On holidays, birthdays, anniversaries, and other special occasions, festive meals are often prepared, including a richer selection of hors d'oeuvres, canapés, pastries, and desserts.

History

Roasted grains, beans, seeds, and nuts as well as fresh fruit have been enjoyed as snacks or a light after-dinner course in all traditional societies. In the Middle East and Europe, where whole grain bread and flour products were the staple food, special sweetbreads were enjoyed on festival days. In ancient Egypt, for example, a tasty bread was made with barley flour, grapes, and figs, and small honey cakes were fashioned in the shape of humans and animals. By the start of modern times each country had distinctive grain-based snacks that were enjoyed frequently in the mornings or afternoons: scones and crumpets in the British

Isles, croissants in Austria and Hungary, strudels and bagels among the Jewish communities of Eastern Europe and Russia.

As the traditional way of eating changed, the demand for extreme yin food-stuffs increased, including sweets, spices, and alcohol, to balance the increased consumption of meat, poultry, and other excessively yang animal products. In the aftermath of the Crusades, sugar arrived in Europe. Originaly considered a dangerous drug and used only for certain medical purposes, it was gradually introduced into festive dishes and later into daily cooking. The sixteenth century saw the development of sugar-based preserves in Italy. In the seventeenth century, chocolate arrived from Central and South America, and the process of making ices and sherbets began to spread from Spain to the rest of Europe. Since then, the use of sugar and other refined sweeteners has risen sharply. In 1800, the per capita consumption of sugar in the West was about 15 pounds. By 1875 this had risen to about 40 pounds. Today, in advanced industrial societies, sugar intake averages about 120 pounds per person.

In the East, desserts were prepared much less commonly than in the West. The daily diet of whole cereal grains and vegetables provided a naturally sweet taste. Meals customarily ended with the serving of tea and pickles or sometimes fresh seasonal fruit or a small amount of dried fruit. The few special dishes made with concentrated sweeteners were flavored primarily with a mild grain-based product such as barley or rice malt.

Snacks and desserts made from whole foods native to the local environment are also the rule in other traditional societies. In the Pacific Islands, rice pudding made with pineapple juice and shredded coconut is popular. In the Sahara, nomads carry date balls made with chopped nuts. The Indians of the southwestern America enjoy pumpkin pudding with sunflower seeds. East Africans fry small cakes made from ground sesame seeds, sea salt, and a little water. The Inuit (Eskimos) make a variety of snacks with cranberries, their principal fruit.

Quality

While snacks and desserts made with whole naturally sweet foods are best, occasionally a high quality natural sweetener is used in small amounts to satisfy the desire for a stronger sweet taste. These products include:

Barley Malt

Barley malt is made by fermenting barley and cooking down the resulting liquid. It has a rich toasted flavor, a dark opaque color, and thick consistency. It is used in pies, cakes, puddings, and other desserts. It is important to obtain the 100 percent variety rather than barley malt that has been mixed with refined corn syrup. A very delicious malt concentrate made from pearl barley and one that tastes like butterscotch is imported from Japan under the name Hato Mugi Malt.

Rice Syrup

Rice syrup is white, transparent, or amber in color and has a much milder flavor and delicate texture than barley malt. It is usually made with a small amount of barley malt. The subtle flavor and light taste of rice syrup are enjoyed on pancakes and waffles, with cooked fruit, in cookies, pies, and baked goods, and in teas and beverages. Rice syrup is also known as rice malt, rice honey, or *amé*. A more liquid form of rice syrup is known as *mizu-amé* (watery rice syrup).

Amazaké

Amazaké is made from fermented sweet rice and a grain starter called *koji*. It is creamy, thick, and delicious. White or beige in color, amazaké may be used as a sweetener for pies, cakes, puddings, and other desserts in addition to being served warm or chilled as a porridge or beverage. When combined with other ingredients and cooked, amazaké gives a thick texture and refreshing, delicious taste. It may be made at home or be purchased at selected macrobiotic natural foods stores.

Mirin

Mirin is a sweet cooking wine made from fermented sweet rice. Like saké, the traditional Japanese rice wine, it is used in cooking primarily as a seasoning but may be added, in small volume, to frostings, sauces, and other sweet toppings.

Maple Syrup

Maple syrup has a sweet, nutty flavor and taste but is much more concentrated than other natural sweeteners. It takes about forty gallons of sap from the maple tree to produce one gallon of maple syrup. Compared to sugar which contains 99 percent sucrose, maple syrup contains about 65 percent sucrose and enters the bloodstream more rapidly than either barley malt or rice syrup. Because of its sucrose content and intense absorption, maple syrup is used very sparingly in macrobiotic cooking. Just a dash in cooking or desserts is usually enough. For those in transition from sugar and other more refined sweets, maple syrup is a good substitute until a taste for the milder and more digestible barley malt and rice syrup is acquired. Maple syrup is graded Fancy, A, B, and C, with C being the most concentrated and requiring the most processing. Imitation maple syrups or those mixed with refined sweeteners should be strictly avoided.

Other Natural Sweeteners

Other traditionally used and commonly prepared natural sweeteners may also be used. In temperate climates, natural sweeteners of tropical origin such as *raw sugarcane, date sugar, chocolate, carob,* and *sorghum molasses* are generally avoided. These products are high in fructose, glucose, or sucrose and can cause elevated blood sugar levels. Most chocolate and carob products, moreover, are usually prepared with refined sugar, dairy milk, hydrogenated oil, or other poor-quality ingredients.

Refined Sweeteners

Highly refined and artificial sweeteners are strictly avoided in macrobiotic cooking. These include all forms of sugar. *White sugar,* also known as cane sugar or table sugar, is made from processing the liquid from raw sugarcane, sugar beets, or other plants containing about 10 to 15 percent sucrose into small white crystals containing about 99.9 percent sucrose.

Modern sugarcane production is one of the heaviest users of chemical fertilizers and pesticides. After harvesting, the cane is shredded and mechanically liquified under high pressure. After straining, the liquid is combined with a small volume of calcium hydroxide (lime) and boiled to remove some of its vitamins, minerals, and other organic nutrients. After most of its water has been mechanically evaporated, the solution is put in a high-speed centrifuge to separate out the sugar crystals from the remaining liquid. The crystals are then bleached with a substance made from charred animal bones. The resulting white crystals, almost pure sucrose, are packaged and sold as table sugar.

Molasses is a by-product of the sugar-making process. It is made from the heavy, dark liquid that remains when the sugar crystals are centrifuged. Molasses contains some of the nutrients refined from sugar but consists of up to 70 percent sucrose, as well as residues from the chemicals used in the refining process. *Blackstrap molasses* contains slightly less sucrose than regular molasses, as does *Barbados molasses,* which is made by boiling the sugarcane down directly into a syrup. *Brown sugar* is simply white sugar combined with a little molasses to give it a dark color and flavor. *Raw sugar, turbinado sugar,* and *blond sugar* are forms of white sugar that have not been subjected to the final bleaching process. They contain about 96 percent sucrose.

Glucose or *dextrose,* the refined sweetener most commonly added to processed foods, is made by treating cornstarch with sulfuric or hydrochloric acid. *Corn syrup* and *corn sugar* are simply glucose mixed with sucrose for extra strength. *Fructose* occurs naturally in fruits, but the kind that is sold as a condensed sweetener is made from highly refined corn syrup or sucrose that has been broken down to simple sugars. *Saccharin* is an artificial sweetener processed from coal tar. *Sorbitol* is made from industrially refined glucose. *Xylitol* is a highly processed chemical obtained from birch trees. *Aspartame,* another synthetic chemical sweetener, has recently been introduced into soft drinks and many other processed foods under the trade name Nutra-Sweet.

Honey

Honey is a natural food that combines both animal and vegetable qualities. The nectar from flowers is primarily sucrose and is refined by the bees into fructose and glucose, two simple sugars that are assimilated rapidly into the bloodstream. Honey can cause a very intense reaction like sugar, and its use is usually discouraged in macrobiotic food preparation. However, pure, unfiltered honey contains a small volume of vitamins and minerals not present in refined sugar and may be used for those in transition to grain-based natural sweeteners such as barley malt and rice syrup.

Varieties

Grain-Based Snacks and Sweets

Roasted grains, puffed grains, popcorn, rice balls, rice cakes, sushi, mochi, and noodles and pasta can all be enjoyed as snacks. Whole grain flour makes nourishing, crispy crusts for pies, strudels, and other pastries, as well as crackers, wafers, biscuits, muffins, pancakes, sweetbreads, and cookies. Sweet rice mochi is very delicious and may be made into waffles or served with a light sweet sauce or fruit topping. Amazaké may be used to sweeten puddings, pies, cakes, and other dishes as well as be enjoyed as a snack by itself. Frozen amazaké is an excellent substitute for dairy ice cream and far better for health.

Bean-Based Snacks and Sweets

Roasted beans are traditionally eaten as snacks, as are boiled or baked beans seasoned with a little barley malt or rice malt. Azuki beans are particularly sweet and are frequently prepared as a snack or dessert sweetened with a grain-based sweetener or cooked with chestnuts or with squash.

Seed- and Nut-Based Snacks and Sweets

Seeds and nuts roasted and seasoned with or without sea salt, tamari soy sauce, barley malt, or rice syrup make excellent snacks. They may also be mixed with raisins, apricots, or other dried fruit. Seeds and nuts are used in cookies, crackers, and as an ingredient in other baked flour products as well as kanten. Tahini and other seed or nut butters may also be used in small volume to give texture and add flavor to puddings and pastries. Chestnuts are very sweet and combine well in special dishes prepared with whole grains, azuki beans, and autumn squashes.

Sea Vegetable-Based Snacks and Sweets

Deep-fried sea vegetable chips, baked sea vegetables, and roasted sea vegetables are all traditionally consumed as snacks. Favorites include kombu chips, hijiki chips, and lightly roasted dried dulse which has a zesty flavor, mild salt taste, and crinkly texture. Sea vegetables may also be added as an ingredient to crackers, cookies, and other baked flour products as well as candies. A delicious, smooth light gelatin, known as kanten, can be made by cooking agar-agar or Irish moss with fresh fruit, dried fruit, seeds and nuts, or barley malt or rice syrup.

Fruit-Based Snacks and Sweets

Fresh fruits, cooked fruits, dried fruits, and fruit kanten are among the most popular and universal snacks and desserts. Fruit may also be used as an ingredient in cookies, muffins, tarts, pies, and other baked flour products. However, it is advisable that fruits, as mentioned in the chapter on fruit, be traditionally grown in the climate region in which they are prepared and be eaten in the season during which they ripen.

Cooking Methods

In preparing snacks, desserts, and festive dishes, macrobiotic cooking avoids the use of sugar, honey, molasses, and other refined or artificial sweeteners, as well as limits or avoids eggs, dairy foods, bleached or unbleached white flour, chocolate, carob, tropical spices, baking powder, and dry or fresh yeast.

To provide a sweet taste, three methods are generally used. The first and most recommended is to regularly prepare dishes with naturally sweet vegetables such as fall and winter squashes, cabbage, carrots, daikon, onions, and parsnips. The second method is to make dishes consisting of fresh or dried unsweetened temperate-climate fruit such as apples, pears, peaches, apricots, cherries, grapes, melons, and berries. The third is to use a good-quality natural sweetener such as rice syrup, barley malt, or amazaké or combine other ingredients with chestnuts, raisins, dried fruit, apple juice, apple cider, or other temperate-climate fruit juice.

For baking, dark sesame oil is used whenever its taste will not conflict with the other ingredients. Otherwise, a lighter oil such as light sesame oil, corn oil, or other unrefined vegetable oil may be used. Kuzu powder or arrowroot flour thickens and is used instead of cornstarch or egg whites in puddings, fruit toppings, and other desserts. For cakes, pies, sweetbreads, pastries, and other baked flour products, a moderately light texture that rises naturally can be obtained by using naturally fermented dough, a sourdough starter, or whole wheat pastry flour. For garnish or a slight spicy taste, a little fresh grated ginger is recommended. Grated orange, lemon peel, tangerine and their juices used in small amounts for taste and flavor provide a slightly sour or bitter taste.

In the West, the introduction of tofu has resulted in the creation of many tofu-based desserts such as tofu cheesecake, tofu ice cream, and tofu whip topping. In the Far East, however, tofu is not traditionally combined with barley malt, rice syrup, or other sweetener. It is recognized that tofu's cooling qualities are naturally balanced by a salty taste, not a sweet one. As a result, tofu is customarily cooked and served warm, rather than prepared raw and eaten cold, except in special cases for cooling and refreshment, usually in the hot summer. The macrobiotic diet does not encourage the use of tofu in sweetened desserts except for those in transition from dishes made with dairy food and sugar.

Special Dishes

There are an endless variety of snacks and desserts. Among those popular in macrobiotic households are the following:

Roasted Seeds and Nuts

Roasted sesame seeds, sunflower seeds, pumpkin seeds, almonds, peanuts, or other commonly consumed seeds and nuts are very delicious and make a satisfying snack by themselves or along with raisins, currants, or other dried fruit. Toward the end of roasting in an oilless skillet or baking in the oven, a little tamari soy sauce or sea salt may be added to make them more tasty and digestible.

Popcorn

Homemade popcorn is very enjoyable. It can be prepared without oil in a pot or saucepan, though a flame deflector should be placed under the pot after the initial kernels have popped. If oil is not used, there is no need afterward to make balance with salt. Popcorn balls can be made by sprinkling regular popcorn with a little sea salt and coating with heated barley malt or rice syrup. Chopped walnuts, pecans, or peanuts may be mixed in. Preferably organic quality popcorn is used rather than the specialty popcorn made from hybrid varieties. Sweet brown rice may also be popped like popcorn and topped with rice syrup, sea salt, or tamari soy sauce very lightly.

Rice Cakes and Crackers

Rice cakes are made from puffed brown rice and sea salt. They are available ready-made in most macrobiotic natural foods stores and often include sesame seeds, buckwheat, millet, oats, or other seeds and grains mixed in. Rice cakes make a crunchy, satisfying snack and may be enjoyed plain or topped with seed or nut butters, natural fruit preserves, or spreads made with miso, tofu or other ingredients. Puffed brown rice cereal, puffed millet, puffed oats, and other puffed grain cereals are also available and may be used now and then as snacks, plain or topped with fresh or cooked fruit. A variety of good quality rice crackers, sweet rice crackers, barley crackers, rye crackers, and whole wheat crackers is also generally available.

Spreads and Preserves

A large assortment of spreads and preserves may be made at home or obtained at the macrobiotic natural foods store. Popular varieties include tahini, hummus, miso-tahini spread, walnut-miso spread, peanut butter, sesame butter, sunflower butter, almond butter, apple butter, apple cider jelly, squash-apple butter, and preserves made from strawberries, apples, peaches, plums, apricots, cherries, blueberries, grapes, and other temperate-climate fruits. If purchasing store-bought spreads and preserves, it is important to obtain only those of good quality which do not include sugar, honey, fructose, hydrogenated oils, preservatives, food colorings, and other potentially harmful ingredients.

Chips and Pretzels

Macrobiotic natural foods stores stock a wide variety of corn chips, potato chips, pretzels, and other snack foods. Unlike most supermarket brands, they do not contain additives, and they use unrefined rather than refined oil. Nevertheless, their high oil content and heavy processing qualify them as very occasional party foods rather than regular snack items. One of the better quality foods in this category is sea vegetable chips, which can be made at home by deep-frying strips of kombu in light sesame oil. Carrots, mushrooms, jinenjo, and other vegetables can also be made into chips. Sea vegetable and vegetable chips imported from Japan are available at selected natural foods stores. Store-bought chips, pretzels, and breadsticks made with cheese, yogurt, spices, honey, yeast, and other ingredients usually not consumed in the macrobiotic diet are generally avoided.

Fresh Fruit

Fresh fruit, in season and locally grown, makes a cooling snack or light dessert. Apples, strawberries, blueberries, peaches, grapes, apricots, pears, plums, melons, and other commonly consumed temperate-climate varieties are enjoyed plain or sliced and prepared in a mixed fruit salad. A touch of sea salt sprinkled on the fruit at the table will bring out its full naturally sweet taste and juiciness. The juice of these fruits may be enjoyed from time to time in moderate volume, especially during the hot summer season or after vigorous physical exercise.

Cooked Fruit

Cooked fruit is simple to prepare and makes a delicious end to the meal. Applesauce may be made at home by simmering fresh apples and a pinch of sea salt until soft and puréeing in a *suribachi* or hand food mill. Other naturally sweet fruits and vegetables can be made into sauce in this way. One of the sweetest is onions. Apples are also enjoyed baked with a sauce made from apple juice, raisins, and kuzu for thickening. Pears may be glazed with a sauce made from apple juice, kuzu, and fresh grated ginger. Fruit compote can be made by simmering sliced apples and pears with raisins or currants, seasoning with a pinch of sea salt, and thickening with a little diluted kuzu. Dried fruit can be substituted for fresh fruit but requires soaking beforehand and longer cooking in order to soften.

Kanten

Kanten is one of the most popular desserts in macrobiotic cooking. It is an all-natural gelatin enjoyed plain or made with sliced fruit, beans, nuts, or seeds dissolved in a sea vegetable gel made from agar-agar. Apples, strawberries, raspberries, nectarines, watermelon, or any seasonal fruit, as well as cooked chestnuts, or fall or winter squash may be used. Azuki beans and raisins are an excellent combination. A few almonds, sunflower seeds, or other nuts and seeds may be added for texture and variety. The agar-agar, which comes in bars, flakes, or powder form, is dissolved with a pinch of sea salt in boiling spring water and/or apple juice, simmered for a short time, and either combined with the sliced fruit at the very end of cooking or poured over the ingredients at the end. After jelling in small molds or individual serving dishes in the refrigerator for less than an hour, it is ready to serve. Kanten may also be made with Irish moss.

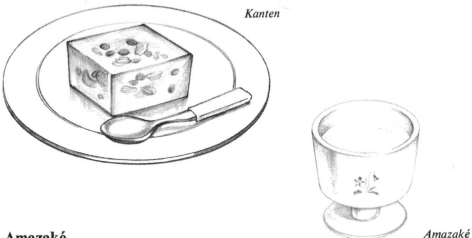

Kanten

Amazaké

Amazaké

Homemade amazaké, a thick, delicious porridge made from fermented sweet rice, may be enjoyed by itself or topped with strawberries, other fresh fruit, or fresh grated ginger. In the macrobiotic natural foods store, ready-made amazaké is usually diluted and at home may be prepared as a beverage or used in cooking as a sweetener. As a warm or chilled drink, it is also very tasty and energizing.

Puddings

Amazaké is also commonly used in making puddings. When cooked for a few minutes with kuzu, it acquires a firm consistency but requires constant stirring to avoid lumping and burning. Sliced fruit, raisins or dried fruit, nuts, and seeds, and squash or chestnut purée may be added to the pudding at the end of cooking. It may be served warm or chilled. Another nice dessert is rice pudding made from cooked brown rice, apple juice, almonds, and a small volume of tahini. After pressure-cooking with a little sea salt, the mixture is transferred to a baking dish and baked. Tahini custard is also enjoyed from time to time prepared with apples, raisins, apple juice, spring water, sea salt, tahini, and agar-agar.

Chestnut Dishes

Chestnuts are very sweet and flavorful. In addition to plain roasting, they may be prepared in other ways and combined with other ingredients. After roasting, for example, they may be puréed by pressure-cooking with several times their volume of spring water and a pinch of sea salt and then be mashed or ground in a hand food mill until smooth and creamy. Chestnut *ohagis*, a traditional Japanese snack, are made by wrapping one tablespoon of the chestnut purée around a teaspoon of cooked mochi dough. The purée may also be placed into different shaped molds and decorated with seeds, nuts, and sliced vegetables. Chestnut purée can also be used to make chestnut twists. These are made by taking a couple tablespoons of chestnut purée, placing them in a cheesecloth, drawing up the ends and twisting tightly. This creates an attractive round, twisted shape. In the Far East, twists made from puréed winter squashes are also very popular. Another customary dish is chestnuts cooked with azuki beans and raisins. Traditionally served over mochi that has been baked or pan-fried, this dessert needs no additional sweetener. The chestnuts, beans, and fruit are prepared by long-time boiling with a strip of kombu or by pressure-cooking. In any of these preparations, either fresh or dried chestnuts may be used. The dried variety is a little sweeter and requires soaking several hours or overnight to soften.

Pancakes, Muffins, and Sweetbreads

With their full nutty flavor and light texture, buckwheat pancakes are a favorite macrobiotic treat. They are enjoyed plain or topped with barley malt, rice syrup, strawberries, blueberries, peaches, or other fresh fruit, or a sauce made from cooked fruit, kuzu, and a grain-based sweetener. Buckwheat flour, as well as other flours, can also be combined with whole wheat flour to make waffles. Sourdough starter, cooked whole grains, or chopped nuts and seeds may be added in small volume to the batter for a distinctive taste. Dark or light sesame oil is usually used for cooking. French crêpes can be made with a batter consisting of pastry flour, spring water, and a little sea salt. After frying on a griddle, the crêpes can be filled with vegetables or fruit, rolled up, and served fastened with toothpicks.

Muffins are also nice from time to time. Popular kinds include corn muffins made with cornmeal and pastry flour; rice muffins made with brown rice flour, whole wheat flour, cornmeal, and cooked rice; apple muffins made with whole wheat flour, whole wheat pastry flour, and diced apples; and blueberry, cranberry, or peach muffins made similarly to apple muffins. Corn or light sesame oil is commonly added to the dry ingredients, along with a little sea salt, and either spring water or apple juice. Additional sweetening is usually not necessary.

A variety of delicious party and festive breads can be made using all natural ingredients. These include raisin bread, rice *kayu* bread (combining cooked brown rice and whole wheat flour), corn bread, corn rice bread, apple bread, and many others. Sesame oil is often added to party breads to provide moisture. Usually additional sweetening is not necessary, though a little barley malt or rice syrup may be added if desired. Doughnuts, bagels, rolls, biscuits, croissants, and other baked products can be made using whole wheat pastry flour.

Cookies

A favorite macrobiotic snack is sweet rice cookies. These large thin round cookies are made with sweet rice flour, whole wheat pastry flour, roasted sesame and sunflower seeds, apple juice, corn or sesame oil, raisins or currants, and sea salt. Other delicious cookies include oatmeal cookies, peanut butter cookies, oatmeal-raisin cookies, raisin cookies, and apple-butter cookies.

Crisps and Crunches

Crisps and crunches are two popular baked desserts made with fruit, nuts, rice syrup or barley malt, and either rolled oats in the case of crisps or granola in the case of crunches. Kuzu is used as a thickener and sea salt is added during cooking as a seasoning. Popular types of crisps and crunches include apple, pear, peach, and blueberry. They are very rich tasting, have a firm, chewy texture, and are a good way to occasionally enjoy rolled oats and granola, which in macrobiotic cooking are not usually prepared as regular morning cereals.

Pies, Tarts, and Strudels

Delicious pies are often served as part of the Standard Macrobiotic Diet and can be made with a wide assortment of fruits and vegetables. In the fall and winter, squash pie is a favorite made with buttercup squash, butternut squash, Hokkaido pumpkin, regular pumpkin, or other hard variety of squash or pumpkin. Barley malt is often used to sweeten squash pie, kuzu is used as a thickener, and chopped walnuts are added on top as a garnish. For this pie and others, a basic pie crust can be made with whole wheat pastry flour, sea salt, corn oil, and cold spring water. For a different texture and taste, rolled oats can be combined with the pastry flour to make an oat crust. Apples, peaches, blueberries, cherries, and other seasonal fruit make wonderful pies. For fruit pies, rice syrup is usually used instead of

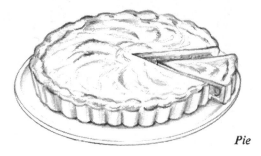

Pie

barley malt and gives a more delicate taste. Amazaké also provides a mild, sweet taste and may be used in place of either seasoning. Tarts and strudels may be made with cherries, apples, raisins, or other fresh or dried fruit.

In addition, vegetable and sea vegetable pies are often enjoyed in macrobiotic cooking. Parsnips, onions, and other naturally sweet vegetables are very tasty baked in a pie crust, while hijiki and arame are enjoyed rolled in dough, baked, and sliced into rounds like sushi. Cooked root vegetables and tofu may be added to the sea vegetable rolls.

Cakes

Several delicious cakes are enjoyed in macrobiotic cooking. One of the most popular is couscous cake. It has a mild, sweet taste and is served with a gelled topping made from strawberries, apples, cherries, or other fresh fruits cooked with spring water, apple juice, sea salt, and agar-agar. A heavier, sweeter dessert is strawberry shortcake. The shortcake may be made with cornmeal, whole wheat pastry flour, sea salt, and both barley malt and rice syrup. The topping is made by cooking the fresh strawberries together with rice syrup, arrowroot flour, spring water, sea salt, and sesame oil. Other fruits such as peaches, blueberries, and pears may be used instead of strawberries. Fluffy lemon cakes, flavorful walnut cakes, and rich fruit-nut cakes can also be made for holidays and other special occasions.

Candy

An assortment of candies made with barley, pearl barley, rice, kombu, or other grains and sea vegetables and sweetened with barley malt or rice syrup may be made at home or be purchased at the macrobiotic natural foods store. Candy made with refined sweeteners, honey, carob, chocolate, and other excessively yin ingredients is avoided.

Nutritional and Health Benefits

Whole grains, beans, vegetables, and sea vegetables contain complex carbohydrates such as starch, cellulose, gums, and pectin. These complex sugars, or polysaccharides, are an ideal way to consume sugar. They are absorbed slowly in the intestines and release sugar into the bloodstream at a slow, gradual rate. In contrast, refined sugar, honey, molasses, and other concentrated sweeteners contain simple sugars such as sucrose, glucose, and fructose. These simple sugars are metabolized rapidly soon after entering the digestive system in the mouth and passing through the esophagus to the stomach. Premature absorption of sugar can create elevated swings in mood, cause insulin flooding and raise blood sugar levels, and overwork the adrenal glands. Excessive consumption of sugar and other refined sweeteners is associated with a wide range of physical, psychological, and mental disorders including tooth decay, hypoglycemia, diabetes, high blood pressure, coronary heart disease, liver disease, pancreatic cancer, breast cancer, prostate cancer, ovarian cancer, and many others.

In the macrobiotic diet, the natural taste of daily food satisfies much of the desire for a sweet taste. Thorough chewing of each mouthful makes foods even sweeter, especially brown rice and other grains. When properly chewed, an enzyme in the saliva begins to turn the starch of grains and vegetables into sugar in a way similar to the fermentation of malt. Among vegetables, the especially sweet-tasting ones such as fall and winter squashes, carrots, parsnips, rutabagas, and onions are served often. Adding a pinch of sea salt to vegetables during cooking makes them even sweeter. Long-time *nishime* style boiling and baking also make foods richer and sweeter to the taste. Properly cooked beans are also naturally sweet and satisfying as are chestnuts.

By eliminating or reducing the intake of meat, poultry, eggs, dairy food, and other extreme yang foods, the desire for concentrated sweeteners gradually declines. As whole foods become the foundation of the diet, a natural sense of taste is restored. The natural sweetness of grains and vegetables is appreciated, and the frequency and amount of snacks and desserts consumed falls sharply. Instead of two or three times a day, snacks and desserts are prepared only once a day or every other day. Chemically, barley malt, rice syrup, and other grain-based natural sweeteners contain primarily maltose, a double sugar that is released into the bloodstream much more gradually than sucrose, glucose, or fructose. As a result, the change from sugar, honey, or refined sweetenings to grain-based sweeteners can contribute to smoother metabolism, reduce blood sugar levels, and have far-reaching effects on mental and emotional behavior as well as physical health. However, barley malt, rice syrup, and similar products are still very concentrated products and should be used only occasionally and in moderation.

Snacks and desserts are an enjoyable part of the Standard Macrobiotic Diet. Observing the distinction between daily food, food for occasional enjoyment, and party and holiday food will contribute greatly to personal health, family and social order, and environmental harmony.

Salt, Oil, and Other Seasonings

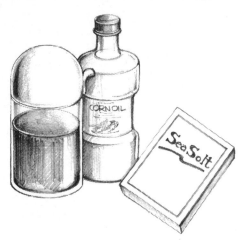

Daily Use

Within the Standard Macrobiotic Diet, a variety of seasonings is used regularly. The seasonings are all vegetable quality, naturally processed. Unrefined sea salt is regularly used in cooking whole grains, beans, and many vegetables. Tamari soy sauce, miso, and umeboshi plums, which have been salted and pickled, are also used frequently to provide a salty flavor or taste. For daily cooking, unrefined dark sesame oil is preferred. Light sesame oil, corn oil, and mustard seed oil may also be used frequently, and other unrefined vegetable oils on occasion. Fresh grated gingerroot, daikon and radish are used in seasoning to provide a pungent taste, and brown rice vinegar, sweet brown rice vinegar, and umeboshi vinegar give a pleasant sour flavor. Mirin, amazaké, barley malt, or rice syrup may be used occasionally for a sweet flavor. A wide variety of other seasonings may also be used from time to time. However, in a four-season environment, herbs and spices are usually avoided or limited in daily macrobiotic cooking and food preparation. Their stimulant, aromatic, and fragrant qualities serve to balance the effects of living in a hot and humid tropical climate but are much too extreme for regular consumption in temperate latitudes.

The use of seasonings should be moderate and adequate for personal needs. The amount of salt in daily cooking will vary according to climate, season, age, sex, and level of daily activity. Slightly more salt is used in colder climates than warm ones and during the autumn and winter than during the spring and summer. Generally no salt is used in cooking for babies under ten months. After that age, a salty taste may gradually be introduced. At age three, a child can receive about one-fourth to one-third the amount of salt of an adult, and until age seven or eight their food is usually prepared separately or set aside prior to final adult-strength seasoning. At this age, the amount of salt and other seasonings may slowly be increased to that of older children or adults. Women usually require slightly less salt than men, and the elderly take less than other adults. The more physically active also take a little more strongly salted food than those who are more mentally inclined.

The frequency and volume of oil consumed will also differ with the individual. Ideally oil and fat are taken in whole form in foods such as whole grains, beans, and seeds. For a person in normal good health, one or two dishes a day may be made with a small amount of unrefined vegetable-quality oil. This could include a side dish of sautéed vegetables or sea vegetables and a sauce or dressing containing a little oil. About once a week, or for holidays and special occasions, deep-fried seitan, deep-fried tofu, or vegetable, fish, or seafood tempura may be prepared. Deep-frying and tempura style cooking utilize large amounts of oil. However, if properly done, foods prepared in these ways are not oily and heavy but crispy and light to the taste. For persons who are ill, oil consumption may need to be minimized or avoided altogether until the condition improves.

History

Salt is essential to life and has been a universal food commodity since ancient times. In most traditional cultures, salt was obtained from evaporated seawater, though in some inland regions it was mined from rock salt deposits or obtained by burning sea vegetables or swamp plants and retaining the crystallized sediment in the ashes. In modern times, highly refined table salt, made with a variety of chemical additives, has largely replaced unrefined salt. In addition to basic salt, different societies used different seasonings. In the Far East, miso, tamari soy sauce, and umeboshi plums were used in a wide variety of cooking and pickling styles, and sesame oil and mustard seed oil were used in cooking. In the Middle East and Mediterranean region olives and olive oil served a similar function. In the Americas, native peoples used oil from corn, sunflower seeds, and other seed-bearing plants.

Quality and Varieties

Some of the major seasonings used in macrobiotic cooking are described below.

Salt

Regular table salt is a highly industrialized product containing about 99.5 percent sodium chloride. While it is made from either sea salt or rock salt, most of the natural trace elements have been removed in processing and magnesium carbonate, sodium carbonate, and potassium iodide have been substituted in their place. Furthermore, dextrose, a highly refined industrial sugar, is customarily added to table salt to stabilize the iodine.

Unrefined sea salt is processed in several ways. Usually it is evaporated from salt water, dried in the sun, redissolved in water, filtered, reevaporated, and crystallized in wood- or gas-heated pans. Unrefined sea salt made in the largely tradi-

Table 18   Salt Composition

Refined table salt has a very different composition than unrefined sea salt. Made from sea salt or mined land salt, refined salt is almost pure sodium chloride to which several mineral compounds, iodine, and dextrose, a refined sugar to stabilize the iodine, are added. In contrast, unrefined sea salt usually contains from 94 to 97 percent sodium chloride, with the remainder consisting of mineral compounds and trace elements. However, the actual percentages vary according to the natural processing method used. This table shows the results of one such test.

Table Salt		Unrefined Sea Salt	
Sodium chloride	99.50 (%)	Sodium chloride	97.51 (%)
Magnesium carbonate,	0.50	Magnesium carbonate	1.51
potassium iodide,		Calcium chloride	0.40
dextrose (sugar),		Potassium sulfate	0.42
sodium carbonate		Fluoride, strontium and boron	0.14
		Trace elements including gold, silver, platinum, lead, tin, radium and about 54 others	0.003

Source: Thom Leonard, et al., "Choosing the Best Sea Salt," *East West Journal,* November 1983.

tionally manner contains compounds of several minerals such as magnesium as well as minute quantities of about sixty other elements naturally found in the sea including gold, silver, and tin. The unrefined sea salt available in North American and European natural foods stores comes primarily from coastal waters off Mexico and Europe. The proportion of trace minerals varies according to the method of processing used, usually from a high of about 3 percent to a low of 0.5 percent (see Table 18).

Good quality sea salt is very delicious. A bit on the top of the tongue should taste sweet and then gradually turn salty. The saltier it tastes, the less trace minerals have been retained. If the tongue contracts immediately, however, it shows that too many mineral compounds, especially those containing magnesium, have been retained. When selecting salt, one with a nice sweet taste is preferable to salty-tasting varieties or crude grey sea salt which contains excess minerals and has not been processed enough. In macrobiotic cooking, iodine is naturally obtained from sea vegetables, which are plentiful in this element, so that there is no need for it to be added artificially to salt.

Tamari Soy Sauce

Soy sauce has been a staple of Far Eastern cooking for thousands of years. It is traditionally made from organically grown soybeans and wheat, good quality water, and unrefined sea salt that have fermented naturally for several years in well-aged cedar vats. Modern commercial soy sauces are a far different product. They are made with defatted soybean meal, chemically grown grains, refined salt, and usually contain monosodium glutamate, caramel, sugar, or other additives and preservatives. Moreover, commercial varieties are artificially aged in temperature-controlled stainless steel or epoxy-coated steel vats to reduce their aging to several months.

In Japan, soy sauce is traditionally called *shoyu*. In the eighteenth century a Swedish botanist mispronounced the bean from which this product came and named it the "soya" bean. In the mid-twentieth century when naturally processed shoyu was reintroduced to the West, further linguistic confusion resulted. Originally George Ohsawa selected the name *tamari* to distinguish natural, traditionally made soy sauce from modern chemicalized soy sauce which was customarily marketed under the name shoyu. The word *tamari* derives from the traditional name for the liquid that rises to the top during the process of making soybean miso. This tamari was used traditionally in specialty cooking and has a deep mellow flavor, rich dark-brown color, and often a mildly thick consistency. Since it was not used in the Far East as a daily soy sauce, Ohsawa did not anticipate that it would be mistaken by Westerners with the wheat-free by-product of the miso-making process. However, about twenty years after Ohsawa popularized tamari soy sauce, a type of wheat-free shoyu was introduced to the natural foods market called *real tamari* or *genuine tamari*. As a result, some people have had difficulty distinguishing between the two products. In daily macrobiotic cooking, "tamari soy sauce" is regularly used, though depending on the distributor it may be labeled as "organic shoyu" or "natural shoyu." Thicker-tasting "wheat-free tamari," also known as "real tamari" or "genuine tamari," is used occasionally, especially as a dipping sauce for tempura, sashimi (raw fish), or other festive or holiday cooking. Wheat-free tamari is also more expensive than regular tamari soy sauce.

Miso

Miso, a fermented food made from soybeans, usually various grains such as barley or brown rice, sea salt, and an enzyme starter called koji, has a sweet, rich flavor and is used in seasoning as well as in the preparation of soup. (Quality considerations and the varieties of miso are discussed in the soup chapter.)

Umeboshi Plums

Umeboshi plums grow in the warmer, southern and middle regions of Japan and are related to the apricot. Traditionally fermented with sea salt and pickled with shiso leaves, umeboshi plums have a tangy flavor, combining a sour and salty taste. They are a very balanced food, give a strong centering energy, and have a wide range of uses in macrobiotic cooking and home cares. Once again, the quality of modern commercially prepared umeboshi plums is very different than that of the past. Their aging is artificially speeded up, and synthetic colorings are often added to give them a deep red color that naturally comes from aging.

Even though the umeboshi plums in the macrobiotic natural foods store are generally good quality, their taste and energy differ widely. Those that have aged the longest are less tart and salty and give stronger energy, especially for medicinal preparations. In recent years, a ready-made umeboshi paste has become available. This product is very convenient to use since it does not require pitting the plums nor puréeing them by hand in a *suribachi*. However, the energy and nutrients they provide are much less than those of umeboshi consumed in whole form. The paste is primarily suitable for party and holiday cooking when larger amounts of food are prepared and convenience is more of a factor.

Oil

Good quality oil is essential to health. Unrefined vegetable-quality oils are processed in different ways and come in several grades (see Table 19). The highest quality oils are pressed from seeds, grains, fruits, or nuts at relatively low temperatures and then minimally filtered and bottled. Rich and cloudy in appearance, they retain the natural aroma and flavor of the whole food from which they are extracted. They also retain the antioxidants and other nutrients that help prevent against rancidity. An inferior type of unrefined vegetable-quality oil is currently produced by solvent-extraction. In this process, hexane, a highly toxic chemical derived from petroleum, is heated at extreme temperatures to extract the oil, destroying most of the nutrients. Some oils in the natural foods store are labeled "cold-pressed" to signify that they are not processed at high temperatures. However, among unrefined oils commonly available only olive oil is truly pressed cold without heating. Moreover, the term "cold-pressed" also has been applied to some refined oils manufactured at moderate temperatures. Because of a lack of industry standards, "cold-pressed" is not necessarily an indication of quality.

Refined oils may also be either pressed or solvent-extracted. However, unlike unrefined oils, they are degummed, washed in a highly caustic solution of lye and soap which removes essential fatty acids, bleached with hydrochloric or sulfuric acid, deodorized, preserved with harmful chemicals such as BHT and BHA, and often winterized (chilled). The result is a bland colorless product that has little or no natural color, taste, aroma, or proper nutrients but one that lasts for a long time on the supermarket shelf and in the refrigerator. Some oils are also hydrogenated to make them solid at room temperature, particularly margarine, potato chips, and fried fast foods. The process of hydrogenation converts the polyunsaturated fatty acids of the original oil to varying degrees of saturated fat. All refined and hydrogenated oils are strictly avoided in macrobiotic food preparation.

The principal types of unrefined vegetable-quality oils include:

1. Sesame Oil. Dark sesame oil, made from pressing roasted sesame seeds, has a rich nutty taste, smoky aroma, deep dark color, and cloudy appearance. It is a superior oil and the one preferred for regular sautéing, pan-frying, deep-frying, cooking tempura style, baking, sauces, and spreads. Light sesame oil has a milder taste, is clearer in consistency, and has less flavor. It is used for making delicate dishes where the strong flavor of dark sesame oil might interfere with the other ingredients. Highly stable and resistant to spoiling, sesame oil should be kept tightly sealed after opening in a dark, cool place or in the refrigerator.

2. Corn Oil. After sesame oil, unrefined corn oil is the most frequently used oil

Table 19   Unrefined and Refined Oil Processing

Unrefined vegetable-quality oils have a flavorful, often nutty taste, deep aroma, and dark cloudy consistency, thereby retaining much of the energy and nutrients of the original seed, nut, or bean. However, there are generally two types of unrefined oils. The recommended type is naturally processed at relatively low temperatures (expeller- or screw-pressed). This type is sometimes referred to as cold-pressed, but this term is also used with some refined oils. The other type of unrefined oil is solvent-extracted with hexane or other chemical and is distilled at extremely high temperatures, which considerably reduces its nutritional value. Refined oils—the family of bland modern cooking and salad oils—are made from crude solvent-extracted oils by further processing at high temperatures. Commercial oil products such as corn or soy margarine are subject to additional processing at high temperatures which further alters their quality. This table lists the major steps in each type of processing.

EXPELLER-PRESSED UNREFINED OIL	*SOLVENT-EXTRACTED UNREFINED OIL*
Cleaning and hulling of seeds, nuts, beans	Cleaning and hulling of seeds, nuts, beans
↓	↓
Cooking (steam jacket) 110° F.–250° F.	Flaking (mechanical rollers)
↓	↓
Expeller "Cold Pressing" 140° F.–160° F.	Solvent extraction (hexane or other oil-derivative) 136° F.
↓	↓
Filtering	Distillation (evaporation) 300° F.
↓	↓
Bottling	Bottling

REFINED OIL	*COMMERCIAL PRODUCTS*
Degumming of unrefined crude oil (oil and water, centrifuge separation) 90° F.–120° F.	Preservatives added to refined, bleached, deodorized oil such as BHA, BHT, TBHQ, citric acid, etc., and defoamers such as methyl silicone
↓	↓
Refining (oil and alkali solution, agitation, centrifuge separation) 140° F.–160° F.	Hydrogenation (saturation with hydrogen)
↓	↓
Bleaching (fuller's earth, filters) 230° F.	Bottling, packing, or winterization and bottling (in some cases, nonhydrogenated oils are cooled and filtered at 45° F.)
↓	
Deodorizing (steam and vacuum) 450° F. +	
↓	
Bottling	

Source: Whole Foods Natural Foods Guide, And/Or Press, 1979.

in macrobiotic cooking in North America. It has a rich corn flavor and smooth buttery consistency. A lighter variety is derived from the corn germ, while a darker one comes from the whole kernel. It is used frequently for sautéing, baking, and in making sauces and dressings. However, because it foams readily at high temperatures it is not used for deep-frying or tempura.

3. **Mustard Seed Oil.** Mustard seed oil is pressed from the seeds of the same plant from which mustard greens are harvested. Though not widely available in the West, tiny mustard seeds are valued in Asia and the Middle East where they are the subject of many legends such as in the New Testament.

4. **Sunflower Oil.** Sunflower oil is a staple oil in the Soviet Union, Canada, and other cold northern environments. It has a pleasant taste, clear consistency, and keeps well. It is used occasionally in place of sesame or corn oil.

5. **Safflower Oil.** Safflower oil is very mild tasting and makes nice light sauces and dressings. It spoils more easily than other oils and is unstable at high temperatures. It is not used so much in daily macrobiotic cooking.

6. **Soybean Oil.** Soy oil has a strong somewhat fishy flavor which some people enjoy but many others find unappetizing. A much more bland-tasting refined soy oil is widely used by the commercial fast food industry.

7. **Olive Oil.** Olive oil has a distinctive light sweet flavor and taste and keeps well without refrigeration for up to a year. It is nice in salads and used occasionally in cooking. Olive oil is the only major commercially available oil that is not processed at high temperatures or high pressures. The highest grades, obtained from the first pressings of the fruit, are called virgin. The second best grades are called pure and are sometimes obtained with the use of chemicals. The oil in olives is primarily monosaturated in quality, which makes it heavier and more fatty than polyunsaturated oils.

8. **Other Oils.** Other unrefined, naturally processed vegetable-quality oils that are traditionally prepared and commonly consumed may be used by those in usual good health for variety and enjoyment from time to time. These include peanut oil, cottonseed oil, linseed oil, almond oil, and walnut oil. Coconut oil and palmseed oil are largely saturated in quality and are avoided in macrobiotic cooking.

Ginger

Fresh ginger is an essential seasoning in macrobiotic cooking. It stimulates the appetite, gets circulation moving, and adds a mild spicy flavor to the meal. The knobby gingerroot may either be freshly grated or minced, or a handful of gratings may be squeezed for their juice. The juice is much more concentrated than the gratings and usually requires only a few drops. Dried ginger powders lack the energy and nutrients of fresh gingerroot and are usually avoided.

Vinegar

Good quality vinegar provides a pleasant sour flavor to dishes and is used frequently in macrobiotic food preparation. The best quality vinegars are naturally processed *brown rice vinegar* and *sweet brown rice vinegar*. These are traditionally made with deep well water, koji (a special rice-based mold that is also used in making saké or rice wine), seed vinegar (mash from the previous year), and cooked brown rice or sweet brown rice that have been mixed together and aged in large earthenware jars. The jars are set outside in a field with their bases buried about a foot deep in the earth and allowed to ferment for six to ten months depending upon climatic and weather conditions. When the mixture is mature, the mash is pressed through canvas sacks in a simple wooden press and filtered through cotton to remove any remaining impurities from the liquid. The vinegar is then bottled and heated to stop the fermentation.

Another type of vinegar regularly used in the macrobiotic kitchen is *umeboshi vinegar*. Umeboshi vinegar, made from the juice left over from pickling umeboshi plums, is also marketed as *ume-su*. Good quality *apple cider vinegar* is much more acidic than grain-based vinegars and is used very occasionally for variety or enjoyment. *Wine vinegars* and *commercial vinegars* containing herbs, spices, and additives are avoided in macrobiotic food preparation.

Mirin and Saké

Mirin, a liquid natural sweetener made from fermented sweet rice, and saké, the traditional rice wine of Japan, are traditionally used in small volume for holiday cooking or other special occasions.

Other Seasonings

Other traditionally prepared and commonly used seasonings may also be used from time to time within the Standard Macrobiotic Diet. These include sauerkraut brine, barley malt, rice malt, grated daikon, grated radish, horseradish, lemon juice, tangerine juice, orange juice, freshly ground black pepper, red pepper, wasabi paste, yellow mustard paste, sesame oil, corn oil, safflower oil, mustard seed oil, olive oil, and saké lees.

Cooking Methods and Special Dishes

In macrobiotic food preparation, salt or other basic seasoning is ordinarily added to foods during cooking rather than at the table. Dishes prepared in this way are much more balanced and digestible. However, just enough salt or other seasoning is used in cooking to meet the minimal needs of each family member. Further seasoning is provided at the table with an assortment of condiments, which may be added as desired. Some of these, such as gomashio, contain roasted sea salt. Some of the ways in which salt, tamari soy sauce, miso, and other seasonings are used in macrobiotic cooking are described below.

Salt

In pressure-cooking or boiling brown rice or other whole grains, a pinch of sea salt is ordinarily used for each one or two cups of uncooked grain. The salt makes the grain sweeter to the taste, chewier, and stronger in energy. While salt is not used usually in miso soups, clear soups, or tamari broth, it may be added to some soup stocks, bean soups, or vegetable soups. In these cases, a little salt is sometimes added at the beginning of cooking and most of the salt is added toward the end of cooking. Slightly more salt is used in cooking soups than in preparing grains.

Vegetables become softer and lose more water when cooked with salt. Raw vegetables may be sprinkled with salt and either marinated or pickled. For cooked dishes, a pinch of salt makes water boil faster. A touch of sea salt may be added to root and ground vegetables at the beginning of sautéing, steaming, and quick boiling. The salt makes them crispier, sweeter to the taste, and keeps their colors clear and deep. A pinch of salt may also be used with the sweeter-tasting green leafy vegetables such as collard greens, Chinese cabbage, and kale. However, salt should be avoided with those that are naturally slightly bitter such as watercress, mustard greens, or daikon greens.

Beans are usually seasoned with salt after cooking about 70 to 80 percent. Otherwise, if salt is added in the beginning, the inside and outside of the beans will cook unevenly. Slightly more salt may be used when cooking beans than grains. Sea vegetables contain sea salt and other mineral compounds and are usually cooked with tamari soy sauce rather than salt. Salt may be sprinkled on top of baked fish to make it crispier. A pinch of salt on fresh melon, berries, or other fruit will bring out their natural sweetness and make them juicier. Seeds and nuts are customarily roasted with a little sea salt or tamari soy sauce which helps to balance their high oil content. Salt is also roasted for making certain condiments such as gomashio.

Tamari Soy Sauce

Though a touch of tamari soy sauce may be added to pressure-cooked brown rice or other whole grains instead of salt, it is more frequently used to season fried rice or fried noodles. It may also be added to a kuzu sauce to put over grains. Tamari soy sauce is the foundation of tamari broth, dashi soup stock, and some clear soups. It is also commonly used to flavor squash soup, onion soup, and other naturally sweet vegetable soups. In bean and grain soups, it gives a slightly stronger taste than salt.

With vegetables, tamari soy sauce is usually added at the very end of cooking and allowed to simmer for several minutes. However, in some styles, such as *ni-shime* style boiling, a mild tamari soy sauce flavor may be added at the start of cooking, especially when the ingredients include tempeh, seitan, or tofu. Tamari soy sauce is frequently used to make a dressing or marinate fresh salads, quick pickles, and a dipping sauce for tempura. Its subtle flavor goes well with either sweet, sour, or pungent tastes.

In some beans, notably yellow and black soybeans, tamari soy sauce brings out a strong delicious taste. A dash may also be added during cooking to azuki beans. Beans are often prepared with a little salt added after cooking about 70 to 80 percent and then flavored to taste with tamari soy sauce for a few minutes before the end of cooking. Sea vegetables are usually seasoned during cooking with tamari soy sauce, especially hijiki, arame, and kombu. Salty condiments such as shio-kombu are prepared with tamari soy sauce. At the table, macrobiotic cooking generally discourages the use of adding tamari soy sauce to cooked foods. However, it is customary to add a few drops to noodles for extra flavor and taste, if necessary. In beverages, a little tamari soy sauce is occasionally added to medicinal teas to create a calming effect and stimulate energy.

Miso

In macrobiotic cooking, miso is used almost daily to prepare miso soup and a wide variety of other dishes. The amount of miso used will depend on the type of miso used, how long it has aged, and its relative saltiness as well as environmental and personal factors. As a rule of thumb, about one teaspoon of undiluted miso is used per cup of liquid or other ingredients. Miso paste is traditionally diluted in a little cold water in an earthenware bowl called a *suribachi*. This grooved mortar and a thick wooden pestle are widely available in different sizes in macrobiotic natural foods stores and may be used for making many sauces and dressings as well as for puréeing miso. Because miso contains live enzymes and bacteria that are beneficial to digestion, it is preferable to add it at the end of cooking and allow it to simmer for a few minutes before serving rather than let it boil. In general, cooking with miso creates a sweeter taste than either salt or tamari soy sauce. For day to day cooking, barley miso is generally preferred, though brown rice miso and Hatcho miso are also used frequently. Red miso, yellow miso, and other misos that have fermented for a shorter time are used occasionally or for special dishes.

For grains and noodles, miso makes savory sauces and gravies. It may also be used instead of salt in seasoning whole grains or in baking. In addition to miso soup, miso may be used from time to time to season bean, vegetable, or grain soups or to prepare broths for noodles. With vegetable side dishes, miso is usually added at the end of cooking. However, for some dishes, such as whole onions, miso is added at the start and allowed to penetrate into the ingredients during cooking. When baking, broiling, and barbecuing, miso may also be used at the start. Miso seasoning also makes tasty salad dressings, sauces, spreads, dips, and sweet, delicious pickles. Deep-fried grain balls seasoned with miso are also very enjoyable.

Miso gives beans, especially kidney beans and soybeans, an extra sweet flavor and taste. It also goes extremely well with tofu, especially as a spread for pan-fried tofu or for making pickled tofu. Though not usually used to season sea vegetables, miso goes well with wakame in soup, salads, and sauces. Miso is used to make many condiments including tekka. It blends well with sweet, sour, and pungent tastes and is often combined with roasted seeds and nuts, with natural sweeteners, with brown rice vinegar or lemon, and with ginger. Spread on top of broiled fish, miso makes a delicious seasoning. It may also be used as a marinade for fish and seafood. Miso is very versatile and has many other uses.

Umeboshi Plums

Umeboshi plums have a wide range of uses as a seasoning and after pitting are ordinarily puréed in a *suribachi* with a little water or cut into small pieces. They may be used instead of salt to season brown rice and other whole grains during cooking and contribute a mild sour flavor and taste. They may also be added raw to soft rice or other cooked grain. A small piece of umeboshi is traditionally added to the center of rice balls and gives them very strong energy and taste. They also make a tangy dressing or sauce for noodles, grains, and vegetables. In macrobiotic households, a little puréed umeboshi or umeboshi paste is spread on corn on the cob instead of butter and gives a zesty, salt taste.

For vegetable dishes, umeboshi are also used in making sauces. They go especially well diluted in a little water or soup stock and combined with scallions and roasted sesame seeds. A beautiful pink dressing is made with umeboshi and tofu. Red radishes and other raw vegetables are often pickled with umeboshi or the shiso leaves with which they are fermented and traditionally packed. In the summertime, umeboshi makes a cooling tea steeped in water by itself or added to bancha tea. Umeboshi and *ume extract*, a concentrate, have many medicinal applications in macrobiotic home care treatments.

Oil

Oil creates outward, expanding energy. Only a tiny amount is needed when cooking. A single tablespoon or just enough to cover the pan is usually enough to sauté a large skillet of vegetables, noodles, or grains for an entire family. For those who must limit their oil intake, oil may be brushed on the pan with a tiny brush. Some foods combine well with oil, including most root vegetables; onions, cabbages, and some round vegetables; some leafy vegetables; hijiki and arame; and tofu, seitan, and tempeh. Other foods do not blend so well, including azuki beans, chick-peas, kombu, and fall and winter squashes, though squashes may be deep-fried. To help digest oil, especially for deep-fried or tempura dishes, a little grated daikon and sometimes fresh grated gingerroot or umeboshi plum are customarily served. For fish and seafood, prepared with or without oil, a stronger condiment such as horseradish or wasabi, the Japanese horseradish, is served in addition to grated daikon.

Ginger

Fresh grated gingerroot adds zest to a wide variety of soups, grain dishes, noodles, and vegetable preparations. It is also used in many sauces and dressings. It is customarily added at the very end of cooking and simmered with the other ingredients for a minute or less before serving. Ginger is also used frequently as a raw garnish. Ginger may also be pickled, used in condiments, and added to beverages. In macrobiotic healing, it has many internal and external uses.

Vinegar

Brown rice vinegar and sweet brown rice vinegar give a delightful sour taste and make excellent sauces and dressings. They are not ordinarily used in cooking or soups, but a touch may be added occasionally to soften burdock or sea vegetables, especially the latter if they are hard and salty. Umeboshi vinegar also makes flavorful dressings and sauces. It is occasionally added from the beginning of cooking to cabbage, cauliflower, and red radishes. Umeboshi vinegar is also sometimes added to noodles and salads.

Mirin and Saké

Mirin or saké may be added from time to time to sweeten whole grains, beans, sea vegetables, and vegetables. Mirin in particular mellows the flavor of excessively salty or overly spicy foods. A touch of mirin added to noodle broths, dressings, sauces, or marinades gives a unique, subtle taste.

Nutritional and Health Benefits

Salt is essential to life. The quality of salt, the amount consumed, and the way salt is used in cooking are paramount questions in the life of an individual, family, community, and culture. In proper volume, good quality natural unrefined sea salt, containing trace minerals and elements, contributes to smooth metabolism, steady energy and vitality, and a clear, focused mind. Too little salt or no salt at all can lead to lack of vitality, stagnated blood, and loss of direction in life. Too much salt can produce hyperactivity, rigid thinking, aggressive behavior, and excessive retention of fluids, leading to kidney troubles and other physical, mental, and emotional disorders.

The poor quality of refined table salt is a major factor in the degeneration of modern society. Compared to the Standard Macrobiotic Diet, the usual modern diet contains about four times the amount of sodium. In addition to the large amount of refined salt used in frozen, canned, and convenience foods and salt added to foods at the table, sodium is consumed in large volume in animal-quality food, including meat, poultry, eggs, and dairy products. Excessive sodium from these sources as well as refined salt is a major factor in some forms of cardiovascular disease and other degenerative conditions.

While unrefined sea salt is much superior to the refined variety, it too can be under- or overconsumed. The style of macrobiotic cooking initially introduced to the West proved over the years to be too salty for most Americans and Europeans.

Japan's climate is much more moist than that of the United States and requires more salt to make balance. Also, because of past meat and other animal-food consumption, most Americans and Europeans already have an excess of sodium and other minerals in their systems and are thus more susceptible to overconsuming salt than Far Easterners. As a result, much less sea salt, miso, and tamari soy sauce are generally used in the West than in the East, and current macrobiotic cookbooks reflect this adjustment.

Like miso, whose nutritional and health benefits are discussed in the soup chapter, tamari soy sauce and umeboshi plums are fermented products. They are high in iron, thiamine, riboflavin, and in the case of miso and tamari soy sauce B_{12}. Like other fermented foods, miso, tamari soy sauce, and umeboshi plums are beneficial to digestion, stimulating the secretion of digestive fluids in the stomach and fostering the growth of healthy bacterial cultures in the intestinal tract. Their saline nature neutralizes acidic foods, improving blood quality and circulation, providing energy and balance, and contributing to physical, emotional, and mental harmony.

High quality oil is also essential to health and longevity. It strengthens cells and capillaries, reduces cholesterol in the blood, and lubricates the skin and hair. High in vitamins A and E and other nutrients, unrefined vegetable-quality oil is flavorful and easy to digest. It is also high in polyunsaturated fatty acids. These are the type needed by the body for smooth metabolism and are naturally found in whole grains, beans, seeds, and in some fish and seafood. In contrast, meat, poultry, cheese, butter, milk, and other dairy foods are high in hard, saturated fat and dietary cholesterol, two substances that can accumulate in arteries and around vital organs leading to heart disease and certain forms of cancer. About 40 percent of the modern diet consists of fatty substances, and the majority of these are consumed in the form of refined polyunsaturated cooking oils, margarine, spreads, and convenience foods containing hydrogenated oils. Whole foods contain natural antioxidants, such as β-carotene and vitamin E, which help prevent their oils from oxidizing. The oxidation of polyunsaturated oils, especially refined and hydrogenated oils, has been associated with damage to cells and tissues, destruction of artery walls, and elevated cholesterol levels. Interestingly, the vitamins A and E, lecithin, and other nutrients taken out of natural oils in the refining process are often sold back to consumers in the form of vitamin and mineral supplements. Like white bread and white rice, refined oil and refined salt are lifeless products and detrimental to human health.

Salt and oil form a natural balance, and their proper use is one of the chief arts of cooking. While completely mastering these basic ingredients may take a lifetime, the macrobiotic cook begins with the best quality ingredients and over time learns to make daily adjustments for the everchanging climate, season, daily weather cycle, age, sex, level of activity, and personal needs and desires of his or her family. As the ancient parables recognized, a tiny seed from which oil is pressed and a grain of salt profoundly shape the lives and destiny of the human race.

Dressings, Sauces, Garnishes, and Condiments

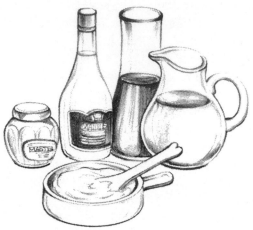

Daily Use

Like salt, oil, and seasonings in general, dressings, sauces, garnishes, and condiments are very important to making balance in the meal. They offer variety to daily cooking and are a simple way to create the five basic tastes. Dressings and sauces add body, texture, and flavor, providing uniqueness to many dishes. Garnishes are frequently used in small volume to balance some dishes, especially for the purposes of providing color and aesthetic enjoyment, stimulating the appetite, and creating easier digestion. Condiments are sprinkled on, or added in small amount to, food at the table. In addition to providing nutritional and energetic harmony, condiments allow for individual adjustments to be made during the meal according to personal taste and condition of health. Condiments are commonly used for grains, soups, vegetable dishes, bean dishes, and sometimes with desserts.

History

Dressings, sauces, garnishes, and condiments are key elements in the cuisines of all traditional cultures. In the past, when less processed food, less unseasonal food, and less food from a different climate was available, these preparations allowed the same food to be served daily in new and interesting ways. In the Far East, miso, tamari soy sauce, umeboshi plums, dried sea vegetable powder, grated daikon, grated gingerroot, and other ingredients were commonly used to add variety to different dishes. In the Near East, roasted sesame seeds, minced onions, sliced scallions, and lemon or lime juice were commonly used for these purposes. In Europe, sauerkraut, apple cider vinegar, and sauces made with whole wheat flour were very popular.

Quality

In macrobiotic cooking and food preparation, dressings, sauces, garnishes, and condiments are usually prepared fresh in the kitchen using the highest quality ingredients. Store-bought dressings and sauces are usually low in nutrients and energy and are preferably avoided, especially those containing unrefined or hydrogenated oils, herbs, spices, preservatives, or other artificial ingredients. Some high-quality ready-made condiments, such as tekka, which take many hours to prepare and keep well for a long time, are available in the macrobiotic natural foods store and are suitable for use, though making them at home is still ideal. Gomashio, the roasted sesame salt widely used as a condiment by many macrobiotic people, is also available ready-made. However, gomashio begins to lose its freshness after about a week on the shelf, so it is highly recommended that it be prepared at home regularly in small amounts rather than be purchased or made in large amounts and stored over a long period of time.

As a thickener for sauces and dressings, as well as soups, stews, and vegetable dishes, a good vegetable-quality starch is recommended such as kuzu powder or arrowroot flour. Kuzu (or kudzu as it is known in the southern United States where it is found in abundance) grows wild in the mountains of Japan and has very deep roots. It is traditionally harvested and processed by hand into a white, chalklike substance. In the kitchen, a small amount of kuzu is diluted in a little cold water, cooked with the other ingredients for a few minutes until it becomes translucent, and stirred gently during cooking to prevent lumping.

When using unrefined vegetable-quality oil for dressings or sauces, only a very small amount is usually necessary. Oil is preferably heated for a few seconds to make it more digestible rather than added raw to other ingredients.

Varieties

Dressings

For salads, marinades, servings of leafy green vegetables, or other dishes, a variety of dressings is commonly prepared. These include: 1) *tamari soy sauce dressings*, combining the natural salty taste of tamari soy sauce with brown rice vinegar, lemon, or ginger; 2) *umeboshi dressings*, featuring a slightly sour and salty taste in combination with minced onions, a little sesame oil, or sliced scallions and parsley; 3) *miso dressings*, featuring a nice sweet and salty taste combined with a little brown rice vinegar, grated ginger, or tahini or sesame butter; 4) *tofu dressings*, creamy preparations made with lightly boiled tofu puréed with grated onions and sesame butter or tahini or with umeboshi plums and sliced scallions or chives; 5) *sesame dressings*, made with roasted sesame seeds, soup stock, brown rice vinegar, and tamari soy sauce. Usually spring water is added to each of these dressings, and there are endless variations that can be made by substituting mirin, umeboshi vinegar, brown rice vinegar, and other ingredients.

Sauces and Gravies

Sauces and gravies make excellent toppings for whole grains, noodles, beans, or vegetables. Among the many varieties, popular ones include: 1) *dashi broth*, a basic soup stock made with kombu and often shiitake mushrooms and tamari soy sauce to which chopped seitan, fu, tempeh, or tofu may be added; 2) *miso sauce*, made with onions, carrots, burdock, or other vegetables sliced fine and sautéed for a few minutes until creamy, seasoned with a little diluted miso, and occasionally garnished with sesame seeds or a drop of sesame oil; 3) *kuzu sauce* made with carrots and onions, fall or winter squashes, or other ingredients, sliced and cooked in a little water until creamy, thickened with a little diluted kuzu, and seasoned with tamari soy sauce and garnished with grated ginger; 4) *sweet and sour sauce*, a delicious topping for seitan, tempeh, noodles, rice, or other dishes made from minced onions, grated carrots, and sliced celery cooked in soup stock, thickened with kuzu, and seasoned with sea salt, tamari soy sauce, brown rice vinegar, and either apple juice, mirin, or a touch of maple syrup; 5) *bechamel sauce*, a rich gravy for millet and other grains made with whole wheat pastry flour or brown rice flour, spring water, diced onion, and tamari soy sauce.

Garnishes

Principal garnishes include: 1) *grated daikon*, used mainly as a garnish for fish and seafood, mochi, buckwheat noodles and pasta, natto, and tempeh; 2) *grated radish*, used similarly to grated daikon; 3) *grated horseradish*, used similarly to grated daikon; 4) *chopped scallions*, used in soups, noodle and pasta dishes, fish and seafood, natto, and tempeh; 5) *fresh grated ginger*, used in noodle and pasta dishes, soup, fish and seafood; 6) *toasted nori*, cut in strips or squares, used in soups, salads, rice and other grains, noodles, vegetables, and other dishes; 7) *bread crumbs*, cut in small cubes and added fresh, dried, or deep-fried, used in soups and salads; and 8) *other traditionally used and commonly consumed garnishes* including wasabi paste, red pepper, freshly ground pepper, and lemon slices.

Condiments

Gomashio, made from ground roasted sesame seeds and roasted sea salt, is the most commonly used macrobiotic condiment. Its salty-bitter taste balances the natural sweetness of brown rice and other grains and vegetables, and it is often added in small volume to soups, salads, and other dishes as well. The proportion of salt to sesame seeds varies from 1: 8 to 1:16 depending on the age and level of daily activity of family members. For very active adults, the generally recommended ratio of salt to sesame seeds is slightly higher than for ordinary adults, while for less active adults and for children the proportion of salt is slightly lower. Gomashio is very delicious, and care must be taken not to overconsume it. A half teaspoon to one teaspoon on a bowl of rice is usually plenty.

Sea vegetable powders are an excellent way to introduce mineral-rich sea vegetables into the meal and are tasty on whole grains, noodles, salads, soups, and other dishes. Those made with nori and dulse are the lightest tasting, kombu and kelp the heaviest, and wakame the saltiest. Sea vegetable powders are prepared by roasting the sea vegetable for about ten to fifteen minutes until dark and crisp and crushing and grinding in a *suribachi* until it becomes a fine powder. They may be combined with roasted sesame seeds for variation.

Tekka is a traditional condiment made of burdock, carrots, lotus root, Hatcho miso, and ginger that have sautéed together for a long time in dark sesame oil and have been cooked down into a concentrated black powder. Since it provides a very strong, concentrated form of energy, tekka should be used only in small amounts and is enjoyed sprinkled on grains, noodles, and other dishes. Since it traditionally takes about sixteen hours to prepare, many modern people prefer to buy ready-made tekka, which comes in small jars in the macrobiotic natural foods store. Tekka will keep up to a year if tightly covered after use.

Umeboshi plums are often used as a condiment at the table, whole or in small slices, or puréed with raw scallions or onions. Their exquisite combination of a sour and salty taste, along with a tangy flavor and bright red color, make them popular at many meals.

Shio-kombu means salty kombu and is a popular condiment in many macrobiotic households. It is traditionally made by soaking kombu sea vegetable in tamari soy sauce for one or two days and then covering with a little tamari soy sauce and cooking over a low flame for several hours. Several roasted sesame seeds are customarily mixed in at the end. Because it is so strong, only one or two pieces are usually eaten at a meal. There is also a much quicker method of preparing this dish in about an hour using a mixture of half tamari soy sauce and half spring water and pressure-cooking.

Shiso leaves, the deep red or purple colored leaves of the beefsteak plant, are customarily prepared with umeboshi plums and are sometimes available packaged by themselves in the natural foods store. Chopped or roasted they make a nice condiment for grains, vegetables, and soups.

Miso with scallions or onions has a nice pungent taste and goes well on rice, other grains, noodles, boiled vegetables, or as a spread for bread.

Nori condiment, prepared by cooking small squares of nori in spring water and tamari soy sauce, gives a nice salty taste. Green nori can also be served at the meal and provides both a bitter and sweet taste.

Wasabi paste or yellow mustard is used mainly to balance the oil and fat in fish and seafood. Occasionally yellow mustard is also added to natto.

Other traditionally used and commonly consumed condiments may also be used from time to time.

Selection Methods

As in preparing main food for the meal, principles of ecological balance should be observed in preparing dressings, sauces, garnishes, and condiments. In a four-season climate, it is preferable to avoid strong curries, chili, hot peppers, and other tropical spices as well as shredded coconut, dates, figs, and other tropical fruits. If extreme foods such as these or common vegetables of tropical origin such as tomatoes, potatoes, and eggplants are desired, especially in hot, humid weather, they can be prepared with strong long-time cooking methods and served in small condiment-sized amounts. However, it is best to avoid these foods altogether.

For regular use, many macrobiotic households keep a variety of condiments on hand at the dinner table for easy access by those who wish them and for individual use in the amount desired. These usually include gomashio dried sea vegetable powders, tekka, toasted nori squares or strips, brown rice vinegar, and tamari soy sauce (which is used primarily in cooking and very sparingly at the table, primarily on noodles). Depending upon the day's menu, the season of the year, personal health and condition, and other factors, a variety of other condiments may be set out for the meal. These are often selected by the cook to balance the meal, especially when there is a lack of sour, bitter, or pungent tasting side dishes. On the basis of the tastes they provide, garnishes and condiments may be selected from the following listings. Note, however, that some items provide two or more tastes.

Sour

Garnishes and condiments that provide a sour taste include sauerkraut, most vegetable pickles, brown rice vinegar, sweet brown rice vinegar, umeboshi plum, shiso leaves, lemon rinds, lime rinds, apple cider vinegar, sourdough bread crumbs, and some wild grasses.

Bitter

Bitter-tasting garnishes and condiments include gomashio, tekka, green nori, dried parsley, wakame powder, dandelion root and their greens, and walnuts.

Sweet

Grains and vegetables are naturally sweet, so this taste is substantially present at every meal. However, the strength and degree of sweetness will often vary with the menu and personal preference. Sweet tasting garnishes and condiments include miso, tekka, miso with scallions or onions, green nori, dried parsley, applesauce, barley malt, amazaké, carrot tops with miso, and green peppers with miso.

Pungent

Scallions, watercress, onions, chives, miso with scallions or onions, grated daikon, gingerroot, mustard, horseradish, and some wild grasses give a pungent taste.

Salty

A slight salty taste is usually provided in cooking with sea salt, miso, tamari soy sauce, or umeboshi plums. Sea salt, miso, and tamari soy sauce are much more digestible cooked than eaten raw and preferably not added to food at the table. For a saltier flavor at the table, gomashio which includes roasted sea salt may be added. Shio-kombu, wakame powder, and umeboshi plums or umeboshi paste are also salty and may be consumed from time to time.

Nutritional and Health Benefits

Garnishes and condiments provide nutritional and energetic balance to the meal. Like salt, oil, and other seasonings, they are a key ingredient in macrobiotic food preparation. Regular lack of a certain taste in cooking can lead to poor health as well as lack of appetite, binging, and other manifestations of imbalance. Consuming condiments in excessive amounts can also lead to disharmony. The frequency and amount of condiments consumed may need to be adjusted frequently to take into account the changing seasons, personal health, and other conditions.

Among regular condiments, gomashio is especially nutritious. It contains a high amount of calcium, iron, and other nutrients and is an excellent way to obtain polyunsaturated vegetable-quality oil in whole form. Also, because they are roasted, the sesame seeds in gomashio are easier to digest. The roasted salt with which they are combined provides a harmonious balance to the oil in the seeds.

In macrobiotic home cares, condiments have many further medicinal uses and may be recommended for consumption over a period of time to help balance specific conditions. In addition to the regular condiments listed in this chapter, there are many others that are made at these times for healing purposes.

Beverages

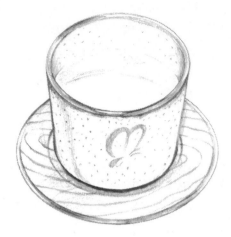

Daily Use

The Standard Macrobiotic Diet includes various beverages for daily, regular, or occasional consumption. The frequency and amount of beverage intake vary according to the individual's personal condition and needs as well as the climate, season, and other environmental factors. Generally, it is advisable to drink comfortably when thirsty and to avoid icy cold drinks. For daily consumption during or in-between meals, commonly consumed beverages include clear, clean spring water or well water, bancha twig and bancha stem teas, roasted cereal grain teas or cereal grain coffee, and other traditionally used and commonly consumed nonstimulant, nonaromatic natural teas made from seeds, leaves, stems, bark, or roots.

History

Throughout history, human communities have evolved around or near sources of good quality water for cooking and drinking. In addition to plain water, a variety of beverages has been traditionally prepared from cereal grains, beans, fruits, vegetables, sea vegetables, and other plants. Tea, originally native to China, has become popular throughout the world. Drinks made from roasted rice, millet, or barley, as well as sea vegetables have also been enjoyed in the Far East since ancient times. In the Middle East and Europe, mineral waters, beer brewed from barley and other grains, and wine, apple cider, and other drinks made from fermented fruit have been staples. In the Americas, beverages made from corn, roasted coffee beans, cacti, and other native plants have been commonly prepared to relieve thirst and contribute satisfaction to the meal.

Quality and Varieties

Water

A source of good quality water is essential for daily cooking and drinking. *Natural spring water* or *deep well water* that is moving and alive (charged with natural electromagnetic energy from the environment) is best. *Municipal tap water* often contains chemical additives such as the disinfectant chlorine, as well as pesticide residues, detergents, nitrates, and heavy metals such as lead. There are several mechanical methods used to filter tap water of impurities, but it is still less preferable to natural spring water that comes up to the earth before it is bottled or clear well water drawn from an underground vein. The natural mineral content of spring water or well water varies considerably. Usually *hard water* containing more minerals is preferred for drinking, while *soft water* containing less minerals is used primarily for washing. Bottled spring waters differ widely in quality, and changing brands may improve the energy and taste of foods and beverages. Spring water may often be ordered in large 5-gallon containers and be delivered directly to the house or be purchased at the natural foods store in 2½-gallon or 1-gallon plastic containers.

Apart from regular spring water, bottled *mineral water* is available in the natural foods store. This sparkling, effervescent water has either natural bubbles or bubbles induced by carbonation. Mineral water is not recommended for regular consumption but may be enjoyed occasionally at parties instead of alcohol or soft drinks. The less carbonated ones and those without additives are preferred. *Distilled water*, from which the minerals have been removed, is stale, low in nutrients, and without energy and is avoided in the macrobiotic kitchen.

Tea

The tea bush grows in China, Japan, India, Ceylon, and other parts of Asia. Bancha tea, green tea, and black tea all come from the same plant but differ widely in their energy, nutrients, and effects. Tea may be made from the buds, leaves, twigs, or stems of the tea plant. The season when these parts of the tea shrub are harvested and the manner in which they are processed determine the quality of the tea.

1. **Bancha Tea.** Bancha tea is picked in midsummer from the large and mature leaves, stems, and twigs of the tea bush. These are called respectively bancha leaf tea, bancha stem tea, and bancha twig tea. Traditionally picked by hand in the high mountains, the bancha leaves, stems, and twigs are roasted and cooled up to four separate times in large iron caldrons. This procedure, as well as the late harvest when the caffeine has naturally receded from the tea bush, makes for a tea containing virtually no caffeine or tannin, especially in the stem and twig parts. Also, unlike other teas which are acidic, bancha is slightly alkaline and thus has a soothing, beneficial effect on digestion, blood quality, and the

mind. It is entirely safe for even infants and small children to drink. In most macrobiotic households, bancha tea is the most commonly consumed beverage, usually served after every meal and in-between meals. Although customarily drunk plain, it may be prepared with a drop of tamari soy sauce, umeboshi plum, or other ingredients for medicinal use or occasionally sweetened with apple cider or a touch of rice syrup if desired. Bancha twig tea is also known as *kukicha tea*, from the Japanese words for "twig tea." Because of some linguistic confusion, green tea sold in the United States and Canada is sometimes mistakenly labeled as bancha. In Europe, bancha tea is often sold under the name "three-years' tea," signifying that the bushes are three years or older.

  2. Green tea. Green tea comes from the early green leaves of the tea bush. It is picked in the late spring and processed by an elaborate method of steaming and rolling. Brought to Japan from China by Zen Buddhists, a thick green tea known as *matcha* become the basis for the Japanese tea ceremony. The higher grades of green tea are prepared from the first, tender young leaves of the plant and contain more caffeine than the harder grades, which are picked later in the season. The naturally bitter taste of green tea goes well with pickles or mildly sweet snacks and is occasionally prepared in place of bancha tea. Good quality green tea is available in the macrobiotic natural foods store.

  3. Black Tea. Black tea, the most popular tea in the West, is prepared from tea leaves that have been fermented, highly processed, and often dyed. It is high in caffeine and tannin, the reddish substance which gives black tea its strong, astringent taste. Also known as *red-leaf tea*, it comes in many types, blends, grades, and flavors including Orange Pekoe and Souchong. There is another type of fermented tea called *oolong tea*, which is made from a combination of black and green tea leaves. It is usually scented with gardenia or jasmine. Black and oolong teas are generally avoided in macrobiotic cooking because of their strong stimulant effects and usual processing with chemicals and other artificial ingredients for conventional commercial purposes.

Roasted Grain Tea

A delicious, calming beverage can be made by roasting whole cereal grains and preparing them like ordinary tea. *Roasted barley tea*, or *mugi-cha* as it is known in Japan, is very cooling to the body and commonly enjoyed during the hotter weather. *Roasted brown rice tea* has a unique nutty flavor. Other grain teas, such as millet tea, oat tea, and buckwheat tea, may also be made in this way. All whole grain teas are suitable for daily use. For variety, they may be mixed with bancha tea in various proportions.

Grain Coffee

Grain coffee provides a nourishing alternative to regular coffee or decaffeinated coffee which is usually processed with chemicals. Grain coffee may be prepared at home from roasted grains, beans, and chicory. George Ohsawa created a popular grain coffee known as *yannoh* made from roasted and ground brown rice, wheat, azuki beans, chick-peas, and chicory root. A variety of grain coffees is available in the macrobiotic natural foods store. Those made with 100 percent cereal grains, wild grasses, beans, and other vegetable-quality ingredients and containing no honey, molasses, or other strong sweeteners and fruit powders are suitable for occasional consumption.

Umeboshi Tea

Umeboshi tea, made from boiling pitted umeboshi plums in spring water, has a nice sour taste. It is very cooling to the body and in summer helps prevent loss of minerals through perspiration. It is generally served cool, though may also be warmed up.

Sea Vegetable Tea

A calm, soothing tea can be prepared by steeping a small strip of kombu, wakame, or other sea vegetable in hot water.

Corn Silk Tea

The yellow silk strands of fresh corn, when simmered in hot water, make a mellow, soothing tea. Enjoyed traditionally by Native American people, silk strand tea is especially beneficial to the heart and kidneys.

Mu Tea

Mu tea is a beverage prepared from either nine or sixteen herbs. It is slightly sweet tasting and very strong. Used originally for medicinal purposes, Mu tea may also be taken from time to time in the colder months to increase strength and vitality. Mu tea contains a small amount of ginseng, an extremely contractive herb that is ordinarily not used in macrobiotic food preparation. However, George Ohsawa, who originally devised Mu tea from traditional Oriental herbal teas, especially those used for the health of women, felt that the other herbs in Mu tea balanced its otherwise extreme energy. In the case of Mu #9 these include peony root, Japanese parsley root, hoelen, cinnamon, licorice, peach kernels, gingerroot, and rhemannia. In addition to these ingredients, Mu #16 also contains mandarin orange peel, cnicus, atractylis, cypress, cloves, moutan and coptis. Mu tea is available prepackaged in most macrobiotic natural foods stores. In serving, it is sometimes sweetened with a little apple juice or rice syrup.

Herbal Tea

In addition to Mu tea, there are a variety of other herbal teas that may be prepared for variety or enjoyment from time to time. These are made from the flowers, leaves, stems, or roots of various plants. Mild tasting ingredients such as dandelion root, burdock root, and lotus root are more suitable than those with a stimulant, aromatic, or fragrant effect such as peppermint, chamomile, or hot, spicy teas.

Juice

Juice made from fresh fruits or vegetables is occasionally enjoyed within the Standard Macrobiotic Diet. However, since juice is a very concentrated product, requiring many fruits or vegetables to prepare a single glassful, it is used very sparingly and in small amounts. Apple juice or apple cider is the most balanced of the fruit juices, though other temperate-climate fruit juice such as grape juice, pear juice, apricot juice, cranberry juice, and others may also be prepared. In the macrobiotic natural foods store, a variety of unsweetened fruit juices is available. Those that are organic, unfiltered, and not made from concentrates are the best quality. Carrot juice, celery juice, beet juice, and juice from leafy green vegetables may also be enjoyed now and then. In addition to their raw nature, which makes them harder to digest than cooked beverages, juices are often prepared with highly mechanized equipment or home juicers that pulverize the ingredients, creating very fragmented energy.

Amazaké

Amazaké, made from fermented sweet rice, is a delicious beverage that is enjoyed hot or chilled. Its thick, delicious taste and strong energy are traditionally beneficial to nursing mothers, babies, and others requiring strength and vitality. It may also be used as a sweetener for pies, cakes, puddings, and breadstuffs. Amazaké may be made at home with rice *koji*, an inoculated grain starter, or it may be purchased in pint or quart containers in macrobiotic natural foods stores. It is often served with a little fresh grated ginger or sliced seasonal fruit such as strawberries or blueberries.

Soy Milk

Soy milk, has traditionally been enjoyed as a beverage in the Far East and is becoming increasingly popular in the West. Several naturally processed soy milks are now available in the natural foods store. Those containing pearl barley, barley malt, and other grain or vegetable-quality ingredients, as well as a small amount of sea salt or sea vegetables as a mineral source, are preferable to those containing honey, chocolate, carob, or other strong sweeteners. Because of its concentrated nature, soy milk is recommended only occasionally and in small amounts. For those in transition from cow's milk and other dairy foods, it may be used more frequently.

Alcoholic Beverages

Light alcoholic beverages that have been naturally fermented and prepared with high-quality ingredients may be enjoyed, if desired, at parties, on holidays, and on other special occasions. Most commercially available beer, wine, saké, and other alcoholic beverages contain sugar and other highly refined ingredients as well as preservatives, artificial coloring, and other chemical additives. For example, the U.S. Department of Agriculture currently allows fifty-two unlisted additives to be included by commercial beer manufacturers including tannin and enzymes to chill the beer, calcium, disodium, ethylene, diamine-tetra-acetate to prevent gushing, propylene glycol alginate to stabilize the foam, and caramel and three coal tar dyes for artificial coloring.

Mild alcoholic beverages with more naturally fermented quality are preferred, such as brown rice saké (the traditional rice wine of Japan), unsweetened grape or plum wine, and beer made without additives or other harmful ingredients. Hard liquor is generally avoided in macrobiotic food gatherings.

Other Beverages

Other beverages that are traditionally prepared and commonly consumed may also be used. Burdock tea, dandelion tea, clove tea, peony tea, and others are included.

Cooking Methods

Besides drinking fresh water, in macrobiotic food preparation well water or spring water is sometimes heated and allowed to cool to room temperature prior to drinking. This process makes it slightly stronger and more soothing to the digestive system.

There are several traditional methods of preparing tea as explained in classic Chinese and Japanese tea books. The simplest is to place several teaspoons of twigs, stems, or leaves in a quart of water, bring to a boil, reduce the flame to low, and simmer several minutes. The longer the tea steeps, the darker and stronger it will become. In macrobiotic kitchens, a large pot of bancha tea is often left to simmer on top of a flame deflector and taken as needed. Fresh twigs may be added to replenish old ones, and old ones also may be reused several times before they lose their strength. A variety of tea kettles made of glass, ceramic, cast-iron, or stainless steel are all suitable for making tea. Because fresh tea is extremely sensitive to its environment and picks up other scents and odors, it should be kept tightly covered in a jar or tin container until needed.

Nutritional and Health Benefits

Up to 80 percent of our blood, other bodily fluids, tissues, and organs consist of water. The quality, volume, and frequency of the liquids we drink are very important factors in our everyday health and vitality. Modern people tend to overconsume beverages of all kinds as well as drink too much milk, soft drinks, fruit juices, and other extreme or highly concentrated fare because of overeating in general, especially the overconsumption of foods rich in animal-quality protein, fat, and minerals, together with foods with high amounts of simple sugars. Stimulant beverages, such as coffee, black tea, and cola drinks, are particularly harmful and have been linked with a wide range of physical and mental disorders including fibrocystic disease, irregular heartbeat, and others.

In addition to helping decompose food substances and facilitating digestion and absorption, liquid forms a natural balance to salt and other minerals in our bodies, and either too much liquid or poor quality liquid can have a detrimental effect on all organs and systems, especially the kidneys and urinary tract. On the other hand, a restriction in liquid intake is also dangerous because it creates dehydration resulting in overall weakness, exhaustion, loss of appetite and energy, as well as contracting the body systems and slowing down metabolism.

In an era of polluted rivers and streams, acid rain, and toxic chemicals and nuclear wastes, finding a source of clean, good quality water is not always easy. For ordinary everyday consumption, bancha twig tea is the most soothing drink. The twig is high in calcium, iron, and complex carbohydrates as well as vitamin A, thiamine, riboflavin, niacin, and vitamin C. When it is boiled or simmered in water, some of these nutrients melt in the tea liquid. Although some of its nutritional elements are reduced by cooking, bancha twig tea can help to decompose and digest whole grains, vegetables, beans, sea vegetables, and other foods generally recommended in the diet. In most traditional cultures, spirit is associated with living waters. A return to clear natural spring water or well water for farming, gardening, cooking, and drinking tea and other beverages is essential for securing the future development of humanity.

Part 3

The Effectiveness of
the Macrobiotic Diet

Principles of Macrobiotic Cooking

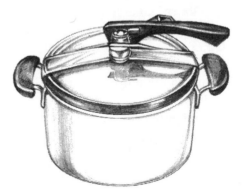

Quality of Foods

In selecting food it is important to obtain the freshest and highest quality natural foods. Growing one's own grains and vegetables is ideal, and many macrobiotic families also make their own miso, tofu, seitan, and bread at home from whole foods. For many other households, however, especially those in a modern urban environment, gardening, farming, and natural food processing at home is impractical, and the local macrobiotic natural foods store, health food store, farmers market, or coop will be the primary source of their daily food.

Applied to food, the word *natural* means food that is whole and contains no artificial ingredients and food that is unprocessed or minimally processed by natural methods. These include cutting, grinding, drying, or pulping, removal of edible substances, and sufficient processing to make the food ready for consumption or cooking. The term *organic*, when further applied to natural foods, is understood to mean food that is grown in soil treated only with organic materials and containing no artificial or synthetic fertilizers, herbicides, pesticides, or other chemicals during food production. Many suppliers have been certified by an organic growers' association, which makes on-site inspections, performs lab tests on soil and product samples, and offers educational guidance to farmers and consumers. While there are no uniform standards for the country as a whole, many of these associations require a minimum of three or more consecutive years of untreated soil for food to qualify as organic. Standards of water quality, air quality, and quality of organic plant starters and natural fertilizers vary considerably. Thus selecting a store to shop at regularly that maintains high standards of natural quality is essential. Whole grains, beans, seeds and nuts, and other nonperishable goods are also available through mail-order from several macrobiotic suppliers.

Organic food is far superior to chemically grown food and should be obtained whenever possible. As noted in the chapter on nutritional value, laboratory tests by scientists at Rutgers University found that inorganic produce contained as little as 25 percent of the nutrients of organic produce, including calcium, magnesium, potassium, sodium, iron, manganese, copper, and other minerals and trace elements.

The harmful effects of chemical fertilizers and pesticides have been more widely recognized in recent years. For example, in 1984 the Environmental Protection Agency restricted the use of alachlor, the nation's most heavily used herbicide, after studies showed it caused tumors in laboratory animals and could threaten human health. Other studies have found that dependence on chemicals for the eradication of crop pests are producing strains of disease-resistent insects and rodents, including immune cockroaches, malaria-bearing mosquitoes, and "super rats" that thrive on rat poison. Between 1970 and 1980 the number of harmful insect species immune to one or more pesticides almost doubled.

Organic foods, however, are not always available, nor can they always be afforded because of their slightly higher price. In this case, the next best available product should be obtained such as "ecologically" or "naturally" grown food cultivated in soil that is in transition to becoming fully organic or treated with a minimum of additives. Inorganic produce should be thoroughly cleaned and properly cooked to reduce potentially harmful pesticide residues and other chemical sprays. Adding a little sea salt to washing and rinsing water can help neutralize these substances.

For better health and vitality, it is preferable to avoid or drastically reduce consumption of all chemically and industrially mass-produced foods including instant foods, canned foods, frozen foods, refined grains or flours, sprayed foods, dyed foods, irradiated foods, and all foods containing chemical additives, preservatives, stabilizers, emulsifiers, and artificial coloring.

Quality of Water and Fire

The quality of the water and fire with which we cook is a matter of supreme importance. A regular source of clean, clear natural spring water or well water is essential for both cooking and for drinking. Municipal tap water that has been chlorinated, fluoridated, or otherwise chemicalized is usually unsuitable for daily drinking and cooking, as is distilled water from which all the minerals have been removed, leaving a stale, lifeless liquid.

The use of fire for cooking is unique to the human species and developed during the ice age. Fire gives energy, vitalizing the physical, mental, and spiritual functions. It is the foundation of human culture and civilization. Over the centuries, however, fire for cooking, technology, and warfare has been misused, and today modern civilization has developed completely artificial forms of energy. Food cooked with electrical heat and microwave radiation retains less harmonious energy and nutrients than food cooked with gas, wood, or other renewable fuels. Electrical heat not only produces excessive electromagnetic charges in the surrounding atmosphere but also is very hard to adjust for delicate cooking and produces irregular energy in the food, contributing to lowered vitality and fragmented thinking. Microwave, which steps up the vibration of the food even more than electric, creates the most chaotic cooking and potentially elevates susceptibility to various degenerative conditions including some forms of cancer.

Wood heat gives the most peaceful, steady source of heat and the most delicious tasting food. However, in a modern urban home, wood is not always practical.

Gas heat is the next best fuel source, providing a clean, even, easily controllable flame. Coal, charcoal, and other renewable fuels are also suitable. Macrobiotic counselors report that the vast majority of cancer patients they met have used electrical stoves, hot plates, or microwave ovens for a long period, and when they change to gas or wood they usually experience immediate improvement in their cooking, the taste of their food, and their energy levels. A small portable propane gas stove for home, office, or traveling can be used in the absence of a more permanent appliance.

Proportion of Cooked and Raw Food

In general, the application of heat—or cooking—energizes food and makes it more digestible. However, the frequency, type, and amount of heat, as well as the proportion of cooked to raw food consumed, significantly affects individual health, consciousness, and behavior. In modern society, food is commonly prepared with extreme cooking methods and in extreme proportions. Meat is grilled, roasted, or subjected to other intensive heating, as are stews and other animal food preparations. Meanwhile, grain and flour products are prepared primarily in hard, baked form, while most vegetable side dishes are overcooked by boiling in large quantities of water or by baking. To balance this heavy, overcooked food, raw salads are customarily served at lunch and dinner, and large amounts of fresh fruit and fruit juice are periodically consumed.

In traditional societies, where whole grains and vegetables are eaten and animal food is consumed in small amounts, a much smaller proportion of raw vegetables and fruits is commonly consumed. Even in hot tropical regions of India and Africa, people cook a majority of daily vegetables and often trek long distances for firewood or other fuel because they intuitively know that cooked food is essential to health and vitality.

In the past, some modern nutritionists expressed concern that cooking, especially long-time boiling, destroys or diminishes some of the nutrients in certain foods. However, lighter cooking methods, including blanching, short-time boiling, steaming, and stir-frying, which are traditionally used in the Far East and in macrobiotic cooking largely retain these nutritional elements. Recent scientific studies, moreover, have begun to identify some of the nutritional benefits of cooking. For example, many legumes, beans, and seeds, including soybeans, peas, and peanuts, contain protease inhibitors that block the action of enzymes necessary to digest protein. Cooking inactivates these inhibitors, allowing the protein to be properly digested. Similarly, nutritional studies have found that, in raw form, cabbage, broccoli, Brussels sprouts, kale, turnips, rutabaga, cauliflower, and some other garden vegetables contain nutrients that interfere with the ability of the thyroid gland to acquire iodine. Lightly cooking these foods makes the iodine available to the thyroid.

In macrobiotic food prepartion, food is served in many styles, ranging from well cooked to moderately and lightly cooked to raw and uncooked. In general, about two-thirds of the daily volume of vegetables consumed each day in a temperate

232 of the Macrobiotic Diet

environment is cooked and about one-third is consumed raw, including fresh salad, marinated or pressed salad, or pickles. A slightly higher percentage of raw vegetables and other uncooked food is prepared in tropical or subtropical regions. Similarly, nuts and seeds are preferably lightly roasted before eating, and fruits are more digestible cooked, though they also may be enjoyed occasionally unheated, in moderate volume.

Use of Salt and Oil

Salt and oil are also central to cooking and play an often overlooked role in shaping human destiny. Good quality unrefined sea salt that is high in minerals and trace elements is essential to human health and development. Modern refined table salt from which most of the compounds and trace elements other than sodium chloride have been removed and to which iodine, dextrose, and other chemicals have been added is a poor substitute. Similarly, unrefined vegetable-quality cooking oils are far superior to refined oils and fats of either animal or plant origin. In macrobiotic cooking, dark sesame oil is generally preferred for everyday cooking, though light sesame oil, corn oil, and mustard seed oil are also used regularly. Other unrefined vegetable oils are used occasionally.

Salt and oil form a natural balance, and their proper use can transform the energy, taste, and texture of foods. Generally, salt is more contractive (yang), while oil is more expansive (yin). With experience, the macrobiotic cook learns to adjust salt and oil according to changing climatic conditions, the season of the year, age and level of activity of family members, and other factors. Generally, much smaller amounts of both salt and oil are used in macrobiotic cooking than in conventional modern cooking, and for better digestion both ingredients are preferably consumed in cooked form rather than eaten raw. (Their use is described in detail in the chapter on salt, oil, and other seasonings.)

Use of Pressure, Time, and Drying

The quality of food can also be changed by the application of pressure, time, and drying. The use of pressure in pressure-cooking, in making pressed salad, and in pickling gives foods more contractive (yang) energy. Longer cooking time in general, baking, and preserving foods by natural means such as drying fruits and vegetables in the sun or wind also makes for more yang fare, through dehydration and contraction. Conversely, foods that are consumed raw or cooked rapidly with plenty of water are generally more expansive (yin). Quick cooking methods include *ohitashi*-style boiling, steaming, and stir-frying.

Quality of Utensils

High quality cookware and utensils will improve the flavor and taste of food, as well as make for more nourishing and satisfying meals. Natural materials such as wood, glass, ceramic, or earthenware and metals such as cast-iron, stainless steel, or enamelized stainless steel that do not interact with food and alter their qualities are recommended. Plastic, teflon, and other synthetic materials, as well as aluminum and asbestos, are preferably avoided. For daily cooking, hand methods of preparation that give more calm, peaceful energy such as the traditional Japanese mortar known as a *suribachi*, a hand mill, and a hand grinder are superior to electric blenders, electric mills, and electric food processors. For parties and other special occasions when an extra large amount of food is prepared, modern time-saving appliances may be used. Proper care of pots and pans, sharpening of knives, and a clean, orderly kitchen will give utensils a longer life and make for more enjoyable cooking.

Preparing and Serving Food

Cooking with simple ingredients is the key to producing meals that are nutritious, tasty, satisfying, and attractive. The cook has the ability to change the quality of the food and thereby influence directly the health and consciousness of the family. Longer cooking, the use of pressure, salt, heat, and time make the energy of food more concentrated. Quick cooking and less salt preserves the lighter qualities of the food. The cook's own consciousness also directly affects the quality of the meal. A calm, peaceful mind is important while preparing and serving food. All internal and external distractions should be put aside during this time.

In general, prior to cooking, sliced foods should be kept separate from each other rather than being mixed to avoid premature interchange of quality. During the cooking process, foods should be allowed to mix themselves as much as possible rather than be frequently mixed and stirred. Excessive use of fire, water, pressure, and time, as well as the excessive use of salt, oil, and other seasoning, should be avoided. The taste of the seasoning should not be evident but should only be used to bring out and enhance the natural taste of the food itself which should predominate.

The same style of cooking and the same type of dish should not be repeated too often. It is preferable to alternate the type of food, change the style of cooking, and vary cutting methods often to prevent meals from becoming repetitive, stale, and uninteresting. However, novelty for its own sake should also be avoided. Meals should always reflect an understanding of the Order of the Universe and maintain harmony with the changing climate, seasons, and personal needs.

Food should be prepared as fresh as possible for each meal and leftovers minimized. Some foods such as leftover rice and noodles are even better the next day boiled, steamed, or fried. However, others such as miso soup and most vegetable dishes rapidly lose their energy after the first day. Whole foods should be used as much as possible. Whole brown rice and whole wheat berries, for example, give centering, more complete energy than brown rice flour, whole wheat flour, cracked wheat, couscous, or other grain products. Hard baked flour products, in particular, are mucus-forming and hard to digest and should not be prepared too frequently.

Meals should offer a full range of tastes. Whole grains and vegetables are naturally sweet, and sea salt, miso, and tamari soy sauce usually provide a salty base

Dietary Modifications and Adjustments

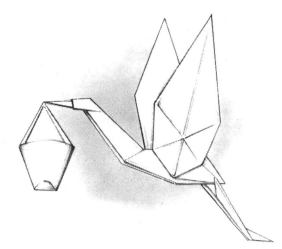

The standard macrobiotic dietary guidelines offer wide latitude for individual choice and variation among normally healthy persons. However, further modifications and adjustments may need to be made according to changing seasonal conditions, as well as the age, sex, and level of activity of family members.

Adjustments According to Seasonal Change

In the temperate regions of the world, the seasons alternate from warm to hot to cool to cold. Just as plants and animals change their qualities and characteristics according to the change in season, so human beings also should adapt to their changing environment. In the past, traditional societies observed seasonal order by eating fresh food in the months or season during which it grew or preserving it over the year with natural methods such as pickling, drying, and smoking. Today, however, advances in transportation, refrigeration, and artificial preservation methods have made it possible to consume any and all kinds of foods year-round. The result has been declining health and vitality as well as the disruption of local ecosystems. If we eat summer products such as yellow squash, strawberries, and cantaloupe in the winter season, we lose our adaptability to the immediate environment. Along with eating food from another climate altogether, eating unseasonal food is a major cause of modern illness. In macrobiotic cooking and food preparation, we adjust our cooking slightly with each season to harmonize changing energy patterns within the body with those in the external environment.

In spring, for example, the energy within our bodies, as within the earth, begins to thaw after the long winter. To assist this process, we begin to use spring foods with upward energy such as sprouts, leafy green vegetables, wild grasses, and types of wheat and barley that have matured over the winter. In addition, we begin to use lighter cooking methods such as steaming, quick boiling, and light sautéing. The amount of salt, miso, tamari soy sauce, and other seasonings may be reduced slightly, and proportionately more short-time pickles and other fermented foods may be prepared.

In summer, nature's energy reaches a zenith as plants ripen in the hot sun. At this time of year, we include more foods in our diet that have active, expansive energy such as leafy green vegetables, sweet corn, summer squashes, and locally grown fruits. More fresh salads are usually served, including vegetable, grain, noodle, and fruit salads, as well as marinated, pressed, and lightly boiled salads. Umeboshi plums, umeboshi tea, and other condiments are often taken to supply minerals that are lost through perspiration in hot weather. While it is preferably to avoid serving foods icy cold at any time, during the summer dishes such as somen or udon noodles may be served cool or chilled. Sushi, kanten, vegetable aspics, fresh cucumbers, fresh melons, and tofu prepared with various garnishes are also very cooling and enjoyable. In general, cooking can be lighter and seasoning can be reduced.

In the autumn, as the atmospheric energy begins to flow downward and recede into the earth, our bodies also begin to contract. At this time we can begin to adjust our diets by including more early fall squashes and root vegetables, hard leafy greens that are often harvested in autumn such as daikon greens, cabbages, and other seasonal produce. Onions, turnips, and other round vegetables may also be served slightly more frequently during this period. Colds, coughs, and other symptoms are often experienced during the autumn as a result of excessive intake of fruits, raw foods, liquids, and salty snack items ingested in the summertime. Slightly stronger cooking methods such as *nishime*-style boiling, long-time sautéing, and *kinpira*-style braising and slightly more salt, miso, tamari soy sauce, or other seasoning can help to discharge this excess as well as help the body adjust to a cooler environment. Slightly more oil can also be used in cooking, and this helps insulate the body during the cooler weather. As the fall weather becomes colder, more rich tasting food can be introduced into the daily menu such as fried or deep-fried foods, grain stews, sweet rice and mochi, bean stews, and thick soups. Longer, more slowly cooked dishes can also be prepared with vegetables cut in larger slices and chunks than during the warmer months. Sea vegetable dishes can become stronger and include more root vegetables, dried tofu, and tempeh. Raw foods can be reduced in the menu and dried or cooked fruits, as well as sweet-tasting autumn squashes, used more often to prepare desserts.

In winter, the energy in the earth is usually frozen and that in the atmosphere is usually watery. Similarly, the energy in the body is very contracted or floating and needs to be sustained by warm, strong food. At this season, cold, cool, and raw foods should be minimized, while slightly more salt, miso, and tamari soy sauce, as well as slightly more oil, can be used in cooking. Deep-fried foods, tempura, long sautéed or *kinpira*-style vegetables, and strong sea vegetable dishes can be served more frequently. Fried noodle and fried rice dishes are very warming, as are strong miso soup and different kinds of vegetable, bean, grain, and seitan stews. *Nishime* dishes, *oden* dishes, and baked dishes can be prepared more often, and fresh grated ginger is used more liberally at this season as a seasoning or garnish to stimulate circulation. Vegetables consist primarily of winter squashes, burdock, daikon, carrots, onions, and other root and ground vegetables that keep well over the winter, as well as pickles that have aged slightly longer and are of greater strength. Sweet rice and mochi are very warming at this time of year and can be used in soups, stews, and as side dishes.

Dietary Adjustments for Man and Woman

While men and women and boys and girls generally eat the same type of food, slight differences in the amount of food consumed and in the proportion of various foods have been observed in traditional societies. Generally, females have smaller and more compact (more yang) constitutions than males and require slightly lighter (more yin) food and cooking methods. Lighter dishes such as salads, fruits, and raw foods are prepared a little more often for women, and they can enjoy sweets and desserts more frequently than men. Ideally, it is preferable for women, who are already yang by nature, to consume a minimum of animal-quality food, which is extremely yang. However, a little white-meat fish or seafood can be taken occasionally if desired. Also, the total volume of food consumed is usually less for women than for men.

Conversely, boys and men are generally bigger and more expanded (more yin) than women and require slightly heavier (more yang) food and cooking methods. They also tend to eat more food and enjoy a wider variety of main dishes. Seitan, tempeh, stews, casseroles, and other strong, dynamic dishes can be prepared more frequently for males, seasoning may be slightly stronger, and raw food, fresh salad, fruit, sweets, and desserts slightly reduced. Fish and seafood may be prepared several times a week if desired.

Dietary Adjustments for Menstruation and Pregnancy

During menstruation, girls and women must be very careful to avoid extreme foods of all kinds. To prevent menstrual cramps and heavy discharges, animal food, salty food, an excessive amount of fruit, and desserts should be avoided or reduced. During pregnancy, it is essential that the woman eat well, since her condition will largely determine the future health and vitality of her child. At this time, once again, all excessively yin or yang foods should be avoided, though a good variety of foods and dishes should be prepared, and the use of tobacco and alcohol is discouraged. If cravings arise, good-quality natural foods may be eaten in greater amounts than usual to satisfy the desire for a sour, bitter, sweet, pungent, or salty taste. Also, for pregnant or lactating mothers, amazaké sweet rice, and mochi are traditionally eaten to provide warmth and energy. *Koi-koku* (carp and burdock soup) is also recommended in small amounts eaten occasionally during this time to give strength and vitality.

Adjustments for Babies and Children

The ideal food for babies is mother's milk, and all of the infant's nourishment may come from this source for about the first six to ten months. At this age, the amount of breast milk can begin to be reduced over the next six months while soft foods are introduced and gradually increased. When the baby's first molars begin to appear, usually around twelve to fourteen months, mother's milk can be stopped and soft mashed foods constitute the baby's entire diet.

The principal soft food given to infants in macrobiotic cooking is a cereal grain milk prepared from brown rice, sweet brown rice, and barley whose nutrients and sweet taste approximates mother's milk, to which sometimes barley malt, rice syrup, or amazaké can be added. It is also sometimes cooked with 1 or 2 percent roasted and mashed sesame seeds. A small volume of kombu may also be cooked together with the cereal grain milk to provide minerals but it may be taken out prior to serving. (This grain milk can also be used as a substitute for breast milk if the mother is unable to lactate.) After five months old, babies may also be given special rice cream, soup consisting of well mashed vegetables, the juice from cooked vegetables, and whole vegetables such as carrots, cabbage, winter squash, onions, daikon, and Chinese cabbage that have been well boiled or steamed and thoroughly mashed.

At about one year of age, harder foods such as well-cooked grains, beans, and vegetables may gradually be introduced and by about two years of age mostly replace softer foods. A square of kombu is often included in cereal grain milk and cooked with other foods at an early age but usually taken out before serving. A tiny amount of very soft, well mashed kombu or a touch of nori, arame, or hijiki may be given to babies, but sea vegetable side dishes are usually not introduced until about one and a half to two years of age.

Since babies are very yang (small and compact) they do not initially require any salt. Before ten months of age, no salt, miso, or tamari soy sauce is usually given to babies in macrobiotic households, though kombu which is high in minerals may be cooked in with the food in small volume and taken out prior to serving. After about ten months of age, only a tiny amount of salt or other seasoning is introduced for flavoring. By the beginning of the third year, a child can receive about one-fourth to one-third the amount of salt used by an adult. Seasoning can then gradually be increased until age seven or eight when it can be the same as for adults and older children, except for salty condiments and seasonings. Until this time, it is the usual practice for young children's and adults' food to be cooked together, but before the final seasoning is added for the adults' portion the children's portion is taken out and served separately. Common dishes may also be seasoned minimally, and older children and adults may add additional seasoning at the table with gomashio and other condiments. A less salty gomashio is usually prepared separately for children. In general, young and elementary school children should not be given too much tempeh, seitan, tofu, and other foods high in salt or sodium. However, moderate volumes of these foods, prepared very softly, may be given from time to time.

Fruit may be given to babies and infants, preferably in cooked and mashed form, in small volume and occasionally. In some cases, cooked apples or apple juice may be given temporarily to adjust for certain conditions. Short-term, lightly seasoned pickles may be introduced at about age five. For beverages, spring water or well water, preferably boiled and allowed to cool to room temperature, bancha twig tea, cereal grain tea, or other traditionally prepared and commonly consumed nonstimulant beverage may be served regularly. Apple juice and amazaké may also be served in moderate volume from time to time.

Dietary Adjustments for Personal Needs

The kinds, amount, and proportion of daily foods may also need to be adjusted to take into account varying activity levels. Persons who work outdoors, do heavy labor, or are physically active generally require stronger cooking, more volume of food, and more variety in their meals than persons who work indoors and are more mentally active. For physically active persons, daily food can be prepared with slightly stronger and longer cooking methods, slightly more salt, miso, and other seasoning, and slightly more oil. Foods such as buckwheat, soba noodles, burdock, and jinenjo mountain potato are very energizing and may be served more often, as well as fried noodles, fried rice, tempeh, seitan, fish and seafood, and deep-fried and tempura-style foods. Slightly more root vegetables and hard leafy greens can also be prepared, as well as long-time, often lightly spiced, pickles.

Persons who work indoors or are more mentally active such as writers, artists, and teachers usually require lighter or more moderate cooking and need to keep well within the standard guidelines. Strong supplemental foods such as fish and seafood, fried foods, fruits, nuts and nut butters, juice, herbal teas, and other stimulants should be carefully controlled and avoided, reduced, or taken only in small volume. In general, the total amount of food consumed is less for more sedentary persons and the cooking should not be too salty. Proportionately more round vegetables may be included, and vegetables may be prepared often nishime-style. Boiled salad is also recommended for those in this category. Sea vegetable dishes are especially important to center the mind, stabilize the emotions, and provide flexibility but should not be overconsumed. Slightly less beans and bean products are also advisable. For mental clarity and aesthetic appreciation thorough chewing is also essential.

Adjustments for Spiritual Development

Food governs all aspects of our growth and development, including those we traditionally call spiritual. While spiritual practice and understanding is inseparable from our daily life and manifests in our character, thoughts, words, and behavior, there are times when individuals or family members may wish to further refine their awareness and develop toward universal consciousness. At these times, meals should be completely of grain and vegetable quality and animal food strictly avoided. For improved meditation, prayer, and self-reflection, all spices, stimulants, and strong pungent foods such as garlic are traditionally discontinued. In general, daily food should be made of the simplest ingredients such as brown rice, miso soup, a small side dish of vegetables, beans and their products, sea vegetables, pickles, and tea. In addition to rice, millet, barley, and corn are good for opening the higher electromagnetic channels, or *chakras*, of the body and mind.

In many cultures, wild foods such as wild grasses, roots, pine nuts, berries, and other foraged foods are valued for spiritual development. However, because of their strong energy and unfamiliarity, they should be prepared only occasionally and in small volume by modern urban individuals. In general, the amount of food consumed can be less than usual. Fasting practiced for a short period or periodically one day a week or once a month is also traditionally observed to develop insight and awareness, as well as provide relief from physical and psychological disorders. In macrobiotic practice, fasts are sometimes taken during which only brown rice or other whole grains are eaten with a small amount of condiments and a comfortable volume of beverages for a period of seven to ten days. These grain fasts, during which each mouthful of food is chewed 100 to 150 times, are very energizing and are ideally undertaken under the guidance of an experienced macrobiotic family member, friend, or counselor. In any case, they should not be prolonged beyond that length of time or serious imbalance could result.

Adjustments for Old Age

We generally have less physical energy when we grow older and require more lightly cooked food, though still well-balanced and a good variety, as well as less volume of food and drink. Slightly less salt, miso, tamari soy sauce, and other seasonings are needed in cooking. Because we begin to lose some of our teeth, food may also be prepared a little softer to aid in chewing and digestion. One or two lightly sautéed dishes using good quality unrefined vegetable-quality oil may also be prepared daily to help circulation. However, for older persons who are chronically ill, oil may need to be avoided or reduced for a short period until the condition improves.

Another concern of the elderly is an adequate supply of calcium. Osteoporosis —a thinning of the bones that increases risk of fractures in the hip, forearm, and spine—is epidemic among middle-aged and older women and also common among older men. To remedy this, many people turn to milk, cheese, and other dairy foods that are high in calcium as well as high-protein foods in general that are said to be good for body construction and renewal. Recent medical studies, however, have shown that excess protein, principally from meat, poultry, cheese, eggs, and other dairy food, intensifies the loss of calcium in the urine and is probably the primary cause of osteoporosis and fractures in later life. Much better sources of calcium, contributing to maintenance and flexibility of bones and joints, as well as arteries and other blood vessels, are kale, collards, turnip greens, and other green leafy vegetables as well as hijiki, arame, and other sea vegetables.

In modern society, the health and activity level of older persons vary so greatly that few other general principles can be recommended, and each case needs to be considered individually.

Making the Transition to Macrobiotics

When starting the new way of eating, it is best to begin with just a few basic preparations, such as pressure-cooked brown rice, miso soup, a few vegetable dishes, bean dishes, one or two sea vegetables, and bancha twig tea. Then, day by day, week by week, the selection of macrobiotic natural foods can gradually be widened and new cooking styles can be introduced. In the meantime, some of the types of foods that have been consumed in the past can still be eaten, including proportionately more salad and fruit, flour products, and fish and seafood. Rather than eliminating certain categories of food from our diet, it is better to initially reduce their intake and then switch to a better quality of intermediate food until the mind and body have readjusted and a taste and appreciation for the new foods are developed.

During the transition period, cravings for some of the foods and beverages previously enjoyed may arise. Rather than suppress these natural urges, it is better to take a tiny volume of the accustomed food from time to time until such cravings diminish and finally go away, as they naturally will. During the transition time, the following table may serve as a guide in substituting better-quality foods for the previous items in the diet (see Table 20).

Table 20

Cravings	Replacement	Goal
Meat	Fish, seafood	Whole grains, beans, seitan, tofu, tempeh
Sugar, molasses, chocolate, carob, and other highly refined sweeteners	Maple syrup, honey	Rice syrup, barley malt, and ultimately natural sweeteners from grains and vegetables
Dairy food, cheese, milk, cream, butter	Organic dairy food, in small volume; nuts and nut butters; soy milk	Miso, natto, tofu, tempeh; seeds and seed butters, in small volume
Tropical and sub-tropical fruits and juices; artificial juices and beverages	Organic fruits and juices	Organic temperate-climate fruit (fresh, dried, and cooked) and cider or juice in season and in small volume
Coffee, black tea, soft drinks, diet drinks	Herbal teas, green tea, mineral water	Bancha twig tea, grain coffee, and other traditional nonstimulant, nonaromatic beverages

The Prevention and Relief of Disease

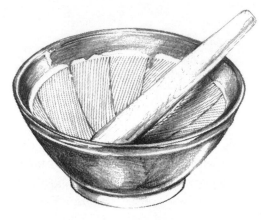

The macrobiotic approach to health is not limited to the relief and prevention of symptoms. It is equally concerned with educating people toward an understanding and practice of a way of life in harmony with the Order of the Universe. Health and happiness are the result of living in harmony with nature, while sickness is the consequence of acting, thinking, and living in a manner that is imbalanced or extreme (see Table 21). The most fundamental way of approaching sickness is to restore ourselves to a condition of harmony with our environment, and the most basic way of doing so is proper eating.

Table 21   A Holistic Approach to Disease

Way of Life	Healthy	Degenerate
Daily Food (primary factor)	Whole	Processed
	Natural	Artificial
	Organic	Chemical
	Unrefined	Refined
	Balanced	Extreme
	Seasonal	Unseasonal
	Locally Grown	Transcontinental
	Home-cooked	Pre-cooked
Environment and Life-style (contributing factor)	Clean	Polluted
	Orderly	Disorderly
	Active	Sedentary
	Real	Synthetic
Outlook (contributing factor)	Peaceful	Complaining
	Grateful	Arrogant
	Flexible	Rigid
	Cooperative	Competitive

If our daily food is in accord with our surroundings, our blood, cells, and tissues—and therefore our emotions, thoughts, and consciousness as well—will also be in accord. Harmony is created through the union of opposites: night and day, summer and winter, man and woman, as well as the balance of countless other complementary phenomena in the universe. Proper eating, combining yin and yang qualities or essential nutritional and energy factors in correct proportion, is essential to maintain physical and psychological health, and without a balanced diet sickness cannot be fundamentally cured.

Sickness is a natural mechanism by which our own bodies seek to restore balance if we continue to live in a disharmonious way. The repeated overconsumption of excessive dietary factors causes a variety of adjustment mechanisms in the organism which progressively develop toward more serious disorders. Since the body at all times seeks balance with the surrounding environment, the normal process is for this dietary excess to be eliminated through normal eliminatory channels, such as the urine, bowl movement, respiration, and perspiration.

After eating or drinking too much improper food, excess accumulates and is released through abnormal discharge mechanisms in the body such as diarrhea, excessive sweating, colds, coughs, fevers, and displays of strong emotions and behavior. Chronic discharge, the next stage in this process, often takes the form of skin diseases. These are particularly common in cases where the ability of the kidneys to properly cleanse the bloodstream has become weakened. If we continue to eat poorly, we eventually exhaust the body's ability to discharge, and an underlying layer of fat develops under the skin and in and around the inner organs which prevents discharge toward the surface of the body.

When it exceeds the body's capacity for normal or abnormal elimination, excess mucus, fat, cholesterol, protein wastes, and other factors accumulate in such areas as the sinuses, the inner ear, the lungs, breasts, intestines, kidneys, and reproductive organs. At first, the swellings and blockages are relatively small, localized, and comparatively harmless such as cysts, stones, and benign tumors or the hardening of peripheral arteries. However, if the diet remains unchanged, the blockages may develop into large, systemic (body-wide), and life-threatening disorders such as cancer, coronary artery disease, diabetes, and other degenerative conditions.

Although there are thousands of seemingly unrelated diseases of the digestive, circulatory, nervous, and reproductive systems, all sicknesses share a common origin and can be classified according to their symptoms and causes into three main categories: 1) those caused by excessive yin—centrifugal and expansive tendencies—or a lack of proper yang—centripetal and contractive tendencies; 2) those caused by excessive yang or a lack of proper yin; and 3) those caused by both excessive yin and excessive yang factors or a combination of a lack of both factors. (See Table 22 for a list of some of the conditions that fall into these three categories.)

Expansive yin qualities (or a lack of proper yang) include dilation, swelling, inflammation, enlargement, loosening, softening, and increased speed, flow, and vibratory rate. Contractive yang qualities (or a lack of proper yin) include constriction, narrowing, tightening, blocking, hardening, and decreased speed, flow, and

Table 22 Yin and Yang Classification of Selected Disorders

	Excessive Yin Origin	Excessive Yang Origin	Combination of Excessive Yin and Yang
Circulatory Diseases	Some low blood pressure	Some high blood pressure	Some high blood pressure
	Some cerebral thrombosis	Some low blood pressure	Some heart failure
	Cerebral hemmorrage	Coronary heart disease	Some cerebral thrombosis
	Valve disorders	Angina pectoris	Cardiomyopathy
	Pulmonary heart disease	Heart attack	Irregular heart beats
	Congenital heart defects	Some heart failure	Rheumatic heart disease
	Some heart failure		Infectious heart disease
			Peripheral heart disease
			Acute thrombosis or embolism
			Aneurysm
			Varicose veins
			Phlebitis
Digestive Diseases	Tooth decay	Appendicitis	Obesity
	Mumps	Duodenal ulcers	Hemorrhoids
	Adenoids	Jaundice	Hepatitis
	Colitis		Typhoid fever
	Gastric pancreatitis		Gallstones
	Peptic ulcers		
	Cirrhosis		
	Dysentery		
	Diabetes		
	Breast cancer	Colon cancer	Lung cancer
	Upper stomach cancer	Prostate cancer	Bladder/kidney cancer
	Skin cancer	Rectum cancer	Uterine cancer
	Mouth cancer	Ovarian cancer	Liver cancer
	Esophageal cancer	Bone cancer	Spleen cancer
	Leukemia	Pancreatic cancer	Malignant melanoma
	Hodgkin's disease	Inner brain cancer	Tongue cancer
	Outer brain cancer		Lower stomach cancer

rate of vibration. On this basis, we can see that disorders involving enlargement and swelling of the body's organs, tissues, or blood vessels are primarily yin in origin and development, while those that involve constriction and tightening of functions and systems are primarily yang. Examples of yin ailments are diarrhea, tonsillitis, adenoids, and mumps. Examples of yang ailments are temporary constipation, appendicitis, and jaundice. Sometimes, both extreme yin and yang qualities are involved, such as high blood pressure which involves both constricted blood vessels and an over-expanded heart.

An overly expanded condition arises from a combination of drinking too many liquids, particularly soda pop, fruit juice, milk, alcohol, coffee, and other stimulants, and eating too many refined foods, fruit, sugar and sugary foods, tropical foods, canned foods, frozen foods, chemicalized foods, and other substances at the extreme yin end of the food spectrum. Conversely, an overly contracted condition arises from a combination of consuming meat, poultry, eggs, hard cheese, and other foods high in saturated fat and cholesterol, too many minerals (especially refined table salt), and other excessively yang substances. A condition arising from both extreme yin and extreme yang qualities involves overconsumption of foods and drinks from both categories. While nearly all these types of foods are eaten in the modern diet, the amount and proportion vary considerably, accounting for the development of different individual conditions.

On the whole, dietary suggestions should be directed primarily toward restoring the individual's excessively yin or yang condition to one that is less extreme and more centrally balanced. To balance a more yin condition (one arising from excessive yin intake or lack of proper yang), the Standard Macrobiotic Diet is recommended emphasizing slightly more yang qualities, such as slightly stronger flavored miso soup, slightly higher overall percentage of whole grains but minimal use of corn (the most yin grain), proportionately more root vegetables, a little less beans but slightly more strongly seasoned, longer cooked sea vegetables with a slightly thicker taste, more long-time pickles, stronger use of condiments, more occasional white-meat fish, and avoidance of raw salads, raw oil, fruit, and desserts.

To balance a more yang condition (one arising from excessive yang intake or lack of proper yin), the Standard Macrobiotic Diet is recommended emphasizing slightly more yin qualities, such as slightly milder flavored miso soup, slightly less overall proportion of whole cereal grains and minimal use of buckwheat (the most yang grain), proportionately more leafy green vegetables, a little more beans and more lightly seasoned, quicker cooked sea vegetables with a lighter taste, more short-time pickles, lighter use of condiments, and avoidance of all animal food.

To balance a condition caused by both extreme yin and extreme yang factors (or a lack of proper yin and proper yang), the Standard Macrobiotic Diet should be followed emhasizing more moderate qualities, including miso soup with more moderate flavor, moderate amount of whole grains and minimal use of both corn and buckwheat, greater emphasis on ground vegetables, beans in moderate volume and with moderate seasoning, moderately cooked sea vegetables with medium taste, more medium-time pickles, moderate use of condiments, and avoidance or minimal use of animal food, raw salad, fruit, and desserts.

In addition to following a more limited form of the Standard Macrobiotic Diet, medicinal beverages or specially cooked side dishes may also be taken depending upon the individual condition. In some instances and under certain conditions, the diet can be further modified to include some other foods usually discouraged in the standard diet such as salmon, tuna, and other red-meat or blue-skinned fish, organic fertilized fowl eggs, caviar, and other fish eggs, white-meat poultry, skim cow's or goat's milk, traditionally naturally fermented cheese and yogurt, unrefined honey, and beet sugar. These modifications are to be made according to individual requirements and necessity. For example, some persons who have received or are currently undergoing surgery, chemotherapy, radiation therapy, or hormone therapy, as well as certain nutritional therapies, may temporarily require proportionately more volume of food consumed, especially protein, complex carbohydrates, minerals, vitamins, or saturated fat of vegetable or animal origin. In practice, the macrobiotic dietary approach is very flexible, always putting the unique needs of the individual above rigid conceptualization.

In addition to dietary modifications, sick persons may also need to receive temporarily for a short period external applications prepared from foodstuffs such as the ginger compress, taro potato plaster, lotus root plaster, or others, depending upon the condition. These traditional home cares are applied directly to various parts of the body to stimulate circulation or help discharge accumulated toxins.

As the body begins to clean itself from many years of improper eating, various physical symptoms may be experienced as accumulated excess comes to the surface and begins to be discharged through the urine, skin, or elsewhere. The elimination of these substances may take the form of colds, fever, headaches, sore throats, constipation, diarrhea, various aches and pains, and mental irritability. Their appearance is a positive sign that the body is beginning to heal itself and return to a condition of more normal equilibrium. However, to make the process more comfortable and control the rate of discharge, medicinal teas and other traditionally and safely practiced home remedies may be beneficial.

In the case of very seriously ill persons, this modified form of the Standard Macrobiotic Diet may need to be followed, depending upon the case, for several months to a year or more. Generally, energy begins to return and pains and aches begin to disappear within about ten days to one month on the new diet. The quality of the blood takes about four months to change, after which time the internal organs begin to heal. Nervous system changes usually take at least nine months to manifest, after which time the person's mental and emotional attitude and basic way of thinking usually begins to noticeably improve. Full recovery may take one, two, or three years or more, depending on the circumstances. In most cases, a wider diet can begin to be adopted after several months as the original condition improves. At this time, supplementary foods such as salads, fruit, desserts, and fish and seafood can usually be introduced in small amounts, and eventually the Standard Macrobiotic Diet with a full range of foods can be adopted.

Persons in generally good health who are making the transition from the modern way of eating to macrobiotics may also experience various symptoms of discharge. Medicinal teas and various home remedies, such as the ginger compress, may also be of value in the beginning to ensure a more smooth transition. Generally, while macrobiotics recognizes that everyone is responsible for his or her own health, it is recommended that seriously ill persons or persons new to the diet see an experienced macrobiotic way of life counselor or medical or nutritional professional trained in this method for direction and guidance.

In addition to a change in diet, macrobiotics recommends a more natural way of life in general, including a moderate amount of regular physical activity and exercise, meditation and self-reflection, and various other physical, mental, and spiritual pursuits to harmonize mind and body, individual and environment, self and cosmos. Dō-in self-massage, shiatsu massage, yoga, T'ai Chi Ch'uan, martial arts, singing, dancing, reading books or poetry out loud, and other activities, especially those that are based on a traditional understanding of electromagnetic energy flow through the body, are very beneficial to health and well-being at all levels.

Macrobiotic Medical Studies

In the last decade, scientific and medical researchers around the world have become increasingly interested in the macrobiotic dietary approach. Their studies are beginning to show that macrobiotics is not only nutritionally adequate but also extremely effective in protecting against and relieving, at least to a certain extent, the degenerative diseases afflicting the rest of modern society. Research is currently proceeding in the following fields:

Heart Disease

Most macrobiotic research to date has been in the field of cardiovascular disease, which is the leading cause of death in modern society. Beginning in 1974, researchers at Harvard Medical School began studying the cholesterol values and blood pressure levels of macrobiotic people living in the Boston area. The researchers found that people eating macrobiotically had among the lowest serum cholesterol values and lowest normal blood pressure levels of any group ever studied in modern society—levels similar to those in traditional societies where degenerative disease was rare or uncommon. Dr. William Castelli, director of the Framingham Heart Study, the nation's oldest continuous heart research project, and a participant in some of the Harvard studies, noted that macrobiotic people have better circulatory systems than conditioned athletes, "The macrobiotic vegetarians we studied, incidently, had a [total cholesterol to HDL cholesterol] ratio of 2.5. Boston marathon runners were at 3.4. These are ratios at which we rarely, if ever, see coronary heart disease." The studies at Harvard Medical School continued over the course of a decade and were published in the *American Journal of Epidemiology*, the *New England Journal of Medicine*, the *Journal of the American Medical Association*, and the *Journal of Lipid Research*. The macrobiotic findings have greatly influenced the medical profession's understanding of the dietary foundation of heart disease and were cited in *Healthy People: The Surgeon General's Report on Health Promotion and Disease Prevention*, a statement of national dietary policy issued in 1979.

In 1982, Dutch medical researchers, supported by the Netherlands Heart Foundation, reported that macrobiotic men and boys had the healthiest hearts, as measured by cholesterol values and blood pressure levels, of all groups studied, including nonvegetarians, semilactovegetarians, and lactovegetarians. Their conclusions were published in *Atherosclerosis*, an international heart research journal.

In 1983, researchers at the Academic Hospital of the Ghent University in Belgium evaluated the blood values of macrobiotic men working at Lima Natural Foods Factory. According to the tests, all the men were very healthy. Their blood pressure and body weights were low, their hormone levels favorable, and they had normal values for proteins, vitamins, and minerals. Overall, however, their cholesterol values were superior to ordinary people. J.P. Deslypere, M.D., one of the researchers, concluded, "In the field of cardiovascular and cancer risk factors this kind of blood is very favorable. It's ideal, we couldn't do better, that's what we're dreaming of. It's really fantastic, like children, whose blood vessels are still completely open and whole. This is a very important matter, deserving our full attention."

In 1984, physicians at Columbia Presbyterian Hospital in New York City reported that patients with angina pectoris, a form of coronary heart disease, significantly improved when put on a macrobiotic diet. In a pilot study that lasted over a ten-week period, eight businessmen suffering from angina and their spouses were trained in macrobiotic cooking and food preparation at the Gourmet School of Natural Cookery. At the end of this period, tests showed that the patients were able to perform better, and three patients experienced the disappearance of all angina symptoms such as difficulty in breathing while walking or climbing steps. In addition to the hospital, the project was sponsored by the New York Cardiac Center.

Cancer

In the early 1970s, the East West Foundation and *East West Journal* began publishing case histories of cancer patients who had overcome their illness by adopting a macrobiotic diet. An annual conference was also organized to bring together doctors, nurses, nutritionists, and other health care professionals, as well as cancer patients, their families, and macrobiotic counselors, to assess the relationship of diet and cancer. These activities, along with many books and magazine articles growing out of these events, had a major impact on public awareness of the relationship of diet and cancer.

In 1982 the National Academy of Sciences issued a report, *Diet, Nutrition, and Cancer*, in which the modern diet high in saturated fat, animal protein, sugar, and chemical additives was associated with a majority of cancers. The report issued interim dietary guidelines calling for substantial decreases in meat, poultry, egg, dairy, and refined carbohydrate consumption and increased consumption of whole cereal grains, vegetables and fruits. The American Cancer Society and the National Cancer Institute issued similar dietary recommendations shortly thereafter.

In 1983, researchers at the Tulane School of Public Health and Tropical Medicine announced plans to study the effectiveness of the macrobiotic diet on cancer patients in the New Orleans area. In 1984, a team of researchers at medical schools and hospitals in Boston, headed up by Dr. Robert Lerman, director of Clinical Nutrition at University Hospital, announced plans to evaluate persons with cancer who had seen Michio Kushi for macrobiotic way of life guidance and compare their subsequent condition of health with data accumulated by authoritative cancer studies.

Radiation Sickness

At the time of the atomic bombing of Nagasaki in 1945, Tatsuichiro Akizuki, M.D., was director of the Department of Internal Medicine at St. Francis's Hospital in Nagasaki. Most patients in the hospital, located one mile from the center of the blast, survived the initial effects of the bomb, but soon after came down with symptoms of radiation sickness from the radioactivity that had been released. Dr. Akizuki fed his staff and patients a strict macrobiotic diet of brown rice, miso and tamari soy sauce soup, wakame and other sea vegetable, Hokkaido pumpkin, and sea salt and prohibited the consumption of sugar and sweets. As a result, he saved everyone in his hospital, while many other survivors in the city perished from radiation sickness.

In Japan, several other macrobiotic survivors of the atomic bombings in Hiroshima and Nagasaki have published accounts of how diet protected or healed them of radiation sickness, keloid tumors, and other serious effects of the bombing. In the 1970s and early 1980s, Japanese medical researchers began investigating some macrobiotic quality foods and reported that miso soup, commonly consumed sea vegetables such as wakame, kombu, hijiki, and arame, and shiitake mushrooms are protective against cancer and heart disease.

Diabetes

Over the years, several case histories were published by the East West Foundation of individuals who had overcome diabetes on the macrobiotic diet. In 1984, a case-control study with diabetic patients in Oregon showed that a macrobiotic diet helped lower major risk factors for this degenerative disorder.

AIDS

In 1983 a group of men in New York City with AIDS (Acquired Immunity Deficiency Syndrome) began macrobiotics. They hoped to change their blood quality, recover their natural immunity, and survive this otherwise always fatal illness. In 1984 immunologists in New York and Boston began to monitor their blood samples and immune reactions. Although these tests are still ongoing and have not yet concluded, preliminary indications are that many of the men have been stabilizing or improving their condition on the diet.

Mental and Psychological Disorders

While many individuals have experienced relief of mental and emotional illnesses by adopting a more balanced diet, so far there have been few scientific studies in this field. One of the first took place at Shattack Hospital in Boston where part of a mental ward was put on a macrobiotic diet. The geriatric patients, many of whom had been institutionalized for many years, experienced positive changes on the new diet. The study was part of a double-blind experiment in which neither patients nor staff were aware of the test, since the macrobiotic foods were made to look and taste like their regular foods. The results of this study are expected to be published in 1985.

Other Degenerative Disorders

During the last decade, the East West Foundation has also compiled and published personal accounts of individuals who have overcome a wide variety of other physical and psychological disorders on the macrobiotic diet including multiple sclerosis, pneumonia, tuberculosis, herpes, kidney stones, fibroid tumors, and many others. In the future, the East West Foundation, the Kushi Foundation, and macrobiotic educational centers around the world hope to cooperate with scientific and medical authorities in supervised clinical experiments to evaluate the possible benefits of the macrobiotic dietary approach for these and other conditions.

Social, Economic, and Spiritual Considerations

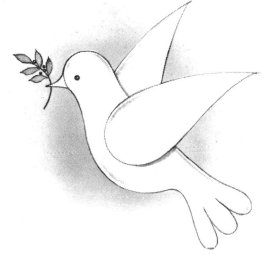

The biological revolution of humanity is peaceful in its entirety and universal in its scope, securing the health and uplifting the spirit of the planet as a whole. Though still in its infancy, modern macrobiotics has already begun to plant the seeds for widespread social and economic change, leading eventually to the creation of one healthy, peaceful world.

During the 1960s, 1970s, and early 1980s, the natural and organic foods movement, actively pioneered and carried out by many macrobiotic people, spread around the globe and began to strengthen family and community life and influence public policy as well as improve personal health and well-being. In this chapter we shall look at a few domains of modern life that have been affected by society's change toward a more healthy, natural way of life, including a more balanced way of eating.

Family

Modern family life has declined steadily during the last several generations, as family members turned away from whole cereal grains—the traditional Staff of Life—and adopted a more refined and artificial way of eating. In addition to a deterioration in the kinds and quality of food consumed, the modern family rarely eats together any more. Sharing the same food is the bond that unites families, creating common blood quality, a common way of thinking and feeling, and a common dream. The disappearance of the family meal is a principal cause of lack of communication and understanding within the modern family today.

The macrobiotic way of life, based on underlying principles of familial respect, has begun to reverse this trend. Parents and children have begun to share common food together again and to cook and eat with one another much more regularly. Deep feelings of love, respect, and common purpose are kindled, and past differences and disagreements are usually put aside, as the new way of life is entered into. In addition to the nuclear family, ties between the generations are generally strengthened. Grandparents and in some cases great-grandparents, if they are still living, are welcomed back into daily family life as the health and judgment of all family members continues to improve.

Man and Woman

The relationship between the sexes has also sharply declined in recent years, and many boys and girls, and men and women, are confused about their sexual identity, their ability to relate to the same or opposite sex, and their place in society. Many sex roles and expectations in modern culture have long been rigid and imbalanced as a result of dualistic thinking caused by excessive animal food intake and other dietary excess. Nevertheless, there are biological strengths and capacities unique to both sexes that have been recognized in traditional cultures and have led to harmony and fulfillment at all levels.

In general, because of her unique role in the creation of biological life and her more practical nature, the woman is the center of the household, while the man, because of his more conceptual thinking and organizing ability, as well as his physical vitality, is more active in the community and society. In practice, macrobiotic education encourages both men and women to engage in cooking or some other aspect of regular food preparation, to share in household responsibilities, and to help bring up the children together. In some cases, the man will have an outside job or career, in other cases the woman, and in still others both will be employed. After becoming macrobiotic, many couples become involved together in some aspect of food production, natural small business activity, or appropriate technology that allows them to work out of their homes or closer to their homes, thereby reducing the split between work and home life that characterizes modern life and is one of the centrifugal tendencies dividing the sexes.

While most macrobiotic men and women eventually marry and have a family, other relationships that are harmonious and based on love and respect are also valued. Some individuals prefer to live together, others to live alone, and still others are gay. In some cases, solitary persons find that a change in their way of eating affects their outlook and they are more attracted to other persons who share a similar dream and way of life.

While attitudes and changes in life-style often take many years to develop and perfect, men and women eating macrobiotically tend to relate to each other more harmoniously than in the past. By eating the same quality food, man and woman develop similar physical and mental conditions, while still maintaining their unique male and female characteristics. Through respecting such similarities and differences, they can establish the most harmonious physical relationship as well as mental understanding, and they become one biologicially, psychologically, and spiritually.

Community

From individual and family practice, macrobiotics has begun to spread out into the community. In addition to thousands of macrobiotic natural foods stores and restaurants, pilot whole foods programs have been established in selected schools, hospitals, nursing homes, and other community institutions in the United States, Canada, Europe, and elsewhere.

For example, in Santa Cruz, California and parts of New York City, local school districts have introduced brown rice, tofu, whole grain bread, and other macrobiotic natural foods in school lunch programs, and these meals have received enthusiastic response on the part of children, teachers, and parents. At Salem Children's Village in Rumney, New Hampshire, dozens of "problem children" who have been unable to adjust to family life, foster homes, or juvenile detention centers have become transformed into happy, healthy youngsters with a holistic program based on whole foods, including macrobiotically prepared food.

In Boston, the Shattuck Hospital set up a macrobiotic food service in its employee cafeteria, and over a two-year period about half of the hospital's one thousand doctors, nurses, and other staff regularly took advantage of its daily luncheon menu. The American Heart Association and other leading medical organizations have revised their dietary guidelines and begun to incorporate brown rice, tofu, and other macrobiotic-quality foods in their menus and recipes. Medical researchers are beginning to study the macrobiotic approach to preventing and relieving degenerative diseases, and pilot programs to put ordinary heart and cancer patients on a macrobiotic diet have already begun or are in the planning stage.

Education

Modern education is in crisis, and most students, parents, and teachers agree that it does not prepare young persons adequately for securing health and happiness in a world of endless change. Traditional values have declined, the gap between theoretical concepts and practical application has widened, and for many school has become a place of confinement and restriction rather than opportunity and discovery.

While macrobiotic education is in its formative stages, individual attempts have been made over the years to set up more holistic nursery schools and kindergartens and introduce macrobiotic principles into ordinary elementary, junior and senior high schools, and colleges and universities. Curricula have been developed based on an understanding of cosmology (the principles of the infinite Order of the Universe), the natural world, and human life, including their practical application in cooking, home cares, massage, yoga, meditation, martial arts, and other disciplines.

In 1978 the Kushi Institute was started in Boston to train and certify macrobiotic cooks, teachers, and way of life counselors. Branch institutes have since opened in London, Amsterdam, Antwerp, Florence, Paris, and Barcelona, and thousands of people have graduated or taken beginning, intermediate, or advanced courses and seminars. In addition, local Macrobiotics International centers around the world offer a wide range of local classes in cooking, philosophy, science, the arts, and healing.

Education, in and out of the classroom, and for all age groups, is a life-long process. In macrobiotics, everyone is considered both a student and a teacher, however experienced or inexperienced, whatever their condition or level of judgment. With intuitive common sense and the simple compass of yin and yang, any aspect of life can be understood without the need for formal training and specialized knowledge. Life is endlessly teaching us about the marvelous order of the universe, and all beings are respected for themselves and the gifts of understanding and insight they have to offer.

Crime and Violence

Crime and violence are major concerns in modern society. According to a macrobiotic perspective, antisocial or aggressive behavior is usually caused by longtime chaotic dietary habits—of course, together with environmental conditions— leading to impaired health and judgment. Often criminals are more active, creative, and natively intelligent than ordinary people. However, they lack a positive, holistic view of life and, in many cases, constructive outlets for their excess energy. On the other hand, many other criminals and violent individuals are extremely sick physically, mentally, and emotionally.

In recent years, macrobiotics has entered a few prison systems and begun to fundamentally change the outlook of prisoners and correction officials. In Chesapeake, Virginia, for example, the Tidewater Detention Center is initiating a macrobiotic food program for juvenile offenders. A preliminary study showed that instances of aggressive behavior and other infractions declined 45 percent following solely the removal of sugar from the inmates' food and snacks. Associate Director Frank Kern has interested the Commonwealth of Virginia in starting a macrobiotic natural foods program at a network of state prisons, hospitals, and nursing homes.

In Portugal, a group of maximum-security prisoners became macrobiotic in the early 1980s under the inspiration of Chico Varatojo, a graduate of the Kushi Institute and then a director of Unimave, the macrobiotic center in Lisbon. Prison authorities allowed Chico and other macrobiotic teaching associates to come to the prison and hold cooking classes and discussion groups and eventually provided macrobiotic natural foods for the inmates to prepare. As result of the change in their way of eating, many prisoners became more tranquil and sociable. These included To Ze Areal, leader of an armed robbery brigade who had fomented revolts and unrest in many prisons, led hunger strikes, and gained the reputation as one of the worst prisoners in all of Portugal. In recognition of To Ze's change in behavior, his sentence with many years remaining was commuted, and he came to the United States to study at the Kushi Institute. Now, back in Portugal, together with other former inmates who are now macrobiotic, he is teaching and guiding many people to greater health and freedom.

Compared to many unsuccessful efforts to reform and rehabilitate prisoners, macrobiotics offers change at the biological level as well as the psychological and spiritual. As this approach becomes more widely recognized, society will understand that crime and antisocial behavior are a sickness and that prisons should be places of education, not punishment. In the future, prisons will be more like health centers where persons will come for guidance and direction, first for inspiration in developing an understanding of cosmology—the Order of the Universe—and human life, and secondly biological and biochemical improvement, from which psychological improvement will follow. From the few macrobiotic prison experiments already tried, we can begin to envision the possibility of reforming the entire modern legal system and changing the practice of restriction and punishment to one of love and understanding—a giant step in the direction of one peaceful world.

Exercise and Sports

Contrary to modern belief, a grain and vegetable diet provides more strength and endurance than a meat and sugar diet. This has been demonstrated by the performance of Olympic and world-class athletes from societies following traditional dietary patterns, as well as by several modern scientific and medical studies. In addition, there have been experiments in which entire sports teams have changed their way of eating.

For example, in 1981 Tatsuro Hirooka took over as manager of the Seibu Lions, a Japanese major league baseball team that finished last place in the season. Hirooka put his players on a macrobiotic diet consisting of brown rice, tofu, vegetables, and fish and told them that animal foods increase an athlete's susceptibility to injuries. Natural foods, on the other hand, he said, protect the body from sprains and dislocations and keep the mind clear. The next year, despite a lot of ridicule from other teams, the Lions won the league championship, defeating their arch rivals, the Nippon Ham-Fighters, a team sponsored by a major meat company, and went on to beat the Chunichi Dragons in the Japan World Series. In 1983 the macrobiotic ball team successfully defended their crown.

Ecology and the Environment

Modern chemical farming has resulted in tragic consequences to the land and natural environment. From an average depth of 36 inches in pioneer times, America's topsoil has declined to about 6 inches in depth today. Meanwhile, as a result of hybridization, crop strains have grown weaker. For example, in 1970, 20 percent of the American corn crop failed when a variety of seed produced in a laboratory proved more vulnerable to blight than the hardy local strains it had displaced. By 1980 70 percent of all folk varieties of wheat and garden vegetables once grown in North America and Europe had disappeared. The remaining seeds face rapid extinction from new corporate patent laws favoring hybrid seed. In addition, chemical pesticides have created new generations of disease-resistant pests, requiring yet further rounds of more powerful chemicals to be applied to the soil. As a result of modern agricultural practices, the United Nations has estimated that one-third of the world's remaining arable land will be lost to desertification in the next quarter century.

Modern patterns of food consumption have also had a tremendously negative impact on wilderness lands, deserts, and other ecosystems. For example, in Latin America, large areas of the tropical rain forests—which supply much of the world's oxygen—have been cleared for beef production, much of which is exported to the hamburger and steak market in the United States, Europe, and other modern societies. One-third of the world's different species of plants and animals are located in these regions and face extinction as a result of modern development.

By changing to a more natural and organic food and agricultural system, the world's farmland could be regenerated. Monoculture would gradually be replaced with mixed crops. Heavy mechanical cultivation would give way to small-scale appropriate technological methods, and chemical fertilizers and insecticides would be retired in favor of organic compounds and wastes. These changes would start building up the tilth of the soil, contribute to the return of plants and wildlife, and purify the air and waterways. In time, this approach would help restore thousands of hardy varieties of seed that have adapted over centuries to local climates and soils but which have been abandoned by the modern food production system and its emphasis on uniform size, shape, color, and taste.

World Poverty and Hunger

In less industrial societies, modern food and agriculture have proved disruptive on an even larger scale than in industrial areas. Cattle-grazing, use of marginal lands, and the export of cash crops have overturned patterns of farming and cultural life extending back thousands of years. In the wake of monocropping—growing one major crop or livestock for foreign export such as coffee, bananas, sugar, tomatoes, cattle, or sheep—tens of millions of families, uprooted from their ancestral lands, flocked to urban metropolitan centers such as San Paulo, Cairo, or Calcutta in quest of employment and opportunity. The vast urban slums created by this exodus from the land offer only poverty, hunger, and emergency relief consisting of infant formula, refined foods, and artificial birth control devices and artificial immunizations that further contribute to disease and destitution.

Growing grain directly for human consumption, meanwhile, would result in greater utilization of land and a more abundant food supply. At the present time it takes from five to ten times as much land to raise beef, pork, lamb, and dairy cattle as it does grains and vegetables. An international economy based on whole foods and organic agriculture would reverse the trend toward concentration of farmland in fewer hands. Hundreds of millions of families living in squalor would return to the lands from which they were driven off and find food, shelter, and meaningful employment. World hunger and poverty, largely the result of modern agricultural dislocations and changing patterns of food consumption, would end and tensions among states, aggravated by competing cash crops for foreign export, would diminish as local communities and regions became more self-sustaining. World population would also stabilize at much lower natural levels as high birth rates—largely a survival mechanism, common to other threatened species as well as humans—returned to normal.

Meanwhile, a few emergency relief agencies, including the United Nation's Food and Agricultural Organization and the International Red Cross have begun to distribute brown rice and other whole grains rather than refined grains in Cambodian refugee camps and other selected areas around the world. These and other positive interim measures should be encouraged until more basic solutions can be achieved.

Energy

The modern food and agricultural system requires enormous amounts of energy, mostly in the form of fossil fuels, to run. About 17 percent of America's energy resources go into producing and operating oversize farm equipment, center-pivot irrigation, chemical fertilizers and pesticides, food processing, food distribution, consumer shopping, food preparation and cooking, and other aspects of industrial food production. The two largest energy users are the meat and meat products industry and the sugar processing industry, followed closely by soft drinks and beverages (see Table 23). This type of system is very wasteful of energy. For

Table 23 Energy Use in Modern Food Production and Processing

The modern food and agriculture system uses vast amounts of oil and other fossil fuels. This includes the energy used in the manufacture of heavy farm equipment, chemical fertilizers and pesticides, and in processing. This table shows the approximate amount of energy that is used each year per capita for selected items in the United States. Note how sugar and meat processing, the two major energy users, roughly balance each other. Energy amounts have been converted into gallons of diesel fuel. Altogether, the average person consumes about a gallon of oil or other fuel per day in the making of their food.

Item	Gallons of Oil/Year/Per Capita
Sugar	88.2
Meat and meat products	89.3
Roasted coffee	6.9
Cigarettes	9.2
Frozen fruit and vegetables	21.2
Beverages	80.6
Agricultural machinery	31.3
Agricultural chemicals	48.7
TOTAL	375.4

Source: Adapted from Maurice Green, *Eating Oil: Energy Use in Food Production,* Westview Press, 1978.

Table 24 Energy Saving from Organic Farming

Organic farming can result in substantial energy savings over conventional farming. This table shows the results of an energy productivity study of organic and inorganic wheat growers in New York and Pennsylvania. The organic farmers used about 30 percent less energy per acre than conventional farmers. However, their yield was 22 percent less, so that the net energy consumption per bushel of organic wheat was about 15 percent less than the wheat grown with chemical fertilizers and pesticides.

Input	Conventional (%*)	Organic (%)
Machinery	29.9	38.9
Fuel	24.3	27.2
Nitrogen	24.2	2.3
Phosphorus	4.9	0.7
Potassium	4.3	0.7
Seeds	25.5	26.6
Electricity	1.5	1.8
Lime	1.1	1.8
TOTAL	115.7	100.0

* Percent of total organic energy inputs
Source: Report and Recommendations on Organic Farming, U.S. Department of Agriculture, 1980.

example, in the Midwest, farmers require from 5 to 12 calories of petroleum for every 1 calorie of food produced. In contrast, traditional societies using labor-intensive cultivation techniques and small, appropriate technological methods can produce 3 to 10 calories of food for every 1 calorie of energy expended. In addition, about 24 percent of all the food produced in the United States is later wasted due to poor and inefficient harvesting techniques, transportation, storage, processing, marketing, and kitchen and plate wastage.

Under a more natural and organic system of food production and delivery, reduced processing and packaging of foods, independence from chemical, oil-based fertilizers and pesticides, and lessened need for heavy farm equipment would result in substantial energy savings (see Table 24). The consumption of local, regional, and seasonally grown food—in accord with macrobiotic dietary principles—would further cut back on food imported long distances and from different climates, thus reducing transportation networks and their resulting pollution and other social costs. The need for less metals, chemicals, petroleum, and other raw materials would further ease international competition and crisis.

Economics

A macrobiotic natural foods diet is very economical and in the long run results in substantial savings in many areas of life. According to weekly market basket surveys, the typical macrobiotic household, for example, spends about 35 to 50 percent less on its weekly food budget of grains, fresh vegetables, and naturally processed items than an ordinary family spends eating meat, dairy foods, highly processed foods, canned foods, frozen foods, and a variety of foodstuffs imported from distant climates. In a pilot program, the U.S. Department of Agriculture introduced a meal plan for low-income families in the Washington, D.C. area calling for more whole grains and their products, vegetables and fruit, and dry beans and nuts and calling for less meat, poultry, eggs, cheese, sugar, and soft drinks. Not only did the meals save considerably on food expenses, but also the new meals were readily accepted, found to be not hard to prepare, and "families in the study felt there was, in some cases, too much food."

In addition, the macrobiotic family generally takes major responsibility for its own health care, requiring little or no insurance payments, medical costs, and pharmaceutical expenses. At the social level, a dietary change in this direction would result in vast savings. In 1984 the American Heart Association estimated that the direct medical costs, nursing expenses, and lost output due to cardiovascular disease came to $64.4 billion annually. As public health improved, the economy would also improve. Government expenses for health and medical care, welfare and disability payments, and other social services—now currently greater than defense expenditures—would substantially drop. The national debt would lower, interest rates would fall, employment would rise, productivity and efficiency would increase, international trade would flourish, and generally people would take more pride and interest in their work. Lowered food costs as a whole for each family would further contribute to an increase in real income, more leisure time, and a general improvement in the quality of life.

Spiritual Development

With the spread of macrobiotics, the dietary contribution to spiritual development is being rediscovered. Although not itself a religion, macrobiotics is the thread that unites the world's traditional faiths. Jews, for example, are finding that Abraham, Sarah, Moses, Ruth, and other Hebrew sages and prophets ate a diet centered around unleavened whole grain bread and that observing kosher dietary principles is a major reason the Jewish community has survived for so many centuries. Christians are finding that Jesus, Mary, the apostles, and the early Christian community also ate primarily grains and vegetables, with occasional fish, and dietary common sense underlies the Gospel teachings. Followers of Islam are rediscovering the Prophet Mohammed's natural way of eating, in harmony with the nomadic desert environment in which he lived. Buddhists are recalling that Siddhartha ate brown rice porridge under the Tree of Enlightenment and as the Buddha later taught principles of right nourishment. Students of Chinese religion and philosophy are finding that Confucius and Lao-tzu also followed a simple macrobiotic way of life.

Today, macrobiotics includes individuals and families from every religion, belief, and persuasion, including humanists and those who are not members of any organized religion. People commonly report that their own philosophical view, spiritual understanding, or traditional religious ties are immeasurably strengthened after they have begun to practice macrobiotics for a time. Depending upon the individual instructors, a wide variety of spiritual practices is taught in macrobiotic centers, including meditation, self-reflection, chanting, and yoga. However, a creed or doctrine would be contrary to the macrobiotic spirit of free belief and inquiry. Religious intolerance, prejudice, and misunderstanding are still causes of division in the modern world. By eating macrobiotic food, the individual naturally begins to develop toward universal consciousness and arrive at a deeper understanding of the meaning of life and death. In the future, macrobiotics will be a major unifying force, helping humanity to recognize and appreciate the common qualities and values that underlie the world's diverse faiths.

World Peace

Since time immemorial the common dream of humanity has been to create a world of lasting peace. From generation to generation, seeds from the harvest have been saved and handed down to plant the following spring. In all previous cultures and civilizations, the connection between nourishment and patterns of war and peace has been recognized. In the Far East, the word for peace—*wa* (和)—combines ideograms for grain and mouth. In the Book of Isaiah, the famous vision of beating swords into plowshares makes use of imagery also derived from cultivating and preparing whole cereal grains.

From the individual who is following a more natural way of living, including a balanced way of eating, peaceful thinking and behavior gradually radiate out to family, friends, the community, and eventually the land and planet as a whole. Our life is governed by the natural order, and when we are in harmony with the larger environment, we also experience peace with once another.

In modern times, as the destructiveness and threat of war have increased, the traditional understanding of the relation between basic nourishment and human destiny has become almost entirely lost. During the last hundred years, various heads of state, scientists, reformers, and spiritual leaders have advanced proposals to reduce conflict and prevent war. However, all of these measures have failed to achieve peace because they have overlooked the underlying determinant in our lives: the physical food that creates our minds and bodies and shapes the way we think, feel, act, and relate to each other.

As we have seen in this chapter, a change to a more natural and organic food and agricultural system will have far-reaching effects in all aspects of modern life, including energy savings, environmental preservation, lessening of world poverty and hunger, and other areas that are often the cause of world conflict and war. In 1981 a panel of the American Association for the advancement of Science evaluated the impact of a change to a whole grain diet on society. According to *Science News*, the scientists concluded that "changes in our eating habits can have significant beneficial effects on everything from land, water, fuel, and mineral use to the cost of living, employment rates, and the balance of international trade" as well as reduce coronary heart disease by up to 88 percent and cancer by 50 percent.

In addition to providing society with good quality food, giving cooking classes, and teaching about a more natural way of life, there are several macrobiotic activities directed specifically at promoting world peace through world health. For example, in Lebanon, following the civil war between Christians and Muslims in the late 1970s, a macrobiotic agricultural project brought together warring factions in one small area of Beirut. Families started a bakery to produce Wise Bread, the traditional whole grain flat bread that had been replaced by enriched white loaves. In Europe, the United States, the West Indies and the Middle East, Macrobiotic Congresses have assembled annually, drawing delegates from many nations and states to discuss ways to promote world peace and security.

At the United Nations, an international macrobiotic society was formed in 1984 and during the first year attracted about 150 members from delegations and staff. Its founder, Katsuhide Kitatani, director of development for U.N. programs in Southeast Asia, healed himself of stomach cancer on the macrobiotic diet. Other macrobiotic chapters are expected to start at UNESCO headquarters in Paris and at the World Health Organization in Geneva. Members of both these groups hope to educate their colleagues as well as begin developing programs based on macrobiotic principles.

Garry Davis, leader of the world citizens movement, has begun to raise dietary awareness among those seeking a more peaceful and secure international order. In 1984, Davis, founder and president of the World Service Authority, invited Michio Kushi to be commissioner of the interim world government's World Health Commission. John Denver, who has long been involved in environmental and peace concerns, began eating macrobiotically in the early 1980s. He credits a change in diet with improving his health and music and has participated in several projects with the Kushi Foundation. Actor Dirk Benedict, filmmaker and actor Terrence Hill, and other noted artists, writers, scientists, educators, and executives are contributing their talents and experience to furthering macrobiotic education and global understanding.

No matter how known or unknown, skilled or unskilled, young or old, healthy or ill, everyone can contribute in some way to building a more peaceful world. From the most distant past to the most distant future, dietary common sense, an understanding of the Order of the Universe, and a spirit of love and respect among family members are the main factors unifying the human race. Under many names and forms, macrobiotics will continue to serve as humanity's most fundamental and intuitive wisdom. Macrobiotics offers a key to restoring our daily health and vitality, a vision for regenerating a divided world, a model for building a planetary family, and a compass for charting our endless voyage through the stars toward freedom and lasting peace.

Appendix: Principles of the Order of the Universe

The Seven Universal Principles of the Infinite Universe

1. Everything is a differentiation of one Infinity.
2. Everything changes.
3. All antagonisms are complementary.
4. There is nothing identical.
5. What has a front has a back.
6. The bigger the front, the bigger the back.
7. What has a beginning has an end.

The Twelve Laws of Change of the Infinite Universe

1. One Infinity manifests itself into complementary and antagonistic tendencies, yin and yang, in its endless change.
2. Yin and yang are manifested continuously from the eternal movement of one infinite universe.
3. Yin represents centrifugality. Yang represents centripetality. Yin and yang together produce energy and all phenomena.
4. Yin attracts yang. Yang attracts yin.
5. Yin repels yin. Yang repels yang.
6. Yin and yang combined in varying proportions produce different phenomena. The attraction and repulsion among phenomena is proportional to the difference of the yin and yang forces.
7. All phenomena are ephemeral, constantly changing their constitution of yin and yang forces; yin changes into yang, yang changes into yin.
8. Nothing is solely yin or solely yang. Everything is composed of both tendencies in varying degrees.
9. There is nothing neuter. Either yin or yang is in excess in every occurrence.
10. Large yin attracts small yin. Large yang attracts small yang.
11. Extreme yin produces yang, and extreme yang produces yin.
12. All physical manifestations are yang at the center, and yin at the surface.

Glossary

Amazaké—A sweet, creamy beverage made from fermented sweet rice.

Arame—A thin, wiry black sea vegetable similar to hijiki.

Arepa—An oval-shaped corn ball or cake made from whole corn dough and baked or fried.

Arrowroot—A starch flour processed from the root of an American plant used as a thickening agent in cooking.

Azuki bean—A small, dark red bean originally from Japan but now also grown in the West.

Barley malt—A natural sweetener made from malted barley.

Bancha tea—The twigs, stems, and leaves from mature Japanese tea bushes; also known as *kukicha* tea.

Boiled salad—Salad whose ingredients are lightly boiled or dipped in hot water before serving.

Brown rice—Whole unpolished rice, containing an ideal balance of nutrients.

Buckwheat—A hardy cereal grass eaten in the form of kasha (whole groats) or soba noodles.

Burdock—A wild hardy plant whose long, dark root is valued in cooking for its strengthening qualities.

Daikon—A long white radish used in many types of dishes and for medicinal purposes.

Dashi—Traditional Japanese soup stock made from kombu broth.

Dry-roast—To toast a grain, seed, or flour in an unoiled skillet, stirring gently until brown or golden and a nutty aroma is released.

Dulse—A red-purple sea vegetable used in soups, salads, and vegetable dishes or as a garnish.

Fiber—The part of whole grains, vegetables, and fruits that is not broken down in digestion and gives bulk to wastes.

Fu—Dried wheat gluten cakes or sheets.

Ginger—A spicy, pungent golden-colored root used in cooking and for medicinal purposes.

Ginger compress—A compress made from grated gingerroot and water. Applied hot to an affected area of the body, it serves to stimulate circulation and dissolve stagnation.

Gomashio—Sesame seed salt made from dry-roasting and grinding sea salt and sesame seeds and crushing them in a *suribachi*.

Hijiki—A dark brown sea vegetable which when dried turns black.

Jinenjo—A light brown Japanese mountain potato that grows to be several feet long and two to three inches wide.

Kanten—A jelled fruit dessert made from agar-agar.

Kasha—Roasted buckwheat groats.

Kelp—A large family of sea vegetables similar to kombu.

Kinpira—A style of cooking root vegetables by first sautéing, then adding a little water, and seasoning with tamari soy sauce at the end of cooking.

Koi-koku—A rich, thick soup made from carp, burdock, bancha tea, and miso.

Kombu—A wide, thick, dark green sea vegetable that grows in deep ocean water. Used in making soup stocks, condiments, and cooked as a separate dish or with vegetables, beans, or grains.

Kuzu—A white starch made from the root of a prolific wild vine. Used in thickening soups, gravies, sauces, desserts, and for medicinal beverages; also known as *kudzu*.

Lotus root—Root of the water lily, brown-skinned with a hollow, chambered off-white inside, used in many dishes and for medicinal preparations.

Macrobiotics—From the traditional Greek words for "Great Life" or "Long Life." The way of life according to the largest possible view, the infinite Order of the Universe. The practice of macrobiotics includes the understanding and practical application of this order to daily life, including the selection, preparation, and manner of cooking and eating, as well as the orientation of consciousness.

Masa—Dough made from whole corn, used in making arepas, tortillas, and other traditional dishes.

Millet—A small yellow grain that can be prepared whole, added to soups, salads, and vegetable dishes.

Mirin—A sweet cooking wine made from sweet rice.

Miso—A fermented paste made from soybeans, sea salt, and usually rice or barley. Used in soups, stews, spreads, baking, and as a seasoning. Miso gives a nice sweet taste and salty flavor.

Mochi—A cake or dumpling made from cooked, pounded sweet rice.

Mu tea—A tea made from a variety of herbs that warms the body, strengthens the female organs, and has other medicinal properties.

Natto—A lightly fermented soybean dish with sticky, long strands and a strong odor.

Natural foods—Whole foods that are unprocessed or minimally processed using traditional methods and un-treated with artificial additives or preservatives.

Nishime—Long, slow style of boiling in which vegetables or other ingredients cook primarily in their own juices, giving strong, peaceful energy.

Nori—Thin sheets of dried sea vegetable, black or dark purple in color, which turn green when roasted; used as a garnish, to wrap rice balls, in making sushi, or cooked with tamari soy sauce as a condiment.

Open-pollinated—Type of traditional Indian corn that is pollinated by the wind as opposed to hybrid corn; also known as standard corn.

Organic foods—Foods grown without the use of chemical fertilizers, herbicides, pesticides, or other artificial sprays.

Pan-fry—To sauté with a little oil over a low to medium heat, stirring occasionally but not so often as stir-frying.

Polyunsaturated fats—Essential fatty acids found in high concentration in whole grains, beans, seeds, and to a lesser extent in fish.

Pressed salad—Salad prepared by pressing sliced vegetables and sea salt in a small pickle press or an improvised weight on a plate.

Pressure cooker—An airtight metal pot that cooks food quickly by steaming under pressure at high temperature. Used primarily in macrobiotic cooking for whole grains and occasionally for beans and vegetables.

Refined oil—Cooking oil that has been chemically processed to alter or remove its natural color, taste, and aroma.

Rice cake—A light round cake made of puffed brown rice enjoyed as a snack.

Rice syrup—A natural sweetener made from malted brown rice.

Sea salt—Salt obtained from the ocean; unrefined sea salt is high in trace minerals and contains no chemicals, sugar, or added iodine.

Sea vegetable—An edible seaweeds such as kombu wakame, arame, hijiki, nori, or dulse.

Seitan—A whole wheat product cooked in tamari soy sauce, kombu, and water; used for stews, croquettes, grain burgers, and many other dishes; high in protein and gives a strong, dynamic taste; also called wheat gluten or wheat meat.

Shiitake—A mushroom, used fresh or dried, for soups and stews and for medicinal purposes.

Shio-kombu—Salty kombu; pieces of kombu cooked for a long time in tamari soy sauce and used as a condiment.

Shiso—Leaves usually pickled with umeboshi plums; also known as beefsteak leaves.

Soba—Noodles made from buckwheat flour or buckwheat combined with whole wheat.

Stone-ground—Unrefined flour that has been ground in a stone mill that preserves the germ, bran, and other nutrients.

Suribachi—A serrated, glazed clay bowl or mortar, used with a pestle for grinding and puréeing foods.

Sweet rice—A glutinous type of rice that is slightly sweeter to the taste and used in making mochi, amazaké, and various dishes.

Tamari soy sauce—Traditional, naturally made soy sauce, distinguished from refined, chemically processed soy sauce; also known as organic or natural shoyu. A stronger, wheat-free soy sauce called real or genuine tamari, a by-product of making miso, is used for special dishes. Tamari soy sauce is used for daily cooking in macrobiotic food preparation.

Tekka—Condiment made from soy miso, sesame oil, burdock, lotus root, carrot, and gingerroot, cooked down to a black powder.

Tempeh—A traditional Indonesian soy-food made from split soybeans, water, and a special bacteria; high in protein with a rich, dynamic taste, tempeh is used in soups, stews, sandwiches, casseroles, and other dishes.

Tofu—Soybean curd made from soy milk and *nigari*; high in protein and prepared in cakes, it is used in soups, vegetable dishes, salads, sauces, dressings, and other dishes.

Udon—Japanese whole wheat noodles.

Umeboshi—A salted pickled plum that has aged usually for several years. Its nice, zesty sour taste and salty flavor go well with many foods and it is used as a seasoning, in sauces, as a condiment, in beverages, and in many medicinal preparations.

Umeboshi vinegar—The liquid that umeboshi plums are aged in; used for sauces, dressings, and seasoning and making pickles; also known as *ume-su*.

Unrefined oil—Vegetable oil that has been naturally processed to retain its natural color, taste, aroma, and nutrients.

Wakame—A long thin, green sea vegetable used in making daily miso soup, as well as salads and other dishes.

Whole foods—Foods in their natural form that have not been refined or processed, such as brown rice or whole wheat berries.

Whole grains—Unrefined cereal grains to which nothing has been added or subtracted in milling except for the inedible outer hull. Whole grains include brown rice, millet, barley, whole wheat, oats, rye, buckwheat, and corn.

Whole wheat—A whole cereal grain that may be prepared in whole form or made into flour. Whole wheat products such as noodles, seitan, fu, bulgur, couscous, and cracked wheat make a variety of dishes.

Yang—One of the two fundamental energies of the universe. Yang refers to the relative tendency of contraction, centripetality, density, heat, light, and other qualities. Yang energy tends to go down and inward. Its complementary and antagonistic force is yin.

Yin—One of the two fundamental energies of the universe. Yin refers to the relative tendency of expansion, growth, centrifugality, diffusion, cold, darkness, and other qualities. Yin energy tends to go up and outward. Its complementary and antagonistic force is yang.

Macrobiotic Resources

Macrobiotics International in Boston and its major educational centers in the United States, Canada, and around the world offer ongoing classes for the general public in macrobiotic cooking and traditional food preparation and natural processing. They also offer instruction in Oriental medicine, shiatsu massage, pregnancy and natural child care, yoga, meditation, science, culture and the arts, and world peace and world government activities. Macrobiotics International Educational Centers also provide way of life guidance services with trained and certified consultants, make referrals to professional health care associates, and cooperate in research and food programs in hospitals, medical schools, prisons, drug rehabilitation clinics, nursing homes, and other institutions. In scores of other cities and communities, there are smaller Macrobiotics International learning centers, residential centers, and information centers offering some classes and services.

Most of the foods mentioned in this book arc available at natural foods stores, selected health food stores, and a growing number of supermarkets around the world. Macrobiotic specialty items are also available by mail order from various distributors and retailers.

Please contact Macrobiotics International in Boston or other national centers listed below for information on regional and local activities in your area, as well as whole foods outlets and mail order sources.

Global Headquarters
Macrobiotics International
Box 568
Brookline, Mass. 02147
800–MACRO–17
(This toll-free hotline for information on macrobiotic programs and services in the United States and abroad is open Monday through Friday, 12 noon to 4 P.M., Eastern Standard Time; at other times or in Massachusetts call 617–738–0045.)

Australia
Australian Macrobiotic
 Association
1 Carlton Street, Prahran
Melbourne, 3181
Australia
03–529–1620

Belgium
Oost West Centrum
 Kushi Instituut
Consciencestraat 48
Antwerpen, 2000
Belgium
03–230–13–82

Bermuda
Macrobiotic Center of
 Bermuda
In-The-Lee, Deepwood
Drive Fairyland,
Pembroke, Bermuda
809–29–5–2275

Britain
Community Health
  Foundation
188–194 Old Street
London, ECIV 9BP,
England
01–251–4076

Canada
861 Queen Street
Toronto, Ontario
M6J IC4, Canada

France
Le Grain Sauvage
  Macrobiotic Associa-
tion
15 Rue Letellier 75015
Paris, France
33–1–828–4773

Germany
Ost West Zentrum
Eppendorfer Marktplatz
13 D-2000 Hamburg 20
040–47–27–50

Holland
Oost West Centrum
  Kushi Institute
Achtergracht 17
1017 WL Amsterdam,
Holland
020–240–203

Hong Kong
Conduit RD. 41A,
Rome CT. 8D
Hong Kong, Hong Kong
5–495–268

Israel
24 Amos Street
Tel Aviv, Israel
442979

Italy
Fondazione Est Ovest
Via de'Serragli 4
50124 Florence, Italy

Japan
Macro Bios Tokyo
1–22–11–106, Uehara
Shibuya-ku, Tokyo
151, Japan
03–753–9216

Lebanon
Mary Naccour
Couvent St. Elie
Box 323 Antelias
Beirut, Lebanon

Norway
East West Center
Frydenlundsgt 2 0169
Oslo 1, Norway
02–60–47–79

Portugal
Unimave
Rua Mouzinha da
Silveira 25
1200 Lisboa, Portugal
1–557–362

Switzerland
Ost West Zentrum
Postfach 2502 Bern,
3001 Switzerland
031–25–65–40

United Arab Emirates
Box 4943 SATWA
Dubai, United Arab
Emirates
040440–031
  (national)
97–1–44–4–0031
  (international)

United Nations
United Nations Macro-
  biotics Society
c/o Katsuhide Kitatani
U.N. Development
Programme
1 United Nations Plaza
New York, N.Y. 10017
212–906–5844

United States
East West Foundation
Box 850
Brookline, Mass. 02147
617–738–0045

For those who wish to study further, the Kushi Institute, an educational institution founded in Boston in 1979 with affiliates in London, Amsterdam, Antwerp, and Florence, offers full- and part-time instruction for individuals who wish to become trained and certified macrobiotic cooking instructors, teachers, and counselors. The Kushi Institute publishes a *Worldwide Macrobiotics Directory* every year listing Kushi Institute graduates and macrobiotic centers, friends, and businesses around the world. The Cook Instructor Service is an extension of the Kushi Institute and is comprised of specially qualified graduates of the Kushi Institute's advanced cooking program. These men and women are available to assist individuals and families in learning the basics of macrobiotic food preparation and home care in their home.

Kushi Institute and Cook Instructor Service
Box 7
Becket, Mass. 01223
413–623–5712

Ongoing developments are reported in the Kushi Foundation's periodicals, including the *East West Journal*, a monthly magazine begun in 1971 and now with an international readership of 200,000. The *EWJ* features regular articles on the macrobiotic approach to health and nutrition, as well as ecology, science, psychology, and the arts. In each issue there is a macrobiotic cooking column and articles on traditional food cultivation and natural foods processing.

East West Journal
17 Station St.
Brookline, Massachusetts 02146
617–232–1000

Bibliography

Books

Aihara, Herman. *Basic Macrobiotics*. Tokyo: Japan Publications, Inc., 1985.

Aihara, Cornellia. *Macrobiotic Kitchen: Key to Good Health*. Tokyo: Japan Publications, Inc., 1983.

Akizuki, Tatsuichiro. *Nagasaki 1945*. London and New York: Quartet Books, 1981.

Arasaki, Seibin, and Teruko Arasaki. *Vegetables from the Sea*. Tokyo: Japan Publications, Inc., 1983.

Brewster, Letitia, and Michael F. Jacobson. *The Changing American Diet*. Washington, D.C.: Center for Science in the Public Interest, 1978.

Brown, Virginia, and Susan Stayman. *Macrobiotic Miracle: How a Vermont Family Overcame Cancer*. Tokyo: Japan Publications, Inc., 1985.

Dawber, Thomas Royle. *The Framingham Study: The Epidemiology of Atherosclerotic Disease*. Cambridge, Mass.: Harvard University Press, 1980.

Dufty, William. *Sugar Blues*. New York: Warner Books, 1975.

Esko, Edward, and Wendy Esko. *Macrobiotic Cooking for Everyone*. Tokyo: Japan Publications, Inc., 1980.

Esko, Wendy. *Introducing Macrobiotic Cooking*. Tokyo: Japan Publications, Inc., 1978.

Fukuoka, Masanobu. *The One-Straw Revolution*. Emmaus, Pa.: Rodale Press, 1978.

———. *The Natural Way of Farming*. Tokyo: Japan Publications, Inc., 1985.

Heidenry, Carolyn. *An Introduction to Macrobiotics*. Brookline, Mass.: Aladdin Press, 1984.

——— *Making the Transition to a Macrobiotic Diet*. Brookline, Mass.: Aladdin Press, 1984.

Hippocrates. *Hippocratic Writings*. Edited by G.E.R. Lloyd and translated by J. Chadwick and W.N. Mann. New York: Penguin Books, 1978.

Hufeland, Christolph W. *Macrobiotics or the Art of Prolonging Life*. Berlin, 1797.

I Ching or *Book of Changes*. Translated by Richard Wilhelm and Cary F. Baynes. Princeton: Bollingen Foundation, 1950.

Ineson, Rev. John. *The Way of Life: Macrobiotics and the Spirit of Christianity*. Tokyo: Japan Publications, Inc., 1985.

Kohler, Jean, and Mary Alice Kohler. *Healing Miracles from Macrobiotics*. West Nyack, N.Y.: Parker, 1979.

Kotzsch, Ronald E. *Macrobiotics: Yesterday and Today*. Tokyo: Japan Publications, Inc., 1985.

Kushi, Aveline. *Cooking for Health: Allergies* (Macrobiotic Food and Cooking Series). Edited by Rosalind Rhodes. Tokyo: Japan Publications, Inc., 1985.

———. *Cooking for Health: Diabetes and Hypoglycemia* (Macrobiotic Food and Cooking Series). Edited by Rosalind Rhodes. Tokyo: Japan Publications, Inc., 1985.

———. *How to Cook with Miso*. Tokyo: Japan Publications, Inc., 1978.

Kushi, Aveline, and Michio Kushi. *Macrobiotic Child Care and Family Health*. Edited by Edward and Wendy Esko. Tokyo: Japan Publications, Inc., 1985.

———. *Macrobiotic Pregnancy and Care of the Newborn*. Edited by Edward and Wendy Esko. Tokyo: Japan Publications, Inc., 1984.

Kushi, Aveline, with Alex Jack. *Aveline Kushi's Complete Guide to Macrobiotic Cooking for Health, Harmony, and Peace*. New York: Warners Books, 1985.

Kushi, Aveline, and Wendy Esko. *The Changing Seasons Macrobiotic Cookbook*. Wayne, N.J.: Avery Publishing Group, 1985.

Kushi, Michio. *The Book of Dō-In: Exercise for Physical and Spiritual Development*. Tokyo: Japan Publications, Inc., 1979.

———. *The Book of Macrobiotics*. Tokyo: Japan Publications, Inc., 1977.

———. *The Era of Humanity*. Edited by Sherman Goldman. Brookline, Mass.: East West Journal, 1980.

———. *How to See Your Health: The Book of Oriental Diagnosis*. Tokyo: Japan Publications, Inc., 1980.

———. *Macrobiotic Home Remedies*. Edited by Marc Van Cauwenberghe. Tokyo: Japan Publications, Inc., 1985.

———. *A Natural Approach: Allergies* (Macrobiotic Health Education Series). Edited by Mark Mead and John David Mann. Tokyo: Japan Publications, Inc., 1985.

———. *A Natural Approach: Diabetes and Hypoglycemia* (Macrobiotic Health Education Series). Edited by John David Mann. Tokyo: Japan Publications, Inc., 1985.

———. *Natural Healing Through Macrobiotics*. Tokyo: Japan Publications, Inc., 1978.

———. *Your Face Never Lies*. Wayne, N.J.: Avery Publishing Group, 1983.

Kushi, Michio, with Alex Jack. *The Cancer-Prevention Diet*. New York: St. Martin's Press, 1983.

———. *Diet for a Strong Heart: Michio Kushi's Macrobiotic Dietary Guidelines for the Prevention of High Blood Pressure, Heart Attack, and Stroke*. New York: St. Martin's Press, 1985.

Kushi, Michio, and the East West Foundation. *Cancer and Heart Disease: The Macrobiotic Approach to Degenerative Disorders*. Edited by Edward Esko. Tokyo: Japan Publications, Inc., 1982.

Mendelsohn, Robert S. *Confessions of a Medical Heretic*. Chicago: Contemporary Books, 1979.

———. *Male Practice*. Chicago: Contemporary Books. 1980.

Ohsawa, George. *Cancer and the Philosophy of the Far East*. Oroville, Calif: George Ohsawa Macrobiotic Foundation, 1971.

Ohsawa, George, with William Dufty. *You Are All Sanpaku*. New York: University Books, 1965.

Ohsawa, Lima. *Macrobiotic Cuisine*. Tokyo: Japan Publications, Inc., 1984.

Oski, Frank A., and John D. Bell. *Don't Drink Your Milk*. Wyden Books, 1977.

Price, Weston A. *Nutrition and Physical Degeneration*. Santa Monica, Calif.: Price-Pottenger Nutritional Foundation, 1945.

Sattilaro, Anthony, with Tom Monte. *Recalled by Life: The Story of My Recovery from Cancer*. Boston: Houghton-Mifflin, 1982.

Tara, William. *Macrobiotics and Human Behavior*. Tokyo: Japan Publications, Inc., 1985.

Trowell, H. C., and D. P. Burkitt. *Western Diseases: Their Emergence and Prevention*. Cambridge, Mass.: Harvard University Press, 1981.

Yamamoto, Shizuko. *Barefoot Shiatsu*. Tokyo: Japan Publications, Inc., 1979.

The Yellow Emperor's Classic of Internal Medicine. Translated by Ilza Veith. Berkeley:

University of California Press, 1949.

Periodicals

East West Journal. Brookline, Massachusetts.
MacroMuse. Rockville, Maryland.
Nutrition Action. Washington, D.C.
The People's Doctor. Evanston, Illinois.

Scientific Articles and Reports

Bergan, J. G., and P. T. Brown. "Nutritional Status of 'New Vegetarians." *Journal of the American Dietetic Association* 76 (1982): 151–55.

Chihara, G., et al. "Fractionation and Purification of the Polysaccharides with Marked Antitumor Activity, Especially Lentinan." From *lentinus edodes* (Berk.) Sing. (An Edible Mushroom), *Cancer Research* 30 (1970): 2776–81.

Diet, Nutrition, and Cancer. Washington, D.C.: National Academy of Sciences, 1982.

Dietary Goals for the United States. Washington, D.C.: Select Committee on Nutrition and Human Needs, U.S. Senate. Government Printing Office, 1977.

Healthy People: The Surgeon General's Report on Health Promotion and Disease Prevention. Washington, D.C.: Government Printing Office, 1979.

Hirayama, T. "Relationship of Soybean Paste Soup Intake to Gastric Cancer Risk." *Nutrition and Cancer* 3 (1981): 223–33.

Iritani, N., and S. Nagi. "Effects of Spinach and Wakame on Cholesterol Turnover in the Rat." *Atherosclerosis* 15 (1972): 87–92.

Knuiman, J. T., and C. E. West. "The Concentration of Cholesterol in Serum and in Various Serum Lipoproteins in Macrobiotic, Vegetarian, and Non-Vegetarian Men and Boys." *Atherosclerosis* 43 (1983): 71–82.

Kushi, L. H., et al. "Diet and 20-Year Mortality from Coronary Heart Disease: The Ireland-Boston Diet-Heart Study," *New England Journal of Medicine* 312 (1985): 811–18.

Mead, M. "In Search of the Sweet Life: A Dietary Approach to Diabetes Mellitus." Reed College Biology Thesis in Cooperation with the Oregon Health Sciences University, 1984.

Sacks, F. M., B. Rosner, and E. H. Kass. "Blood Pressure in Vegetarians." *American Journal of Epidemiology* 100 (1974): 390–98.

Sacks, F. M., et al. "Plasma Lipids and Lipoproteins in Vegetarians and Controls." *New England Journal of Medicine* 292 (1975): 1148–51.

———. "Effect of Ingestion of Meat on Plasma Cholesterol in Vegetarians." *Journal of the American Medical Association* 246 (1981): 640–44.

———. "Lack of an Effect of Dairy Protein (Casein) and Soy Protein on Plasma Cholesterol of Strict Vegetarians: An Experiment and a Critical Review." *Journal of Lipid Research* 24 (1983): 1012–20.

Schoenthaler, Stephen S. "The Effect of Sugar on the Treatment and Control of Antisocial Behavior." *International Journal of Biosocial Research* 3 (1) (1982): 1–9.

Skoryna, S. C., et al. "Studies on Inhibition of Intestinal Absorption of Radioactive Strontium." *Canadian Medical Association Journal* 91 (1964): 285–88.

Tanaka, Y., et al. "Studies on Inhibition of Intestinal Absorption of Radio-Active Strontium." *Canadian Medical Association Journal* 99 (1968): 169–75.

Teas, Jane. "The Dietary Intake of *Laminaria*, a Brown Seaweed, and Breast Cancer Prevention." *Nutrition and Cancer* 4 (1983): 217–222.

Yamamoto, I. et al. "Antitumor Effect of Seaweeds." *Japanese Journal of Experimental Medicine* 44 (1974): 543–46.

About the Authors

Michio Kushi was born in Kokawa, Wakayama-ken, Japan in 1926. In 1949, after studies in political science and international law at Tokyo University, he came to the United States. Inspired by George Ohsawa's dietary teachings, he began his lifelong study of the application of traditional philosophy and medicine to solving the problems of the modern world.

In the early 1960s, Michio Kushi and his family moved to Boston from New York and founded Erewhon, the nation's pioneer natural foods distributor, to make organically grown whole foods and naturally processed foods available. During the last twenty years, he has lectured around the world on diet, health, philosophy, and culture and given personal dietary and way of life counseling to thousands of individuals and families. In 1971 his students founded the *East West Journal* to provide macrobiotic information, and in 1972 the East West Foundation was started to spread macrobiotic education and research. Today there are about 500 local and regional macrobiotic centers throughout the United States, Canada, and Europe and in parts of Latin America, the Middle East, Asia, and Australia. In 1978 Michio and Aveline Kushi founded the Kushi Institute, an educational organization for the training of macrobiotic teachers, counselors, and cooks, with affiliates in London, Amsterdam, Antwerp, Florence, Paris, and Barcelona. As a further means toward addressing problems of world health and world peace, the Kushis established Macrobiotic Congresses of North America, Europe, and the Caribbean which meet annually and draw delegates from many states.

In recent years, Michio Kushi has met with government and social leaders at the United Nations, the World Health Organization, the White House, and many foreign capitals. His seminars and lectures on a dietary approach to cancer, heart disease, AIDS, and other disorders have attracted thousands of doctors, nurses, nutritionists, and other health care professionals. Medical researchers at Harvard Medical School, Tulane University, the University of Minnesota School of Public Health, Ghent University, and other universities, hospitals, prisons, and schools are currently pursuing research on the effectiveness of the macrobiotic diet. In 1985 he was elected general president of the International Confederation of Natural Medicine Associations, an association of 300 natural medical and health care organizations with international headquarters in Madrid, Spain.

Michio Kushi has published over a dozen books including *The Book of Macrobiotics*, *How to See Your Health: Book of Oriental Diagnosis*, *Natural Healing through Macrobiotics*, *The Cancer-Prevention Diet*, and *Diet for a Strong Heart*. He lives with his wife Aveline and several of their children in Brookline, Massachusetts, and has a retreat center in Becket, Massachusetts, located in the lovely Berkshire Mountains.

Aveline Kushi was born in 1923 in a small mountain village in the Izumo area of Japan. At college she was a star gymnast, but her athletic career was cut short by World War II. During the war she taught elementary school in her mountain district and after the war became involved in world peace activities at the Student World Government Association near Tokyo directed by George Ohsawa. In 1951 she came to the United States and married Michio Kushi. Along with her husband, she has devoted her life to or flavor to the meal. It is important, however, that the other tastes—sour, bitter, and pungent—also be available at each meal in side dishes, garnishes, or condiments. Lack of foods providing these tastes can create imbalance, cravings, snacking, eating out, and binging.

At the table, dishes should be arranged beautifully to accentuate the natural colors of the food. A variety of colors in the meal, different serving bowls and dishes, and changing garnishes frequently will stimulate the appetite, add flavor, and enhance the enjoyment of the meal.

During meals, food should be eaten in an orderly and relaxed manner. A moment of silent meditation, prayer, or grace may be observed to thank God or the infinite universe for the food that is about to be eaten and dedicate it to the creation of health, happiness, and peace. We may also wish to express our gratitude to the plants and animals who have given their lives that we may live, as well as the farmers, distributors, merchants, cooks, and others who contributed their hard work to bringing us good quality food.

Thorough chewing is an important aspect of macrobiotic dietary practice. Chewing allows us to utilize more fully the energy and nutrients of the food. One of the best ways to ensure that the food we eat is properly digested is to chew each mouthful well, until liquified, up to fifty times or more. Generally, family members may eat regularly two or three times per day, as much as they want, provided the proportion of food is generally correct and each mouthful is thoroughly chewed. However, it is best to leave the table feeling satisfied but not full.

Cooking is the supreme art—the art of creating life and maintaining health, happiness, and peace. In the beginning, it is important that everyone, however experienced in some other style of cooking, take macrobiotic cooking classes in order to taste and see the food actually prepared and have a standard against which to measure their own efforts. Then gradually, as the fundamentals are learned, the cook can begin to experiment and start using his or her own intuition as a guide.

spreading macrobiotics. As co-founder of Erewhon, the *East West Journal*, the East West Foundation, the Kushi Institute, and the Kushi Foundation, she has taken an active role in macrobiotic education and development.

During the last twenty years in the Boston area, many thousands of young people have visited and studied at her home in order to change their way of life in a more natural direction. She has given countless seminars on macrobiotic cooking, pregnancy and child care, and medicinal cooking for cancer, heart disease, and AIDS patients. She has been instrumental in arranging visits to the United States by teachers and performers of such traditional arts as the Tea Ceremony, Noh Drama, and Buddhist meditation.

Aveline has written and illustrated several books including *How to Cook with Miso*, *The Changing Seasons Cookbook*, and *Aveline Kushi's Complete Guide to Macrobiotic Cooking for Health, Harmony, and Peace*. The mother of five children and the grandmother of five, she resides in Brookline and Becket, Massachusetts, and with her husband spends about half the year teaching abroad.

Alex Jack was born in Chicago in 1945 and grew up in Evanston, Illinois, and Scarsdale, New York. His interest in the Far East developed at age eleven when he accompanied his father, a minister, to an international peace conference in Japan. During the mid-1960s Alex served as a civil rights organizer in the South, helped set up an arts festival with atomic bomb survivors in Hiroshima, and reported from Vietnam and Cambodia. He adopted a natural foods diet while studying philosophy and religion at Banaras Hindu University in India in 1965.

After graduating from Oberlin College with a degree in philosophy, he became involved in writing, editing, and small-press publishing. In 1975 Alex Jack joined the staff of the *East West Journal*, serving as editor from 1979 to 1982 and writing extensively on diet, nutrition, and health. Over the years, his work has also taken him to the Soviet Union, China, and many European countries.

Alex is the author or coauthor of seven books including *The Cancer-Prevention Diet*, *Diet for a Strong Heart*, and *Aveline Kushi's Complete Guide to Macrobiotic Cooking for Health, Harmony, and Peace*. He resides in Brookline, Massachusetts.

Index